CRIMINAL EXPERIMENTS ON HUMAN BEINGS IN AUSCHWITZ AND WAR RESEARCH LABORATORIES

Twenty Women Prisoners' Accounts

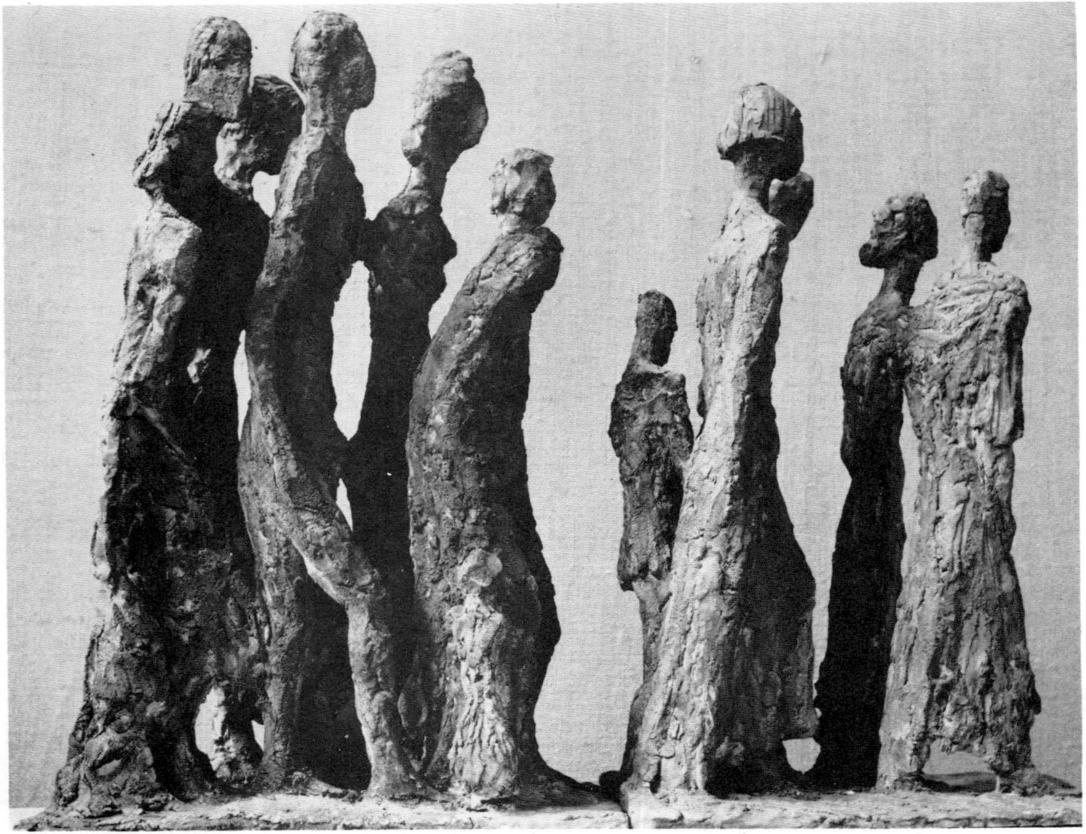

Photo of the sculpture "Der Todesmarsch" (the death march),
used by kind permission of the sculptor, Wanda Ladniewska.

CRIMINAL EXPERIMENTS ON HUMAN BEINGS IN AUSCHWITZ AND WAR RESEARCH LABORATORIES

Twenty Women Prisoners' Accounts

Compiled, translated and edited by
Lore Shelley

MELLEN RESEARCH UNIVERSITY PRESS
San Francisco

Library of Congress Cataloging-in-Publication Data

Criminal experiments on human beings in Auschwitz and war research laboratories : twenty women prisoners' accounts / compiled, translated, and edited by Lore Shelley ; foreword by Yehuda Bauer.
p. cm.
Includes bibliographical references and index.
ISBN 0-7734-9884-2
1. Holocaust, Jewish (1939-1945)--Personal narratives.
2. Auschwitz (Poland : Concentration camp) 3. Human experimentation in medicine. I. Shelley, Lore, 1924- .
D804.3.C75 1992
940.53' 18--dc20 91-40557
CIP

Editorial Inquiries:

Mellen Research University Press
534 Pacific Avenue
San Francisco
CA 94133

Order Fulfillment:

The Edwin Mellen Press
P.O. Box 450
Lewiston, NY 14092
USA

Printed in the United States of America

To the memory of Allegra and the other twenty-nine anonymous women of Block 10 in Auschwitz who were gassed in the concentration camp of Natzweiler-Struthof in August 1943 for the planned skeleton collection of Prof. Dr. August Hirt, Director of the Institute of Anatomy at the University of Strasbourg

Table of Contents

Illustrations of Renée Duering

Foreword

Lore Shelley's book presents us with the Auschwitz inferno from an angle that is different, and in a real sense, new. The twenty personal accounts in the book are not just haphazardly collected. They deal with a number of issues, and they are checked for accuracy, as far as possible, against the known development of the camps that together made up the Auschwitz complex. They try to present, basically, the female experience in the camps, and deal with both general issues that were common to all inmates, and also with gender-specific problems. Not only the victims appear in the accounts—also some of the perpetrators appear, of course through the eyes of the inmates. The perpetrators are both male and female, and some of the relationships between them, hierarchically and gender relations within the same level, contain some important insights. But the main problem of course is that of the inmates—how they lived, how they managed to survive, what were the main problems they had to confront in their struggle for bare existence.

Another new element is the fact that Lore Shelley's fascinating book deals with a number of sub-camps that were within a general area around the chief three camps of Auschwitz (Auschwitz I, the headquarters camp; Auschwitz II, Birkenau, which contained the gassing complex, the women's camp, the Gypsy camp, and the Czech families camp, among others; and Auschwitz III, Monowitz, the industrial center). It deals with agricultural experiments, with forms of industrial slavery, and details the specifics of each such sub-camp through the experiences of the victims. Nor are the testimonies one-sided within themselves. Jews and non-Jews, women from different European countries, all of them participate with their personal stories. Together, they make up a mosaic which has historical as well as psychological interest in the first degree.

We do need more such books—they deal with the problems of oral testimony in a way that enables us to approach the latter with a cross-check and verify the testimonies. In the absence of trustworthy and reliable German documentation, oral testimonies are a most important element in supplementing our knowledge, and whatever written material survived can serve not only as a reference point to the witnesses' stories, but can also be corrected by them, if there are converging testimonies in sufficient number.

Lore Shelley has made another important contribution to our knowledge of that darkest period, so far, in human history.

Yehuda Bauer
Hebrew University, Jerusalem

Preface

> The tens of thousands of survivors' testimonies stand in lieu of written documentation; they are central to our knowledge. Without the survivors we are nothing. They are the link between us and the Jewish life that was destroyed; they are the testimony and the proof; they saw their fellow Jews die. We should treat them and their experiences with the utmost respect—for this, after all, is the basis of all the "lessons."
>
> — Yehuda Bauer

Auschwitz does not require any introduction. It stands for the complete negation of everything man has accomplished, achieved and created since the dawn of mankind.

More than forty-four years have elapsed since the Russian Army liberated the camp and the world caught a glimpse of what had been going on behind the electrified wires. Many events have not yet been recorded and we are trying, at the eleventh hour, to fill in some of the missing pieces of the mosaic.

After the publication of *Secretaries of Death*, the story of some of the inmates who worked in the office of the Political Section of Auschwitz, narrated by thirty-one of my co-prisoners and myself, I was approached by a number of friends who asked that I produce a similar description of other Auschwitz work details. I decided to exclude the FKL (women's camp in Birkenau), about which a vast literature exists, and to restrict the accounts to women who worked in Auschwitz and Rajsko. I contacted or visited more than one hundred and fifty persons in different countries and encountered, in many instances, extreme reluctance to touch upon the deeply traumatic events of the past which were often unmitigated by the passage of time. In addition, quite a number of potential contributors and actual participants passed away since the inception of the project. Thus, the compilation of stories was a truly arduous feat, but eventually, fifty reports were obtained, of which twenty are presented in this book.

We have attempted to describe a few non-Birkenau based women's work details through eyewitness accounts. The stories are often of an extremely personal nature and contain many varied recollections, insights and reactions.

Some of the contributors focused on the pre-Holocaust period, depicting the deterioration of conditions, the narrowing of options, the seemingly inexorable course of events; some dwelled on the dehumanizing Birkenau inferno, on happenings they were ill-equipped to portray because our human vocabulary is simply devoid of adequate terms; a few attempted to tell about, or sometimes only enumerate, as many of those that had perished as they could remember, to tear them out of the anonymity of the Six Million, to give them a face, a voice and a name and to enact a sort of roll call of the dead; some concentrated on recounting simple survival, some on helping others, sabotage, resistance or solidarity among inmates; some recalled the terrible letdown of the liberation period after the initial euphoria had subsided when most of the outside world proved to be unable and unwilling to emotionally assist the survivors, so marked by their experience that total integration into everyday life was a semblance; others wrote about the post-Holocaust era, the psycho-social adjustment problems and the difficulty in coming to terms with a world that had not changed in the direction many of us in camp had idealistically hoped it would.

Some of the women are accomplished writers while others are eloquent in their inarticulateness. Each contributor was unrestricted as to contents, emphasis, structure or format of her story and I tried to preserve the uniqueness of every memoir in terms of style, expression and terminology, refraining similarly from value judgments, comments, assessments or corrections.

The contributors are a widely heterogeneous group with regard to age, education, religious background, occupation, nationality, political and ideological outlook, lifestyle, affiliation and other characteristics, comprising Jewish women from various European countries—now dispersed over four continents, as well as former political prisoners. Even in Auschwitz their experiences were vastly different. Some worked in offices, others in agriculture, research, photography, design, camp hospitals or were used as guinea pigs for pseudo-medical experiments. However, all of them were fortunate enough that, eventually, they managed to fulfill—however inadequately—at least the lowest level of Maslow's hierarchy of needs. Otherwise, they would not be here to tell their stories.

The accounts offer different points of view and perspectives which frequently pertain to the same occurrence—almost in Rashomon fashion. At the same time, they complement, corroborate and resemble each other closely, describing identical atrocities and identical horrors. They lend credence to some scholars' belief that "eventually a consensus version of Holocaust history may emerge from these personal accounts" (Hartman). Hopefully, they forever disprove some academic historians' narrow view that survivor memoirs can never serve as primary material for history.

Acknowledgments

I wish to express my gratitude to a number of people who helped me put this book together.

Edita Maliarova, Grete Roth and Lili Duschinsky served as coordinators for the contributors in Czechoslovakia, Dr. Marie-Elisa Cohen did the same for those in France, while Menahem Rafalowitz served in this capacity in Israel.

Hermann Langbein of the Comite International des Camps in Vienna supplied information about the SS personnel of Auschwitz.

Kazimierz Smolen, Director of the Panstwowe Muzeum Oswiecim Brzezinka, generously allowed me to copy archival material.

Linda Breder and Jan Pessl translated material written in Slovakian, Irene Miller translated from the Czech language, Mila Muller from Polish, and Miriam Silberschatz and Miriam Ofer from Hungarian.

Dr. Erich Kulka and Dr. Jacques Stroumza provided documents from the Wiener Library and from Yad Vashem. Jerry Dubin furnished the sheet music for the Auschwitz Song. And Nina and Mark Lees tirelessly and devotedly typed the manuscript.

I would like to thank Mrs. Hatty Minney for her permission to reprint excerpts from *I Shall Fear No Evil*, by R.J. Minney, William Kimber publisher, London, 1966.

This study would not have been possible without the assistance of my husband, Sucher Shelley.

Introduction

Quien mira lo pasado
Lo porvenir advierte.
Lope de Vega

The concentration camp of Auschwitz was formed in May 1940 in the vicinity of the Polish town of Oswiecim, located in the Voivodeship of Cracow, 60 km. west of Cracow and 30 km. south-east of Kattowitz.

It became the largest concentration camp in the German system comprising approximately 135,168 inmates at one time according to a document smuggled out of camp by the Resistance movement on August 22, 1944: Auschwitz I had 15,971 male prisoners; Auschwitz II had 19,424 male prisoners, 39,234 female prisoners and 30,000 unregistered Hungarian Jews in transit, while Auschwitz III had 30,539 male prisoners (Czech, 1989, p. 860).

Auschwitz had been designated by Himmler as the stage for the execution of the "Final Solution" of the Jewish problem.

After the cessation of the killing centers working under the code name of Operation Reinhardt, i.e., Treblinka, Sobibor and Belzec, and the discontinuation of Majdanek and Chelmno, Auschwitz became a gigantic death factory.

It is estimated that approximately 1.6 million people died in Auschwitz, about 1,350,000 of them were Jews. Of these, it is believed that about 1,345,000 were gassed (1,323,000 of them Jews) while about 255,000 found their death through hunger, disease, work, torture, shootings, hanging, phenol injections and pseudo-medical experiments (Bauer, 1989, p. 7).

In Auschwitz more persons were killed than anywhere ever before at one place on this planet. That's why the term Auschwitz became a symbol for men's organized inhumanity toward their fellow-men.

Auschwitz had been purposefully planned as a place where prisoners were exterminated. The work and living conditions in camp were such that a young, strong and healthy person had the chance of surviving from a few weeks to about a few months, provided he or she was not selected for the gas chambers, did not fall ill, did not have an accident, was not experimented on and did not attract the attention of a prison functionary or an SS man. Nevertheless, there were survivors and the women in this volume are all survivors. What accounted for this survival? In 1974–75, three Polish researchers, Jagoda, Klodzinski and Maslowski, asked former Auschwitz prisoners, most of them Polish political prisoners, the reason for their survival. They came up with a number of factors believed by them to have been responsible for their outlasting the camp:

Psycho-physical ability to resist (inurement of body and mind) was named by 65.5%; 60.6% cited attitudes which had a positive influence on survival (such as belief in survival, religiosity, closeness to relatives, trust in the ultimate victory of good over evil, even a desire for revenge); 59.4% reported the help received from co-prisoners; 55.6% listed heightened self-preservation instincts, presentiment and instinctive avoidance of danger, slyness, spontaneous willingness of risk-taking and good adaptation to camp conditions; 36.3% stated work conditions favorable for survival; 33.7% mentioned chance; 25.6% knowledge of German; 17% referred to medical help received or other factors.

The editor investigated attitudes of Jewish Holocaust survivors in 1981, and obtained the following self-reported reasons for survival:

- 73.8% believed that chance (also termed "luck", "destiny", "miracle" or "coincidence") was the principal ingredient responsible for survival, agreeing with two well-known survivors:

> "Even Solzhenitsyn...would not have survived if he had not been set free by those who rule the Gulag Archipelago."
> (Bettelheim, 1979, pp. 287–288)

> "For Lustig, survival or death was more often a matter of chance than of choice."
>
> (Sherwin, 1979, p. 27)

- 49.5% of the respondents believed faith enabled them to survive the camp.
- 26.8% stated that coping skills helped them to survive.
- 26% asserted that friends assisted them in surviving.

Additional factors mentioned were: the will to survive, special capabilities, youth, survival for some purpose, resistance, type of work in camp, and psychological removal.

Most of the participants of this volume lived outside the main camp, isolated from their fellow-prisoners and survived precisely because their living and working conditions were atypical for Auschwitz and incomparably better than those of the women in Birkenau. Quite a number of them belonged to the resistance movement in camp. A few of them succeeded in saving human lives and others were able to smuggle out information about Auschwitz to the Polish underground which was transmitted to the government in exile and broadcast by the BBC in London.

Finally, I would like to point out that this book contains accounts of survivors about their personal Auschwitz experiences; it does not comprise an overall vision of their camp universe (the make-up of the SS-state, the geography of the camp, the camp structure, the SS-murderers, etc.). It has been said that the Holocaust is not one story but many, not one history, but rather six million or more case studies. To truly comprehend these dark years, we would need nothing less than to trace the individual experience of every survivor. Thus abandoning the general view of the anyway too gigantic whole in favor of an essential detail establishes the right of the individual not to be overlooked and conforms to John Ruskin's view of obtaining the facts right from the source: "The only history worth reading is that written at the time of which it treats, the history of what was done and seen, heard out of the mouths of the men who did and saw."

Part One

BLOCK 10

BLOCK 10

Auschwitz was not only a death factory, it also served as an experimental station for a new crime envisaged to be perpetrated against many millions of people. Since the capacity of the gas chambers and crematoria was not sufficient for the planned annihilation, it was decided to recruit the help of medical science. Professor Carl Clauberg and Dr. Horst Schumann received orders to devise a method of mass sterilization of those nations destined for biological destruction through experiments performed on prisoners.

Both men started their "research" in the fall of 1942 in Block 30 in the women's camp in Birkenau and moved to Block 10 in the Stammlager (the men's camp) in Auschwitz in early 1943. Their "research material" consisted of approximately four hundred Jewish girls. After a certain time the "consumed material" would be returned to the women's camp in Birkenau and replaced by "fresh material" from the newly arrived transports.

Other SS physicians who performed medical experiments on the inmates of Block 10 were Dr. Edward Wirths and Dr. Bruno Weber.

All inmates of Block 10 were Jewish except for the crew of the brothel, which consisted of German black-triangled and Polish prisoners who came from time to time to be examined for venereal diseases.

In March 1943, Magda Blau-Helliger, destined to become the first block-elder of the experimental Block 10 in the men's camp, was transferred from

Birkenau to Auschwitz, together with her crew of room seniors, most of them veterans of the first RSHA transports from Slovakia.

The first guinea pigs to arrive was a transport of 100 Greek women with prison numbers around 41,500-41,600. In April 1943 a transport of 110 women with numbers 42,500-42,600 was admitted to Block 10. From the end of April 1943 until June 1943, and also for the month of October 1943, the number of personnel and patients (the official designation of the guinea pigs) can be seen from an official list that was rescued. On June 29, 1943, the patient pool was increased by 65 women from Berlin, prison numbers 47,400-47,500. On July 21, 1943, 70 women from France with numbers around 50,300 were added. An additional transport from France with 50 women carrying numbers around 52,300 arrived on August 2, 1943. Subsequently, three transports from the Netherlands followed—40 women with numbers around 56,000 in August and 100 women on September 16 and 23, 1943, with numbers around 62,400-62,500 and 63,100-63,200. All these prisoners had been chosen directly at their arrival right from the ramp for Block 10 by Dr. Wirths, the SS-Physician-in-Chief of Auschwitz.

Occasionally, some women with children were housed in Block 10, such as the wives of the Jewish bacteriologists from the Weigl Institute in Lwow who arrived around February 1943 and worked for the Institute of Hygiene, namely Drs. Ludwik Fleck (100967), Bernhard Umschweif (100969) and Jacob Seeman (100968). Not only were the wives admitted, Ernestine Fleck (34967), Natalie Umschweif (34966) and Anna Seeman (34965), but also the children, Karol Umschweif, born September 4, 1938, prison number 103796 (now living in Israel) and Bronislaw Seeman, born December 12, 1932, prison number 103793 (now living in Texas). The third and youngest child was Peter Dattel, born on July 29, 1939, in Berlin, who came with his mother, Ruth Dattel, with Transport 39 from Berlin in June 1943 (mother and son now live in Cologne, Germany).

In addition, Sylvia Friedmann-Vesela, Prof. Clauberg's nurse, who had arrived with the first Slovakian transports in the spring of 1942, had her mother, Prizka Mouchova-Friedmann—shipped to Auschwitz two years later from Hungary—transferred from the C-camp in Birkenau to Block 10.

In the summer of 1944 all the women of Block 10 were moved to Block 1 of the camp extension. Since there was space for 400 women, Clauberg requested and received additional guinea pigs from Birkenau. On January 18, 1945, the occupants of the experimental block were evacuated, together with the rest of the camp.

Clauberg trained an SS-man, SDG Buehning—a former hairdresser—in the method of sterilization through intrauterine injections[1] and the medical laymen performed these sterilizations for about half a year. In addition, Clauberg relegated the execution of the procedure to the chemist of the Schering factory, Dr. Goebel[2]. Both of these men worked independently during Clauberg's absence, although a salpingography should never be performed by non-medical personnel.

The injections were extremely painful, caused high fever and inflammations. Some women even died as a result of them. When the experiments were completed, many of the guinea pigs were returned to Birkenau to be gassed and fresh raw material for research arrived. A large number of the surviving guinea pigs were not only unable to conceive as a result of these experiments but were mentally and physically crippled by them. On pages 11-12, I exhibit the copy of a letter sent in 1988 to the husband of one of these human wrecks by Dr. Horst Witzel, Chairman of the Board of the Schering factory in reply to a request for compensation of the harm done by their former employee, Dr. Goebel.[3]

The letter denies and refutes the responsibility of the Schering factory for the criminal activities of its former employee, points only to Clauberg's animal experiments (although the chemical substances for sterilization purposes he received from Schering contained novocaine—an analgesic which would have been superfluous for animal experiments that were performed under a general anesthetic), does not at all address the fact that Auschwitz concentration camp and Prof. Clauberg were valued customers who ordered large quantities of preparations from Schering and states that juridically the deadline for filing claims had expired long ago anyway.

NUMBER OF PRISONERS IN BLOCK 10

for the months of May, June and October 1943

TAG	MONAT							
	APRIL		MAI		JUNI		OKTOBER	
	P.	H.	P	H.	P.	H.	P.	H.
1	—	—	22	242	39	225	67	395
2	—	—	22	242	39	225	67	395
3	—	—	22	243	39	136	67	395
4	—	—	22	243	39	137	67	395
5	—	—	22	245	39	135	64	394
6	—	—	67	200	39	137	64	394
7	—	—	67	200	39	135	64	364
8	—	—	39	228	39	135	75	394
9	—	—	39	228	39	134	68	394
10	—	—	39	228	35	135	68	394
11	—	—	39	228	35	135	68	394
12	—	—	39	228	35	235	69	394
13	—	—	39	228	35	235	69	394
14	—	—	39	228	35	235	68	394
15	—	—	39	228	35	235	67	394
16	—	—	39	228	35	235	67	394
17	—	—	39	228	35	235	67	394
18	—	—	39	228	35	235	67	394
19	—	—	39	228	35	234	68	394
20	—	—	39	228	35	234	67	394
21	—	—	39	227	35	234	67	394
22	—	—	39	227	35	234	67	394
23	—	—	39	227	35	234	67	389
24	—	—	39	227	35	234	67	388
25	—	—	39	226	35	240	67	388
26	—	—	39	226	35	240	67	388
27	—	—	39	225	35	240	67	388
28	—	—	39	226	35	240	67	388
29	—	—	39	226	35	240	67	389
30	22	242	39	225	40	300	67	388
31	—	—	39	225	—	—	67	387

P — Pfleger (nursing personnel; also inmates).
H — Haeftlinge (prisoners)
(from Sehn, pp. 20–21)

Letter from Dr. Horst Witzel of the Schering Co.

SCHERING

Dr. Horst Witzel
Vorsitzender des Vorstandes

Schering Aktiengesellschaft

Postfach 65 03 11
D-1000 Berlin 65
Telefon: (0 30) 4 68-22 13
Telex: 1 82 03-0 sch d

Für Besucher:
Berlin-Wedding
Müllerstraße 170-178

Berlin, den 8 März 1988

Sehr geehrter Herr

Ihre Schreiben vom 01. und 26. Januar sowie vom 20. Februar 1988 habe ich erhalten. Sie werden verstehen, daß die Prüfung der mir überlassenen Unterlagen und der Angaben über Ihre Frau Gemahlin einige Zeit in Anspruch genommen hat. Ich habe unter anderem auch Auskünfte des deutschen Bundesministeriums für Finanzen erhalten, bei dem Ihr Entschädigungsverfahren bearbeitet wurde; daher erübrigte sich eine Anfrage in Arolsen.

Außerdem habe ich mich anhand verschiedener Unterlagen zu den von Ihnen gegenüber der Schering AG erhobenen Vorwürfen sorgfältig informiert. Ich habe unter anderem auch Schriftstücke eingesehen, die im Rahmen des Strafverfahrens gegen Clauberg im Jahre 1956 angefertigt worden sind. Schließlich habe ich noch Gespräche mit ehemaligen Mitarbeitern der Schering AG geführt, die während des Krieges in unserem Hause tätig waren.

Ich komme nach wie vor zu dem Ergebnis, daß die Schering AG für die Experimente von Clauberg und Goebel in Auschwitz weder verantwortlich gewesen ist noch einen Nutzen davon gehabt hat. Clauberg war seinerzeit Chefarzt einer Klinik in Königshütte, und es war bei der Schering AG bekannt, daß er dort auch Tierversuche durchgeführt hat. Goebel wurde mit der Zubereitung von Präparaten für diese Tierversuche beauftragt. Ende 1943/Anfang 1944 ließ er sich von der Schering AG beurlauben und ging zu Clauberg. Übrigens war Goebel nicht "Chef-Pharmacist" bei der Schering AG, sondern er war Apotheker im Hauptlabor. Leiter dieses Labors war Professor Walter Schoeller, den ich nach dem Kriege noch persönlich kennengelernt habe. Er war ein aufrechter Mensch und hat sich stets schützend vor seine Mitarbeiter gestellt die aus rassischen Gründen verfolgt wurden.

-2-

Wie aus zahlreichen Unterlagen hervorgeht und durch Aussagen heute noch lebender Personen belegbar ist, hat die Schering AG ihre jüdischen Mitarbeiter vor den nationalsozialistischen Machthabern unter anderem dadurch in Sicherheit gebracht, daß sie ins Ausland, insbesondere zu unserer damaligen Tochtergesellschaft in den USA, versetzt wurden, damit sie dort weiterarbeiten konnten. Als Beispiel für den Leumund des Unternehmens sende ich Ihnen einen Ausschnitt aus dem Buch "Klettern in der Großstadt" von Jochen Köhler (erschienen im Wagenbach-Verlag 1981) der für sich spricht.

Aus dem Schicksal Ihrer Frau Gemahlin lassen sich keine Ansprüche gegen die Schering AG ableiten. Bei rein juristischer Betrachtungsweise wären solche Ansprüche im übrigen auch verjährt

Somit sehe ich auch keine Möglichkeit, Ihren Forderungen nach materieller Kompensation für Ihre Frau Gemahlin durch die Schering AG zu entsprechen.

Mit verbindlichen Empfehlungen

[signature]

CHAPTER ONE
Beginnings in Block 30 in Birkenau

Dr. Margita (Manci) Schwalbova
Bratislava (Czechoslovakia)

I was born on September 22, 1915, in Lipt. Mikulas, Czechoslovakia.

In March 1942, I was sent as a prisoner to Auschwitz concentration camp and in August 1942, I was transferred to Birkenau.

In the fall of 1942, the camp administration was looking for a woman to work as nurse and x-ray technician. She was required to have experience in this field and to be of "Aryan" descent. Since they were unable to find an experienced woman who also complied with their "racial" requirements, I was ordered to do the work in Block 30.

After my transfer to Block 30, I met Prof. Clauberg for the first time in November or December 1942. He tested my operational knowledge of the x-ray apparatus which, incidentally, was a diagnostic model.[4]

There were two divisions in Block 30, one belonged to Dr. Schumann and the other one to Dr. Clauberg. Clauberg's section consisted of two rooms. One contained a gynecological table and a diagnostic x-ray apparatus, the other room contained the beds for the women who were used for experiments. As far as I know, they obtained the women by proclaiming in camp that they were looking for young nurses. The girls who applied were, consequently, assigned to be human guinea pigs.

I noticed a small bottle with some liquid during the absence of Dr. Clauberg and attempted to read the label. There was only a number, so that I could not determine the contents or the composition of the liquid.

Shortly after I started to work for Clauberg, Sylvia Friedmann, a nurse, was transferred to Block 30. It was her task to take care of the women who were used for experiments. She had to keep a record whether or not the human guinea pigs experienced pain, fever and disturbances in their menstrual cycles after the experiments.

I had to operate the x-ray apparatus in the following way: either during or after the procedure, Dr. Clauberg gave a sign and I activated the x-ray apparatus so that he could check the results of his experiments through x-rays. He injected some liquid into the vagina of the woman by means of a Jeannette syringe. I knew that these experiments were painful because the women moaned. However, since it was dangerous—here, as well as in other parts of the camp—to express pain openly, the women made a tremendous effort to control themselves and moaned only instead of giving free vent to their pain. After the experiments, the women had fever, shivers, bloody vaginal discharges and vomited.

I remember that Dr. Clauberg visited the block on a weekly basis and, as far as I know, he appeared in civilian clothes, whereas all other physicians were always in their SS uniforms. I had the opportunity to observe that the women felt mentally more at ease during those intervals when Clauberg was absent. The closer the day of Clauberg's visit approached (and these days were known to us, I believe he came on Tuesdays or Thursdays), the more they exhibited signs of anxiety and fear. This anxiety was a clear indication that Dr. Clauberg's experiments did not only affect the women physically and mentally, but had a profound effect on their nervous system. These human guinea pigs knew through the nursing personnel and through rumors that they were used for sterilization experiments or for artificial insemination. Both of these possibilities filled them with fear. Insemination would have meant a death sentence. The camp administration sent pregnant women to the gas chambers; and if a child should have been born, they would have gassed mother and child. Understandably, they were horrified at the thought of being sterilized because it was clear to them that their human dignity was being violated.

Nobody was allowed to leave Block 30. This applied to me, the nurses and, of course, the women who were used for experiments. I only managed to go illegally to the Revier (camp hospital). It meant that everything which happened in the block was kept a secret from all other prisoners.

The first women who occupied the beds in Block 30, and were experimented on by Dr. Clauberg, were all from a transport of Dutch Jewesses. In addition, there was one woman from Slovakia among them as well as a few others.

The experiments were also shown to members of the SS. I recall, for example, that SS-woman Mandel, the SS commandant-in-chief of the women's camp, was present at a demonstration.

I also know that the male prisoner, Frantisek Prazak, visited Block 30 to see Dr. Schumann. He had the possibility to learn about Clauberg's experiments. Besides, Jiri Beranovsky[5] came to do repairs; he was in charge of the proper functioning of the installations.

SS-physician Dr. Vetter had ordered me to keep guard at the entrance to the sick bay (and Block 30 belonged to the hospital complex). He especially assigned me this task because, otherwise, I would not have been able to leave Block 30. In this manner, the nursing staff of the Revier had opportunity to have contact with me. Anyway, in the evenings, I went on my own to the Revier. Thus, I could discuss my observations in Block 30 with them.

Polish prisoner physicians from the men's camp also visited Block 30 illegally. I remember that they advised me not to transfer to Block 10 (during the time when that block was being prepared for Clauberg's women). They believed that the SS would sooner or later execute all those who had been witnesses to their deeds. Well, I did not go to Block 10. I was claimed by the Birkenau Revier to perform medical services. As x-ray operator, my medical training had not been utilized, while it was very much in demand at the Revier.

In approximately March 1943, when the preparations in Block 10 in the men's camp in Auschwitz had been completed, the women, together with Sylvia Friedmann, were transferred to Block 10. There the experiments continued on a large scale.

Dr. Adelaide Hautval, a French prisoner psychiatrist, had been in Block 10 in Auschwitz where she had been assigned to assist Dr. Wirths. He removed the procreative organs of healthy young women for cancer research purposes. Dr. Hautval refused to assist. Dr. Wirths was surprised and told her, "... it concerns inferior human beings, completely different from us." Dr. Hautval replied, "Herr Hauptsturmfuehrer, I consider you also to be different from me; that still does not authorize me to sterilize you." Subsequently, Dr. Hautval was returned to Birkenau and we were afraid for her life. To refuse the execution of an SS-man's order was synonymous with a death sentence. We, therefore, put Dr. Hautval into the Revier and fed her sleeping pills so that she was never conscious when Dr. Wirths visited the Revier.

I remained in the Revier of Birkenau and tried to take care of the patients and to rescue as many as possible from extermination. This was only feasible through a team approach. Initially, my colleagues in the Revier were German political prisoners, most of them communists, who had been already imprisoned for many years: Aurelia, called Orly, Reichert,[6] Emmy Thom, Anny Blumauer, Gertrud Frinke[7] and the nun, Angela Autsch.[8] From Czechoslovakia, there were the physicians or medical students: Ena Weiss, Edith Bock, Greta Reisfeld, Zlattner and the nurses: Gruenberger, Teichner and Skripsky. Later on, transports from all over occupied Europe arrived and additional personnel was admitted to the Revier: for example, the women doctors: Zdenka Nedved, Margita Ernyei, Danielle Casanova, May Pollitzer, Adelaide Hautval, Liubov Jakovlevna Alpatovova, Olga Nikiticna Klimenkova, Irena Konieczna, Jadwiga Wengierska, Jadwiga Hewelkova, Alina Tetmayerova, Francuska Rose, Mari Erdelyova; and the nurses: Olga Boryszpolowa, Eva Neumann and others. All of them, without exception, gave all their energy, knowledge and courage to the battle to save human lives.[9]

Let me conclude with one incident: One day a transport went to the gas chamber. The selected women had been placed in open trucks and next to them, spread-eagled, stood Dr. Mengele. A young girl, almost a child, crept up to him, pointed to a woman on the truck—her mother—and asked for her life. She stared at him with large dark eyes. Since Dr. Mengele did not move, she asked, "Don't you have a mother yourself?" Dr. Mengele gave a sign to the closest SS-man, and he threw the girl on the truck to the mother. After a while, the transport started for the gas chamber.

Why did I insert just this particular occurrence at the end of my memoirs? I have pondered a lot about how I managed to survive Auschwitz, which was extremely difficult, especially for a professional healer. Most certainly, the fact that I could work as a nurse helped me to survive. In spite of the paradox of having a hospital in an extermination camp—the Revier personnel, nevertheless, had the feeling that our work made sense, that we could help those that suffered and that we could save lives—not only because of medication but also because the Revier was one of the principal centers of organized resistance and solidarity. The most distressing feeling was that of powerlessness: when a young comrade was dying from pneumonia in front of your eyes, because you had no medication for her; when you saw a woman go to the gas chamber simply for suffering from scabies, because you did not have any ointment to cure her; when you stood next to a woman who gave birth to a child in this hell, who was gassed the following day together with her baby; when, in your arms, a human being, a mere child, died from hunger or grief or incomprehension of this warped world…

It has to be emphasized that every attempt at saving co-prisoners condemned to die—whether through hiding, exchange of files of living inmates with those already deceased (to seemingly comply with the prison numbers appearing on the selection lists), clandestine abortions, etc.—required great, personal courage since betrayal would have meant sure death for the one who initiated this attempt. From where did we derive the strength and courage for these deeds? It was our endeavor to be true to ourselves, to fulfil our humanitarian mission, even in this inferno, but also the knowledge that together with you and next to you there were women of many nationalities, each one of them determined to remain a human being in the death camp.

❖

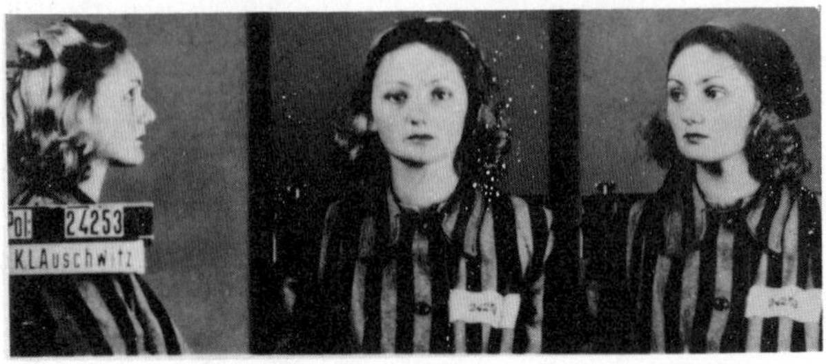

Sonja Fritz (née Fischmann)

Vienna (Austria)

I am the child of a mixed marriage. My parents were very young when I was born; my mother was 20 and my father 23. My mother descended from an old Christian family; the grandfather had been a country lawyer. The ancestors had been peasants in Kaernten (Carinthia, an Austrian province) for many generations. My father's family, which was quite large, came from Czenstochova in Poland. He had five sisters and two brothers. They were Orthodox Ostjuden (Eastern European Jews). My grandfather wore a caftan and my grandmother a "scheitl" (wig).

My parents had marital problems, but there is no point in belaboring them. Suffice it so say that my mother had been ready to compromise. She had converted to Judaism and had married according to Mosaic law. But there were unbridgeable differences. My mother had a very difficult life and the marriage did not last long. I grew up in Kaernten with my grandparents, who loved me very much. My mother remarried, whereas my father never recovered from the separation.

I practiced religion to please my father to whom I was very attached.

I never forgave my mother for having left him. We did not have a good relationship after the war, perhaps because my father perished in Bergen-Belsen. She could not display her feelings, and we never really communicated with one another. Moreover, Auschwitz had changed me and I was no longer the same person I had once been.

My mother died three years ago, and today I regret having done her an injustice. She also was not spared the emigrant's lot. Her second husband was also Jewish, and was similarly executed by the Germans.

On the day Hitler's army marched into Austria, my mother had to leave her house quickly. Lacking in control, as was sometimes her way, she had chided a Nazi. In addition, my father left his apartment on that same night and moved in with me. I was still going to school at that time and was not yet persecuted, but I freely volunteered the fact that my father was Jewish.

My father was a partner in a business and was about to liquidate everything. During the "Crystal Night" (i.e., the "Night of Broken Glass" in November 1938) he was still at home but, immediately afterward traveled to his sister in Paris. My mother had sent French visas to both of us. I did not want to live with my mother, while my family thought I would be better off if I stayed. Everybody believed that the trouble would be short-lived. A well-known attorney assured us that nothing would happen to me.

In the meantime, I was in contact with my father and sent him whatever packages I could throw together.

A few months later I joined a childhood friend in Milan, Italy, and we were married in Rapallo. I had to ask for permission of the Reichssicherheitshauptamt (the Supreme Office of the Gestapo in Berlin) because we were both Mischlinge (half Jewish). Furthermore, I was still a minor. Since it was so easy to arrange a trip to occupied Paris, I visited my father there. On my return to Austria, I was arrested for the first time. As a result of all the excitement, I had a miscarriage. When I finally had liquidated everything and packed my belongings to escape, I was arrested a second time in July 1942, one day before my scheduled departure. After three months of imprisonment by the Gestapo, and with the aid of three lawyers, I was fortunately taken into protective custody instead of being deported with a Jewish transport. The charge: suspicion of espionage, which was ridiculous, but better than being shipped with a RSHA (Reichssicherheitshauptamt) convoy. All the assurances, oaths and petitions of my relatives were to no avail. I was incarcerated in numerous prisons. The last one was located in Prague, which is why I arrived in Auschwitz on November 11th with a Czech transport. The Husta Hundestaffel (dog squad) was waiting for us and chased us like cattle to Birkenau.

Birkenau in 1942: It was indescribable. There was no light and no water. Nor were there any toilets. We walked through the gate, and I thought I had entered an insane asylum. We were ordered to go to the Sauna. The inmates clubbed us and shouted in a language we did not understand. (It was Slovakian).

The entire camp was nothing but a morass. These worn down skeletons were not human beings. It was hell. We received neither food nor drink, and everything we had was taken away from us. Anyway, there was not much to take since we came from prison in contrast to the other transports that arrived with all their belongings and where money and gold was sewn into many a hem. One of the beasts kicked me to the place where the tattooing occurred. I received number 24-253, which I still took in stride. Only when a sadistic woman approached to shave my hair did I refuse. She called SS-man Hustek-Erber of the Politische Abteilung (camp Gestapo) and he saved me because I was a protective custody prisoner. I was given a dress and a jacket which were made of cellulose so that they acted like a sponge when it rained. The underpants reached my knees, while I had to hold them together because they lacked an elastic waist band. Wool stockings and wooden clogs completed the wardrobe. On the dunghill I found a rusty container and later a sort of spoon. This is how I arrived at Block 16, a German block, in the company of criminals and prostitutes. We slept two in a bed with dirty straw, the rats crawling all over us that night. At 4 a.m. I was ordered to fetch a heavy caldron. Carrying it with my forty kilos, I lost my clogs in the mud. In the morning, we marched out to work in the plant nursery of Rajsko. In the evening, when I stood in line to get my soup and a piece of bread, I received nothing but beatings. They always told me that I had already gotten my portion.

We only had candlelight so that one could not distinguish the faces of different inmates. Thus, I lived from cabbage which I stole in the nursery. My feet were encrusted with blood and wool; I was unable to walk in the wooden clogs. I gathered all my courage, went to the clothing warehouse and requested a pair of stockings. Fraenzi Schmidt, supposedly the former secretary of Czech President Benes, was the warehouse Kapo. She kicked me viciously. I sat down in a corner and started to cry bitterly. One inmate took me to the Revier (camp hospital). I was ashamed to show my feet, which I had not washed for so long. I received paper bandages from the physician, Enna,[10] and her assistant, Manci Schwalb, who were very nice to me. They told me to return the following day for new bandages, but I did not dare come back since I had nothing to reciprocate with. Luckily, they found me after two days and decided to look for a job for me that did not require marching out into the cold. At that moment, SS-physician Dr. Schumann entered the room and informed us that he needed somebody in his new block #30. I was deloused and told to heat the barrack on the following morning. At that time, nobody knew what kind of block it would be.

Out of excitement, I could not sleep all night. Maybe I would sleep in a room from now on. I racked my brain trying to figure out where I would obtain coal in order to heat the barrack. I asked many inmates. The consensus was that I would be able to "organize" them in the vicinity of the kitchen—I did not even know yet the meaning of the word "organizing". Whenever I approached the kitchen, I was driven away. But, finally, I managed to get a bucket with a few coals. I ran back to Block 30, jumped over a ditch and landed with my coals in the mud. Underneath me, I could feel the stiff corpses which had been thrown in at night. I was desperate. A Russian with a group of male prisoners was already waiting in front of Block 30. I poured out my troubles to him. Just looking at me, he burst out laughing and he proceeded to rectify everything amazingly quickly. It happened to be my birthday and the few coals constituted the most beautiful present.

Dr. Schumann ordered me to take a helper. Thus Kazia, a very young Polish girl, joined me. I am still in touch with her, and she named a daughter after me.

Later Manci Schwalb was added to our staff, and finally, Ria Hans.[11] Manci worked up front in the ambulance. I do not remember where Ria worked.

Block 30 was a wooden barrack and belonged to the Revier (hospital complex). Inside there was a bedroom for prisoners, a waiting room and an adjacent room with two Siemens x-ray apparatuses. Across from these machines, there was a small booth, insulated with lead plates to protect from radiation, with glass windows from where Schumann could operate the x-ray apparatuses.

Dr. Horst Schumann was approximately 35 years old. He always wore an Air Force uniform and his behavior was reserved, cool and correct. He had no social relations whatsoever with the prisoners. I rarely spoke to him. Nevertheless, he was polite and attempted to grant me certain favors, for example, by placing bread and cigarettes into the wastepaper basket, which I had to empty. I did not accept these "presents" and returned them daily to the x-ray table; a gesture which he seemed to ignore. Soon he discontinued this behavior.

A day in Block 30 passed more or less in the following way:

The previous day, Schumann would give an order to the Arbeitseinsatz (work allocation office) to deliver one hundred young and healthy men or women to his block the next morning. Early the following day the block elder would arrive with the prisoners. In the beginning, even the personnel did not know, and the prisoners never knew, what kind of "treatment" Schumann provided. There were rumors that it consisted of prophylactic measures to combat typhus. The entire procedure was highly confidential. That's why access was forbidden to all unauthorized inmates and even to the SS while prisoner staff had to sleep in Block 30. Moreover, Schumann was afraid of camp diseases. In the morning, when he arrived I had to report the number and nationalities of the prisoners to him. Then the prisoners would undress in the waiting room. I had to record all the prison numbers, make a list, and bring each inmate individually to the treatment room. There were different gadgets attached to the x-ray machines for men and for women. The prisoners were told to stand on a stool between the two x-ray apparatuses so that their profile was turned toward the booth where Schumann was sitting. From his cubicle, Schumann turned on the current. The irradiation had to operate from both sides. The procedure lasted a few minutes. That's why during the course of several hours, a large number of inmates could be sterilized. The x-rays were intended to destroy the reproductive organs. Another side effect was, as I found out later, the extreme burning and suppurations of abdominal tissue.

I remember that women were often nauseated and vomited after having undergone irradiation. Once I asked Schumann whether I should help these women and perhaps give them some water, but he refused. After the treatment, the prisoners were returned to their blocks.

More men than women were sterilized.

Zbiszek and Slezak,[12] two Polish male prisoners, instructed me in sabotage techniques. They showed me how to switch off the water. Without water, there was no electric current. They themselves were afraid. The program was: at first, the Jews and Gypsies, and later the Poles. That was not a heroic deed. Moreover, I did not even realize the damage. Fortunately, Schumann had full confidence in me, or pretended to. It just so happened that at times I could not find the mechanics, although they were next door, and on those occasions the machines did not function and the sterilization did not take place.

Daily kommandos of male prisoners from Auschwitz and Birkenau, all kinds of specialists came who took care of our installation and who returned to their respective camps in the evening. They could circulate freely, and, of course, lots of things happened. In connection with this state of affairs, I was denounced when I was seen talking to a Polish inmate. As punishment, I had to kneel at the gate all day and the Pole was transferred to the KL-Flossenbuerg. This was completely ridiculous since I could admit any prisoner I wanted to Block 30, whereas the SS-women were prohibited from entering.

I worked for Schumann from November 25, 1942 until February 1943. Sterilization took place only during the month of December, because on December 20 we fell ill with spotted typhus. Kazia caught it two days before me, then I, and Schumann did not even return home. He remained in the hospital in Kattowitz.

In January, Professor Clauberg arrived. Sylvia Friedmann, a Slovakian Jewish prisoner, was his assistant.[13] She established a ward for surgical sterilization in our block according to the orders of Dr. Wirths who had been a student of Dr. Clauberg. I had a lot of contact with him and consider him to have been one of the meanest criminals, a cold sadist. After the war, he hung himself. It is still puzzling to me why his activities were couched in silence; did they want to protect his family?

I would like to add that immediately after my liberation and return to Vienna, I gave my deposition to the courts at a time when Dr. Schumann was still living in Halle. Only much later did he flee to the Sudan, Nigeria and to Ghana where he became a sort of Dr. Schweizer in the jungle. Dr. Schumann was protected by the authorities until the Kwame Nkrumah government fell and he was extradited to Germany in 1966. Indeed, Schumann was already involved with murder before he came to Auschwitz, having participated in the euthanasia projects. Because of deteriorating health, he was released without having stood trial for his sterilization and castration experiments. He died in 1983.

I never saw Schumann again although his patients, as well as I, were later transferred to Block 10. After the typhus, I was very weak. My vision was affected and I did not hear well and it took a long time for me to recuperate. I owe my life to Kazia's mother. She provided me with food since she worked in the Kleiderkammer (clothing warehouse). Under different circumstances and without assistance I would not have survived in camp. Kazia and her mother were both released as Volksdeutsche (ethnic Germans).

In February 1943, Dr. Wirths took me as his secretary to Block 10 in Auschwitz. During that period, Dr. Samuel (a Jewish prisoner physician) was working there. He attempted to do as little as possible. Another inmate doctor, Adelaide Hautval, a French woman, refused to work for Wirths. I was present when she declined. She was the daughter of a minister and cited her religion as a reason for her refusal. Many years ago, I saw her again in Paris.

I remember very well the transports that came from Greece. Some of the staff of Block 10 had to go to the ramp to help shave the hair of the new arrivals. The poor Greek girls had spent a long time in the cattle cars and their hair was full of lice and so infested that we got blisters on our hands. The first transport of Greek girls went directly to Block 10 and they gave us so many olives that we got indigestion.

Dr. Wirths performed the most inhuman experiments and I had to be present as well as note down everything. I was very unhappy in Block 10, and I had a sinister feeling about Wirths.

In the meantime, Block 30 in Birkenau had been transformed into a dental ward. Dr. Danielle Casanova,[14] a French prisoner dentist had died and the secretary had been fired. I asked the Kapo to request me as a replacement via Maria Mandel, the chief SS-woman. It worked; I left Dr. Wirths' patients' files behind and was picked up early one morning to be taken to Birkenau. When Wirths learned about my scheme he came himself and placed me in the punishment detail, which was located in Buna at that time. Again Enna (the Jewish Slovakian inmate physician) helped me. She had good connections with SS Dr. Rhode. I was released and allowed to return to Birkenau; only when Dr. Wirths visited the camp did I have to disappear.

In the late fall of 1943, I had to go to Vienna for my trial. SS-man Hustek-Erber made me take an oath in civilian clothing that I had heard and seen nothing while I was in Auschwitz. When I arrived in Vienna, they threw me in jail. I was the first prisoner with a tattooed Auschwitz number that they had ever seen. Therefore, I was a big sensation. Even the director of the prison called me to his office.

Well, at the trial I was acquitted, but "als juedisch versippt" (being related to Jews) I had to remain in protective custody until the end of the war. Thus, back to Auschwitz I went. In order to justify the whole procedure, it was discovered that on the date in question (Stichtag) I had been registered as a Jewess (professed the Jewish faith), hence, according to the Nuernberg racial laws, I was a "Geltungsjuedin" (considered Jewish).[15]

Nevertheless, I was supposed to get certain privileges. Consequently, on my return in February 1944, I was transferred to the Stabsgebaeude in Auschwitz and became the secretary of camp commandant Liebehenschel. I only worked for him, but I shared his antechamber with SS-Unterscharfuerer Herpel and Ackermann, two illiterate cretins. I was picked up every day at the Stabsgebaude with an Austrian inmate, Enni Laibel, by an SS-man, Gwendolin Kiefer, who was a Volksdeutscher, and taken to the Kommandantur (command post). I had to carry his food utensils and he walked behind me with his rifle. Herpel was in charge of arriving RSHA transports. All operations were supposed to be very hush-hush, because foreign radio stations had already frequently been broadcasting the news and partisans attempted to block the rails.

I typed letters and took care of the Bunker-book for the SS alone. For example, those SS-men who stole too much gold were put into the Bunker.

In May or June 1944, I was sent to the punishment kommando in Birkenau to work in road construction because I had written letters which had been smuggled out of camp through SS-woman Edith Nestroy. Her apartment had been searched, and the SS had found large quantities of jewels she had received from a Polish prisoner. Unfortunately, a letter for me, which she had intended to give me the following day, was also discovered.. It was addressed to "Little guinea pig" and SS-adjutant Zoller ran around screaming, "I'll find out who this guinea pig is!" Two days later, SS-woman Nestroy confessed my name in the bunker and Zoller was gleeful. Official whipping had already been forbidden by Berlin. Otherwise, he would have executed it with delight on my person.

For Unterscharfuehrer Ackermann, I had to write identification cards for all SS-personnel, I never managed to fully differentiate between the different ranks. Once, somebody threw his I.D. in my face and prophesied that I would soon be admitted to his work detail. He was SS-man Mokrus from the punishment squad, and sure enough, a short while later I landed in his kommando. You cannot imagine how joyfully he greeted me every morning when we marched out and how jubilantly he made me work in the swampy ditches.

In November 1944, I was transferred to Ravensbrueck where I worked in a Siemens factory. In the spring of 1945, when we were marched to Malchow, I escaped.

When I returned to Vienna after the war, all my friends came to see me. One of them was Anton Jakl, born in Southern Tyrol, whose wife was a Jewess from Berlin. His mother-in-law had been gassed in Birkenau. They wanted an eye-witness report on Auschwitz and asked me to visit them.

We met in his office on Wallner Street, and I told them everything I knew. Suddenly, Jakl grew very reflective and said to me, "It's funny, indeed, but not too long ago a man was assigned to live on my estate." That was during the time when there were already bombs in Vienna and people were evacuated to the countryside.

I cannot remember the name of the village where the estate was situated, but it was in Lower Austria, as can be ascertained from the police file.

Jakl went on telling me that this man frequently received boxes from Upper Silesia. Now, I started to get interested because Auschwitz was situated in Upper Silesia and the SS had acquired many possessions which the inmates had brought with them to Auschwitz. They would send home to their families everything they could lay their hands on. Since I had worked in the Commandant's office and issued the identity cards for the SS men, I knew practically all their names.

When Jakl told me the name "Grabner," I was flabbergasted. The name of SS-Untersturmfuehrer (Lieutenant) Maximilian Grabner was anathema to all of us in Auschwitz since he was the dreaded chief of the Political Section (the Auschwitz Gestapo). We were terribly afraid of him. He was from the same area of Vienna where I had lived. I never could have forgotten his name.

Even though Jakl described a man who had grown a full beard, it was clear that despite his effort to disguise himself, this was the same individual. The coincidence seemed unbelievable.

At that time, the Chief of the Austrian State Police was Dr. Duermayer, a former Auschwitz inmate. I thought to myself that if I reported what I had heard, nobody would believe me. Everyone would laugh at me or think I was hallucinating.

I asked Jakl to contact Dr. Duermayer at Police Headquarters. After I convinced him how important it was, he went to see Dr. Duermayer and, as far as I can remember, they went together to Jakl's estate where Dr. Duermayer arrested Grabner.[16]

Postscript

It was very difficult for me to speak about Auschwitz even now, after 46 years, but I know that eyewitness accounts cannot be published without the participation of former prisoners. However, I seriously doubt that people who were not in the camp will be able to understand. Let's, for example, take the case of the sisters Zimmerspitz, Slovakian Jewesses, who were block elders in the notorious block 25, the gathering point for the gas chamber. I had to go to Block 25 twice, and saw how the Zimmerspitz' were beating their own comrades whom they let starve. When the trucks arrived to pick up their cargo and transport them to the crematoria, the Zimmerspitz' whipped these poor women as they climbed into the trucks. On these occasions, there always was "Blocksperre" (general curfew), only we who worked in the Revier could circulate. It is simply impossible to write about these events—normal human beings will never be able to grasp them.

CHAPTER TWO
Personnel

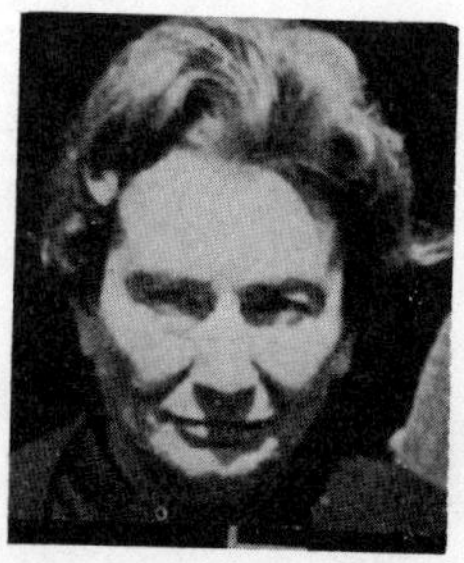

Dr. Alina Bialostocka (née Brewda)
(London, United Kingdom)

Out of superstition, my mother registered my birth on June 14, 1905, although I was actually born on June 13. I was born in Warsaw, the former Polish capital which, at the time, was the headquarters of the Russian Governor-General who ruled this western province of the Tzar from the former Palace of the Polish Kings.

Both of my parents were dental surgeons, and I grew up in a flat in an attractive historical section of the town. There were two brass plates on the front door, two separate surgeries and a common waiting room full of patients with gumboils and toothaches. The odor of iodoform pervaded the air and the flat was vibrant with the buzz of dental drills and the recurrent gargle of the mouthwash.

By the time I graduated from high school, Poland had become an independent state. Since early childhood, I had always intended to study medicine; however, because of the *numerus clausus* I had to wait a year until I could start my studies. Anti-semitism was prevalent at the university and all Jewish students were informed that we could not operate on Christian corpses for the anatomy course. Since Halachic law prohibits the use of Jewish corpses, we were in a predicament. After much begging, we finally obtained some bodies of babies from the Jewish Foundling Home for dissection purposes. In the summer of 1930, I received my medical degree; subsequently, I specialized as a gynecologist and obstetrician.

In October 1940, approximately one year after the German invasion of Poland, we were moved to the Warsaw Ghetto and in April 1943, during the uprising, and while the ghetto was still burning, I was transported to Maidanek. Here I again worked as a gynecologist. Dr. Rindfleisch, the SS physician in charge of the entire camp was so pleased with my work that he sent glowing reports about me to general headquarters in Berlin. In August 1943, Standartenfuhrer Dr. Enno Lolling, Deputy Inspector-General of medical services in all concentration camps, came especially to Maidanek to talk to me.[1]

He informed me that I was being transferred to a most important post at the SS-Lazarett which was the main female hospital in Auschwitz. I told him I did not want to go. He was furious. "Why?" he asked.

"Because in Auschwitz I shall have my head shaved, I will have my arm tattooed with a number—and later, if I am unable to continue to work, I shall be sent to the gas chamber."

"That's a lie," he said. "We don't do things like that. It is just a lot of ridiculous, malicious gossip."

I asked if he could guarantee that this would not be done, and he said, "Of course."

The following morning, Oberaufseherin Ehrlich accompanied me from Maidanek to Auschwitz.

True to Dr. Lolling's promise my hair was not shaved. However, I received the tattooed prison number 62761—but they did not add the triangle that all Jewish prisoners in 1943 received underneath their numbers.

A few days after my arrival in Birkenau, I was sent to the experimental Block at the men's camp in Auschwitz.

Block 10

On the steps of Block 10, I saw three small Jewish boys playing; they were about eight, six and four years of age. I was astonished to see Jewish children at Auschwitz, for Jewish children were sent to the gas chamber the moment they arrived. Children were useless in the labor force and, in any case, the Germans were resolved on stamping out the Jewish race.

I discovered later that the children: Bronek Seeman, Karol Umschweif, and Peter Dattel lived in Block 10 with their mothers, two of whom were the wives of scientists. The scientists themselves lived in another part of the camp, since Block 10 was exclusively a women's block.

The moment I entered the block, I noticed that all the windows had been boarded up: there were wooden boards on the outside and iron bars on the inside. None of the other blocks in the men's camp had their windows boarded and barred. The boards, placed at a slant, let in a narrow strip of light at the top. No other light entered the Block, which was lit entirely by artificial lighting.

Looking about me, I thought at first that I must be in a brothel. I saw a number of half naked girls, not one of them Jewish, walking about in silk nightdresses or in their underwear. I learned later that these girls were in fact prostitutes and had been brought to Block 10 for tests for venereal disease.

I was taken along the corridor to a small dormitory on the ground floor and was told the staff slept here and that I was to sleep here too. There was room for about twenty-five of us, all prisoners of course. Two of them were doctors, but they were not employed as doctors; the others were nurses and laboratory workers, all of them Jewish. I met one of the two doctors and we became friends. Her name was Slavka (Dorota) Kleinova.

During my first days in Block 10, I took a tour of inspection, saw the numerous laboratories and learned about some of the experiments that were in progress under the supervision of various German doctors: Dr. Willy Frank, for example, had a dental laboratory; Dr. Bruno Weber was in charge of the bacteriological laboratories where blood, sputum and sweat tests were being carried out. Slavka Kleinova worked for him and so did Dr. Hans Muench who was quite a kind man and one of the few SS doctors to survive the criminal trials after the war. He had run away, but was caught. I was ill and bed-ridden in Warsaw at the time of his trial in Cracow, but I made a deposition from my sick bed and Muench said afterwards that I was responsible for his being acquitted. I suppose what I said helped.

I heard about Dr. Maximilian Samuel, a German Jew, who did experiments for Dr. Wirths, but I was unaware of the type of experiments he performed. Nobody seemed to know exactly. He had been a senior lecturer in gynecology at Cologne University and had been brought to Auschwitz as a prisoner to work in Block 10 for SS Standortarzt Dr. Edward Wirths.

I also heard about Professor Carl Clauberg and the four rooms he used on the ground floor, but nobody seemed to know what he did in these rooms.

Dr. Schumann's activities, as well, were clouded in secrecy.

The four hundred-odd women guinea pigs all lived on the second floor. They were of many different nationalities, but the Greek girls were extremely young, between sixteen and nineteen years of age. They were divided up among the doctors. There were Dr. Wirths' "specimens;" Clauberg's women who had a caustic fluid injected into their uterus'; Dr. Weber's sputum and blood guinea pigs and the Greek girls who belonged to Dr. Schumann. The latter all had deep x-ray radiation burns on their bodies, since their ovaries had been irradiated and their skin was covered with suppurating blisters and ulcers.

The prostitutes were the only ones who were not Jewish. There were twenty-five of them. Brothels had been set up in every concentration camp because of the prevalence of homosexuality among the men, but only "Aryan" prisoners were allowed to visit these girls. Some of them were Poles and Russians, others were German; they were all prisoners.

While the prostitutes were in Block 10, the secret sterilization experiments of Clauberg and Schumann were brought to a complete standstill. So it was impossible for me to discover what was really being done. Such secrecy made me realize that everyone who discovered the truth about these experiments would one day have to be put to death, besides of course, the top SS doctors who carried them out.

About three weeks after my arrival on Block 10, chief SS doctor Edward Wirths came to the block. He was a young man, but extremely good-looking with penetrating blue eyes.

He addressed me as "Frau Doktor," for which I was grateful. It gave me a sort of status in the eyes of the Block officers, especially the two SS women; and after that they all began to treat me with respect. If any of them dared address me familiarly as "du" ("thou"), I immediately called them on it.

"I am not 'du' to you," I said. "Remember, I'm Frau Doktor to you, as I am to Dr. Wirths. If any of you try to beat me or ill treat me, I'll have you thrown out of the Block." They used to speak of me as "Dr. Wirths' property."

Dr. Wirths told me that he was going to order Dr. Samuel to give me the key to the operating theatre in Block 10. He said he wanted me to take over a colposcope from Berlin that Dr. Samuel was using and that I must do for him what Dr. Samuel had been doing.

Then he added, in a loud voice so that all the senior Block officials and the SS women could hear, that I was to be the medical head of Block 10, under his direct orders and that I was entrusted with the general medical care of the occupants of the Block. "If there is anything you need," he said, "ask me for it. Don't let anybody come into the Block hospital apart from Clauberg, Frank and Weber. Every other person, including SS-men, must produce a written permission from me before they can be allowed to enter, and you must ask for it."

When Dr. Samuel brought me the key to the operating room, he unlocked the door and I followed him in. It had a couch, a table, a stool, a standard lamp, a case of instruments, and a colposcope on a stand. I asked Dr. Samuel what it was used for. He did not answer, but told me that my arrival meant death for him. He was an old man, he said, and had now become superfluous. He explained that the SS had forbidden male prisoner-doctors to treat female prisoner-patients, a rule which I already knew. It was sometimes ignored and had been waived in his case, he said, because of the work he was doing. But, as a male gynecologist, he was useless now and as good as dead already, because he was a Geheimnistraeger, a secret carrier, meaning that he would have to be exterminated.

He then began to tell me a little about the experiments. Dr. Wirths, he said, wanted to learn more about the earliest stages of cancer in the cervix of the womb. He had for that purpose between fifty and eighty women prisoners in Block 10, all of them over the age of thirty-five and up to the age of sixty-five. Dr. Wirths had brought a special instrument, a colposcope, from Berlin to examine the cervix. When something irregular was observed, Dr. Wirths or Dr. Samuel operated and removed the cervix, which was then sent off to Berlin for further examination.

Dr. Schumann's Experiments

Towards the end of October 1943, the prostitutes left. The place had been turned into something like a slave market with the Commandants from surrounding camps having come and inspected them to make their selection.

Shortly afterwards, a very tall officer, dressed in a grey Luftwaffe uniform, whom I had not seen before, came to Block 10. He asked me if I was the prisoner-gynecologist. I said, "Yes," and I asked him who he was. He said he was Dr. Schumann. I then told him of Dr. Wirths' instructions that I must not let anyone come into the Block without his written authority.

He brushed that aside and asked me how long it would take to set up a proper operating theatre in Block 10 as this was only a makeshift one. I realized that this was their second approach to me, for Wirths had already asked me to take over the "machine from Berlin" from Dr. Samuel and to perform the work that Samuel had done. I did not know what to say to Schumann, so I simply said, "I don't know—about three months."

Some minutes later, Schumann asked me whether I could remove ovaries. I said I was an obstetrician and not a surgeon gynecologist. He said I lied. He then asked me how long it would take to remove an ovary. I replied, "About one and a quarter to one and a half hours." He said, "You are lying. Our gynecologist here does the operation in eight to ten minutes."

Although I had deliberately exaggerated the time, I found it impossible to believe that anyone could remove an ovary in eight to ten minutes. He then left without further comment.

Dr. Horst Schumann was about thirty-seven years old and had a hideous scar across his face. He had been working at the Grafeneck Euthanasia Institute and had been moved to Auschwitz by Himmler to carry out the sterilization experiments by x-ray and by castration.

Early in November 1943, Dr. Schumann came into the Block and said briskly, "Come with me," and took me across to Block 21, the men's hospital.

As I entered, I heard a girl screaming. I went with Dr. Schumann into the ante-room of the operating theatre and saw one of the Greek girls from my Block being held down on a special table by two male prisoners in white coats. The girl was held in a suitable position to receive a spinal injection. She kept on screaming. Other Greek girls were also present.

Dr. Wladyslaw Dering, a Polish, non-Jewish prison doctor, who had been on the Warsaw University faculty with me and had married a fellow student of mine, was there too, washing his hands. Dr. Schumann asked me to calm the girls and left.

I went up to Dr. Dering and said, "Do you realize that these girls have had irradiation quite recently?" He said, "I know." I asked him what he was doing and he said, "Oopherectomies." He then went into the theatre and I followed him because the girl on the operating table was screaming and crying and trying to release herself. Dr. Dering put on his gloves and the table was tilted to form an angle of about thirty degrees, with the patient's head downward, which is the lithotomy position.

I sat on a stool by the girl's head and tried to comfort her. Dr. Dering then proceeded to make abdominal incisions and told me to keep the girl quiet. I told him, "What do you think you are doing? This is a young girl, she has already had irradiation of the ovary, so why do you have to operate?" He did not reply.

He cut the peritoneum, and used forceps to lift up the uterus. He then put the forceps between the tube and the ovary and cut off the ovary, only one, putting it in a specimen basin beside him. The operation took about ten minutes. I had never seen this done so quickly before. I had carried out a few operations of this kind in the past, but, according to the technique prevalent at that time in Poland, half an hour was the minimum time necessary.

The girl was then carried out on a stretcher by the two male prisoners and Dr. Dering went and gave the spinal injection to the next girl, who also began to scream.

During the course of that afternoon, ten girls received operations. When they brought in the Greek girl whom I knew as Bella, one of the two girls who already had an operation scar on the abdomen. I said to Dr. Dering, "I suppose you know that one of her ovaries has already been removed. You are not going to make this girl a female eunuch, are you?" He replied, "That's not your business." He had earlier admitted that he had also removed the testicles of certain young male prisoners. They were, of course, Jewish, just as all these girls were.

The ten girls came back from Block 21 restless, crying and screaming. I, with the help of Slavka Kleinova, looked after them. We had nothing to treat them with and had to steal some morphium from Professor Clauberg's room, but there was not enough. Dr. Kleinova and I sat up all night with the girls. Bella died that night and another girl, Buena, died two or three days later from "shock after the operation." The wounds of the others were not healing, the skin was not growing together and there were suppurations, even many months after the operations had been performed.

Ampler details of this heinous Nazi plan for the mass sterilization of Jews were supplied in the course of a trial in the Royal Courts of Justice in London in April and May 1964. Dr. Dering, by then in medical practice in London, and decorated O.B.E., claimed that he had been libeled in a book called *Exodus* by Leon Uris, which in a single sentence referred to Dr. Schumann's attempts at sterilizing Jews by x-ray and castration, and Dr. Dering's role in the process.

Together with my fellow prisoner physicians Dr. Kleinova and Dr. Hautval, as well as eight of the surviving Greek girls and six castrated Jewish male prisoners, I appeared as witness for the defense. The case largely concerned Dr. Dering's activities and behavior while performing such operations at Auschwitz.

It was stressed that not only was he known to have been anti-Semitic, it was also obvious he neglected to give a general anaesthetic to his Jewish victims; a humane gesture that would have alleviated their suffering. The Register of operations clearly showed that general anaesthetics were available and had been given again and again to other prisoner patients.

Giving their verdict, the jury awarded Dr. Dering one half-penny as damages—the smallest coin in the realm. But cost of the defense, amounting to about £16,000 were awarded against him.[2]

Professor Clauberg

Professor Carl Clauberg played a prominent and personal part in the experiments in Block 10. A tiny man, by 1943 he was thick set, had a crooked nose and not much hair. He dressed in civilian clothes that were not only odd, but some thought even laughable. He wore a small Tyrolean hat sporting a feather, and breeches laced all the way up to the knees. He sometimes drove up to Block 10 in a car with his mistress seated beside him and their two small children in the back.

From the very beginning of his medical career he had conducted research into the female sexual hormones and, in his first interview with Himmler, in Berlin in March 1940, he discussed various ways of sterilizing women. Himmler was particularly interested in achieving this without a surgical operation and provided funds for testing by means of injections into the oviducts. The initial tests were made on animals, but a year later, at a further interview with Clauberg, Himmler agreed that in the future experiments should be made on human beings. They planned to use women prisoners from Auschwitz because it was near enough to Clauberg's clinic in Koenigshuette, Silesia, for him to travel back and forth.

Himmler emphasized the need to find a method of sterilization that could be carried out without the knowledge of the victims.

Clauberg began the experiments in December 1942, at Birkenau. He found the huts unsuitable and inadequate and decided to use them for his x-ray work only, requesting that one of the blocks at Auschwitz be especially adapted for his tests. Thus, Block 10 in the men's camp was rebuilt for Clauberg's guinea-pigs on a plan devised by Clauberg, and was put into operation in early 1943.

During my stay in Block 10, about half of the four hundred women were Clauberg's patients. I had been especially instructed by Dr. Wirths to stay away from his guinea-pigs. I only knew that they had a caustic fluid injected into their uterus' while, simultaneously, x-rays were taken to ascertain the blockage. The pain caused by these sterilization experiments must have been tremendous, and the screams of the women could be heard throughout the entire block. Sometimes, even the SS women came to me and asked what Clauberg was doing to these women to make them scream so horribly.

Once or twice, I was called by Clauberg's nurse, Sylvia Friedmann, a Slovakian Jewess, because women were in shock after the injection. I distinctly remember that one woman was lying on the x-ray table and the instruments were still inside her vagina or uterus. I used to administer morphium in cases like these.

From other prisoners, I heard time and time again that Professor Clauberg behaved brutally while giving his injections. Sylvia, herself, used to hit those women who resisted instinctively or who screamed too loudly. It was incomprehensible to me that so little consideration was shown to these guinea-pigs, some of whom were virgins. I talked to Sylvia about it and asked her not to hit. She answered that I should tell the women that they should not scream or resist, then she would not have to resort to beatings.

Ever since I had arrived in Block 10, the Slovakian Jewish Block Elder Margit and her deputy Magda had disliked me. I finally succeeded in stripping her of her authority over me.

In January or February 1944, Dr. Wirths asked me whether everything was okay in the block. I told him that everything could not be okay as long as the patients were beaten by Block Elder Margit. The same day, Dr. Wirths demoted Margit. He declared that there was no need for a Block elder, and that I should fulfill this function. He told Margit that it was not necessary any more for her and her deputy to take the roll calls. That deprived them both of their authority. I produced my patient list whenever it was required for inspection. The secretary of the Block, the Slovakian Jewess Rozana, with whom I shared a room, signed it and the SS-wardens took the report on bicycles to Birkenau because technically, as women, we belonged to Birkenau.

I had taken this step in full cooperation with the underground organization of Auschwitz.

Underground Activity

Dr. Kleinova, who had served in the Spanish Civil War as a doctor in the International Brigade and had joined the French Resistance movement at the very beginning of the German occupation of France, belonged to an Auschwitz Underground movement. She told me about the group. Sixteen of the girls in Block 10, who had in fact worked with Kleinova in the Resistance movement in France, also belonged. She added that they could be trusted absolutely; there was not one traitor among them. I decided to join Kleinova and her friends in their underground work.

The network to which Kleinova belonged, and with which I became associated, was an international group consisting of men and women of all nationalities. It was known as the Auschwitz Fighting Group. One of its principal leaders was Hermann Langbein, a young Austrian, who, like Kleinova, had served in the Spanish Civil War in the International Brigade.

I first met Langbein in November 1943, and we became firm friends. He was Dr. Wirths' secretary and made it possible for me to have access to the SS-dispensary and I was able to "steal" essential drugs that were needed for the girls in Block 10.

Another member of the underground was Josef Cyrankiewicz, a Polish prisoner who became Prime Minister of Poland after the war.

The Underground movement was extremely well organized. None of us knew too much about what was going on—only enough for the work to be carried on if one or another of us was caught. I supplied details of what I had learned to Kleinova and she passed it on, together with other information to certain helpers outside the camp. For example, names of the chief SS offenders were sent to London via Cracow so that they should be broadcast by the B.B.C.

In response to an appeal from the Resistance group, I was able to help the Kapo in charge of the most valuable section of Canada, namely the storehouse in which the gold and jewelry were kept.

I had been performing abortions on Jewish girls for I knew that all pregnant Jewesses were sent straight to the gas chamber. Pregnant "Aryan" girls were secretly brought to me from time to time, among these was the girlfriend of the

Kapo in charge of the gold and diamonds storehouse. He was a Pole from Silesia, but like all other Silesians, he was classified as a German.

Cyrankiewicz asked me to end the pregnancy of this girl as the Kapo was helping the Underground by stealing diamonds and other gems, which the underground needed to buy weapons and ammunition.

I suggested that they should take the girl to the operating theatre in the men's surgery in Block 21, which was opposite our Block, and get her operated on there for appendicitis. Then, at night, they could have her brought across to me since ours was the only women's block.

This they did. After the appendix operation, the girl was brought to Block 10. I found she was an "Aryan." I performed the abortion on the floor of the small laboratory Kleinova had upstairs with Slavka assisting.

While I was engaged in doing this, I heard a knock on the door. We were both startled. Was it the SS? I asked Kleinova to go cautiously to the door and see who it was. She found it was one of our night nurses who had been looking after the girl I was now operating on. The nurse was almost in tears. She said, "My patient has disappeared. She was under my care. I don't know what Dr. Alina will do to me."

I then went to the door and said, "I will try and find her for you." I told her not to worry anymore, but to go to bed and I would look after the girl myself. When I had finished, Kleinova and I carried her back to the ward downstairs.

In The Bunker

One day, at the end of July 1944, suddenly and without any warning, I was taken off to the Gestapo. I was not questioned but was sent straight away to the Bunker in Block 11. Hardly anyone came out of that place alive.

I was put into a minute cell with just a bunk and a tiny bucket for use as a toilet. There was no water at all. I had to take out the bucket once a day, with a guard in attendance, and wash it in a communal wash room.

For two days I was given nothing to eat or drink. No warden came to see me. On the third day, the chief warden, called the Kapo of the Bunker and known only by the name of Jakob, came to my cell. He was a huge man who had once been a professional wrestler. He arrived jangling the keys of the cells. The door was swung open and, to my astonishment, I saw this giant, hairy man standing before me with a dish of prunes. The prunes, he said rather sheepishly, had been sent by the girls in Block 10.

Surprisingly enough, Jakob also worked for the Underground movement. Although he wasn't exactly a member, he knew of our activities and never disclosed anything. He helped us in fact, though, if someone was caught and Jakob was told to hang him, he had no choice but to carry out the order, and he did.

Jakob was a very simple man. He used to come to my cell whenever he was able, which was generally after the evening Roll Call, and sit and chat with me to cheer me up.

Once he told me in his broken Polish, "Pani doktorka, is it worth it to give your head for four hundred Jewish tochusse?"

However, on the seventeenth day of my solitary confinement, Jakob opened my cell door accompanied by a male SS officer and a Ukranian prisoner who was the Bunker doctor. Jakob began to remove the card with my name on it from the door and told me that I was being released.

I never really found out why I had been in the Bunker. Upon my return, Dr. Wirths said, "Do you know why you were sent to the Bunker? This will teach you not to write love letters."

"I never wrote any love letters," I replied.

"Yes, you did," said one of the SS officials with emphasis. That, I suppose, was a sort of face-saving remark.

Shortly after my release, I was transferred to Birkenau where I worked as a seamstress for nearly four months. On December 18, 1944, I was sent back to the new women's camp in Auschwitz and worked once more as a physician in the hospital together with Dr. Kleinova.

One month later, on January 18, 1945, Auschwitz was evacuated. We were first sent to Ravensbrueck and later to Neustadt-Glewe. It was not until May 8, 1945, that the moment of liberation finally came with the arrival of the Russians.

I returned to Poland, but had a coronary thrombosis which required me to stay in bed for seven months.

Friends, however, arranged for the Government to give me a monthly allowance to pay for my room and for other small necessities. In addition, every month I was sent twelve pounds of English marmalade, thirty cans of sardines, two bottles of vodka, five bottles of Russian champagne and a thousand American cigarettes. That was the ration allowed to senior Ministers by the Government. This had been granted me, I was told, because of my Underground work at Auschwitz.

In February 1947, I emigrated to England. I met some friends I had known in Warsaw. Among them was a Polish lawyer, Szymon Bialostocki, whom I had first met when I was three years old and he was eight years older. We were married in London on March 3, 1948.

I kept up my gynecological practice until a few years ago when I had to undergo a mastectomy and the removal of my uterus and ovaries. It took me a long time to recuperate.[3]

❖

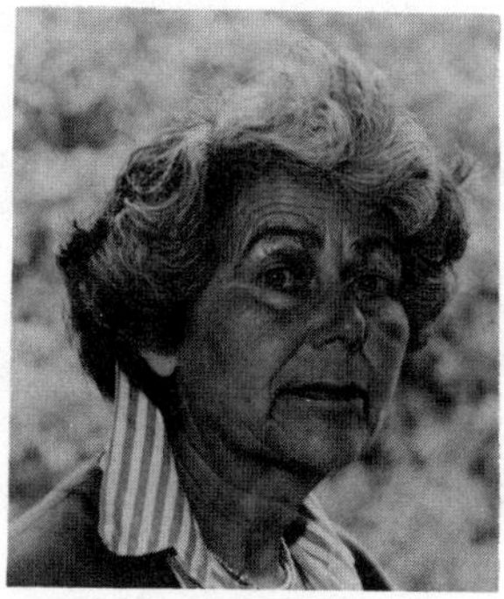

Ima Spanjaard (née van Esso)
Haarlem (Holland)

I was born in Amsterdam on September 10, 1920. My father was a physician and my mother had studied geography. Both belonged to the first group of very enthusiastic Zionists. As a matter of fact, that's how they met. They worked in all kinds of committees as long as I can remember. My two brothers and I received a religious education. It did not do too much for me except that I do know the basics very well and do not need to find my "roots" for which everybody is looking nowadays.

My eldest brother, Dr. Benjamin Ben Assa followed in my father's footsteps. In 1945, he became a well-known physician for the Bedouins in the Negev desert. He passed away, but his widow and four married children are living comfortably in Israel.

My youngest brother, Philip van Esso worked illegally in the well-known resistance group of Joop Westerweel,[4] who was murdered in 1944, and after whom a forest was named in Israel after the war, was brought to Drancy and later exterminated in Auschwitz.

I tried to escape but the organization was betrayed just across the border in Belgium on its way to Switzerland. I was taken to St. Gilles, a prison near Brussels, where I stayed for a month.

There, I was one of three women in a tiny cell. The first thing I did was to divide the little food that I had with me in three, and offer a share to each of the others. The first thing they did was to refuse it. I understood only later that they received packages from Belgium they didn't want to share.

I was twenty-two but still an innocent child, and I cried day and night because of this rejection and because of my longing for my mother.

Out of anger, I spoke to them exclusively in French—school French which I had learned only to translate—until in desperation, they exclaimed, "For God's sake, speak in German!" I was butchering their language. There was a sphere of misery and hate in the cell.

After that I was in a concentration camp in Mechelen for half a year. The one advantage of those periods of captivity was that they gave me a thorough preparation for Auschwitz. For the people who came from Westerbork (a camp in the Netherlands) the transition was too great.

At the time, I was engaged to Louis Micheels,[5] a medical student in his fifth year. And, as on each train there should be a doctor, he was appointed as such. And I functioned as nurse. During the previous year, I had been a dentist's assistant as I had been obliged to break off my studies at the conservatory. There we were, in the most horrible railway-carriage among the most miserable cases of illness and disease.

On April 21, 1943, I arrived in Auschwitz and received the prison number 42646. There was a need for guinea pigs and nurses for Block 10. Since my fiance and I had been termed "Red Cross Medical Couple" of our transport, I called myself a nurse and was selected for Block 10.

Block 10 was the only women's barrack in the men's camp of Auschwitz; downstairs were surgeries and upstairs dormitories each for 150 women. On one of these two wards we remained in quarantine. That meant six weeks in complete isolation without any activity whatsoever.

Right away it appeared that Branco van Thijn, a Dutchwoman whom I had befriended during the transport, was a highly qualified apothecary and presently she was allowed to come downstairs to the so-called "Plegestube" with forty beds. Branco wanted me down there very much, because she felt lonely among all those Polish-speaking people.

Finally, Branco arranged for me to be allowed to sleep downstairs. That's what I call protection. After that I had all sorts of jobs, outside the block as well as inside, amongst others in the typhus lazaret of the SS. I had to clean their rooms and to light the stoves. But as an upper class child who was accustomed to central heating and three maidservants, I had never tried to light a fire, let alone with the help of wet reeds and wet pieces of paper which I had to find outside. Because of the smoke which inevitably developed, the sick Krauts became so furious that they threw their pisspots at my head. This only lasted for ten days. When I came back, Branco saw to it that I became a nurse. It was my job to administer injections, both subcutaneous and intramuscular ones. However, I didn't know how to do it. I only knew how to do things in a sterile way, because as a dentist's assistant I had been used to sterilize things by boiling them in water. Branco taught me how to do it and she did this so calmly and reassuredly, being convinced that I could do it too, that in fact I could. Coming from a medical family, I seemed to have a natural propensity to do something medical in a relaxed way.

Later I was chosen as anesthesiologist for the portio vaginalis operations.

What I had to do was shown to me just once; tying up the arm, finding the vein and then administering as little evipan as possible. The patient then is under sedation right away.

I am still ashamed of it to this very day; but I speak about it now to school classes of the Athenaeum in Holocaust courses.

▼

Below I tell a little about life and people in Block 10.

The SS-Doctors of Block 10

Prof. Carl Clauberg

Although he was feared a lot, he was not the worst. He had a sanatorium of his own in nearby Koenigshuette which facilitated his coming to see his guinea pigs in Block 10 as often as possible. There were rumors that he had bought the women. Sylvia Friedmann, his nurse, tried to bribe him with cigarettes and by knitting him pullovers. Trees Soetendorp, a comrade of mine, told me that he gave her "die Spritze" (an injection) and the following day while looking at her x-ray, he exclaimed "Bezaubernd, entzueckend" (charming, exquisite). Later on she was incapable of having children.

Dr. Horst Schumann

He was one of the worst. Five or six days after my arrival, he inspected us during roll-call. He chose forty of the youngest and best looking girls. I was among those he had selected. But I had told Hélène Frank that my husband was a doctor. Hélène informed Magda, our block-elder that I was a nurse and thus I managed to get out of the experiment.

Schumann had the women sterilized by x-rays in Birkenau so brutally that they were all burnt. At first six, and later on ten were operated on. Their ovaries were removed to ascertain whether or not the previous irradiation had sterilized them properly. Two of the women were operated on twice. It was Dering who performed the operations on the ten women, all with the same instruments in three hours. Some of the women died because of perforated intestines. Others were looked after by Hélène Rosenthal, our only genuine nurse. They suffered for half a year with horrible pains. Upon their recovery, they were sent to Birkenau to work with the Aussenkommando (to do heavy outside work).

I even remember some of the girls names: Mazal, Buena, Gilda, Dora, Bella, Rachel and Lea.

About twenty years ago, I was a witness against Dr. Horst Schumann. They worked about a year on his case. Then he fell "ill"—and that was the end.

Dr. Eduard Wirths

Wirths did cervical "cancer" experiments. While in 1944, in approximately 60 per one million examined women cancer was detected, Wirths removed (or had removed) the portio vaginalis in three hundred young women between the ages of 16 and 25 in Block 10 in Auschwitz.

After the war, Wirths was interrogated by Colonel Draper from the United Kingdom. The colonel told him:

"I now shake hands with one of the men responsible for having murdered four million people. Go back to your cell and think it over. Tomorrow we'll continue." That evening, Wirths tried to commit suicide by hanging. He was discovered and died two days later.

In December 1974, Rolf Orthel, a Dutch movie director, made a film about Wirths to show how a normal student could end up as SS-man in Auschwitz.

Orthel interviewed the father, the wife and three grown-up children of Wirths. His best friend related that as students they had been compelled to join the SS or quit studying. Wirths signed up but his friend refused and the only field of study open to him was theology. He pursued the course although he was absolutely not interested in religion.

Hermann Langbein, who—as inmate—had been Wirths' secretary in Auschwitz, also took part in the film. Langbein had known Wirths very well and had informed him in the end that there existed an underground movement in camp with contacts to England, and that Wirths was on their black list.

Two women of Block 10 participated in the movie: my friend Friedl Couvée and I. I was very sharp, telling Orthel that as an individual I thought Wirths to be both a gentleman and a bastard, but Friedl was soft and more or less philosophical.

The movie received a lot of prizes in Western Europe. Orthel showed it to the Wirths family in Germany. Then, at last, the widow said, "Now I know and understand what happened. I will no more defend my husband."

Dr. Goebel

SS-Obersturmfuehrer Goebel (a Ph.D., not an M.D.) was an assistant of Clauberg. We called him the "chemist of lemonades and tooth paste." He was feared.

I had a non-Jewish inmate friend, Vladimir Hanak, a Czech sportsman, who had to treat Goebel with massages. He insisted that he needed somebody to help him with the "Schroepfkoepfchen" (cupping glasses) against his severe cold—the somebody was I. So, again a subterfuge for me not to serve as Clauberg's guinea pig.

The Inmate Doctors of Block 10

Dr. Adelaide Hautval

Heidi Hautval was already in Block 10 when I arrived. She was a real heroine. This distinction—so often abused—truly belonged to her.

Adelaide Hautval was born on January 1, 1906, at Hohwald in Alsace, as the youngest of seven children. Her father was a clergyman. She received her

M.D. degree at the University of Strassburg and worked in neuro-psychiatric institutes and hospitals until her arrest.

Adelaide Hautval reached Auschwitz in January 1943, because, while in prison in Bourges for an infringement of the permit regulations in crossing into the occupied zone of France, she had insisted on wearing the yellow star as a protest against the Gestapo's treatment of French Jews who were thrown into prison with her. She was branded *amie des juifs* and told that, as she liked Jews so much, she had better share their fate. In Auschwitz she was asked on at least five occasions to help with the experiments in the notorious Block 10, and each time refused to do so. On one occasion when Dr. Wirths of the SS asked her how it was that as a psychiatrist she could not see that Jews were different from herself, she replied, "I can see several people who are different from me, beginning with you."

She explained once to a Polish Jewish doctor, Dorota Lorska, "The Germans will not allow people who know what is going on in Block 10 to get in touch with the outside world. So the only thing that is left is to behave, for the rest of the short time that remains, as human beings." In fact, she fully expected to be punished after her confrontation with Wirths. A German political prisoner, who was in charge of the allocation of work, advised her strongly to accept Wirths' order that she should work for him, since an execution squad instructed to deal with special offenders was coming to the camp the next day and she would almost certainly be on the list. Dr. Hautval said that she could not work for Wirths whatever the consequences, and awaited the arrival of the squad in as calm a frame of mind as possible. However, during the night the German colleague managed to arrange for her to be smuggled to Birkenau. To Adelaide Hautval this "escape" was merely a sign of the relative unimportance of her gesture of defiance and she did not like to talk about it to anyone. That her own courage could ever be sufficient to influence others seemed to her highly improbable.[6]

In 1964 a trial took place on account of Dr. Wladyslaw Dering, a Polish GP with a practice in Finsbury Park. He himself brought an action for libel against the author and publishers of the novel *Exodus*. He claimed that he would be identified with the "Dr. Dehring" mentioned in the novel, who was described as having carried out 17,000 experimental operations on Jewish inmates of the Auschwitz concentration camp "without anesthetics." Although the number of operations had been grossly exaggerated, it was shown—through the able defense led by Lord Gardiner—that Dr. Dering (himself a prisoner in the camp because of his membership in the Polish underground) *had* carried out about a hundred and thirty of these operations at the request of the SS and that, when young Jewish men and women were the patients involved, he had been careless to the point of brutality.

The doctor's main plea of justification in the witness box was that to have refused the Nazis' orders to operate would have been to risk almost certain death, and it was over this question of justification through fear that the testimony of Adelaide Hautval was to have a crucial effect.

Ever since reading about the trial, Hallam Tennyson, then the BBC's Assistant Head of Radio Drama, had wanted to produce a radio program with her. But he waited until Dr. Dering's death in 1969. Then he embarked on a protracted correspondence which lasted for over a year. Adelaide Hautval displayed extreme reluctance to meet him. She was opposed to the war crimes trials, had taken part in the Dering libel action against her will and only agreed in the end because she thought it would have been unfair if he would have been awarded heavy damages. Most important of all, she expressed a deep-seated antipathy to personal publicity. After all, it wasn't an action being brought against Dr. Dering, but an action being brought *by* him *against* others, she said. I saw that it was important that the truth should be known. And now I can see the Dering case did in fact demonstrate very clearly what can happen to a man, an ordinary man, an ordinary doctor. Perhaps even a good doctor, because I believe Dr. Dering was basically a good doctor. This process of degradation is progressive. You agree with a certain principle and you carry on in the same way without even letting yourself see where it's leading you. I'm sure that all the terrible things done in the world begin with small acts of cowardice.

The so-called "experiments" carried out at Auschwitz had absolutely no value at any time for humanity in general. Anyone who worked in Block 10 must have known from the beginning that the Nazi program was aimed at the mass sterilization of Jews and nothing else. One would have to be incredibly naive not to have realized this. The concentration camps were the centers of slave labor for the maintenance of the Nazi war effort. It was for that reason that the Nazis carried out experiments in sterilization. They wanted to find out what was the minimum dosage to prevent the "slave races" from propagating while still retaining their capacity for work. They even thought of finding out how to sterilize people by installing x-rays at the factory gates, so that each worker would receive a sufficient daily dose as he or she clocked in without even being aware of what was happening to them.

Adelaide Hautval maintained that along with the horror and the degradation there was an enormous amount of heroism, of daily acts of courage and devotion. What she did was nothing. And besides, she had the luck to be able to refuse, it was certainly not due to herself, but simply because she had an instinct which told her that there were more important things in life than saving one's own skin.

On July 17, 1987, Heidi wrote to me:

> Nobody could live during the nightmare years who in some instants was not forced to break with the rules of traditional behavior. To be or not to be, that was the question. All of us, including myself, were sometimes in situations in which we had to make abnormal decisions. The impossibility of living without "dirty hands" belonged to that phenomenon.

Unhappily for all of us, Adelaide Hautval died on October 12, 1988, at the age of 82.

Dr. Slavka Kleinova (Dorota Lorska)

Slavka worked together with her two friends Dédé Lerner and Perelka; all three of them are not alive any more. She was well liked by everybody, always tried to help others by listening to them or talking to them in the evenings in her tiny laboratory. She certainly was a lesbian so her influence on us, at that time not at all aware of any kind of homosexuality, exuded a kind of beneficial radiance. Even Blockaelteste Margit trembled with excitement when she was invited. Slavka was a communist and so were her friends. They came from France and had all been arrested at the birthday party of one of them. They had a different way of belonging to the world: their religion was being communists.

Dr. Alina Brewda

Dr. Brewda was also our Blockaelteste for some time. She was clever and quick, but cool and not interested in us, the lower people. As a Blockaelteste she often was more or less drunk, saying, "What can I do when people give it to me."

She lived in luxury. I remember one evening after 6 P.M. when the two SS-women guards had already gone home and the house door was locked from the outside. I had to ask something of Dr. Brewda and knocked on the door of her little room. She was dining with two or three others. The table was elegantly set with a white tablecloth and delicate china dishes (white with pink flowers). There was a tantalizing fragrance of good food, animated conversation and rosy-colored cheeks. Dr. Brewda suddenly became furious at me for having glanced at this concealed corrupt opulence.

Dr. Maximilian Samuel

Dr. Samuel worked in Block 10 as a gynecologist. The women who had known him from Cologne were very positive about him. Still, he was a good surgeon—let's say that was the best thing about him.

His assistant was Fella Pleskowska from Warsaw, a charming woman who died in 1972 in Tel-Aviv. I met her there after the war. Tragically, her daughter, who had been living in hiding, was denounced and deported to Birkenau, where she perished. Fella never recovered from this loss and took her own life.

Dr. Samuel had to write a book for Wirths, but was murdered, nevertheless, after its completion. Wirths showed him his portio vaginalis operation and later Samuel performed them for him, approximately thirty altogether. At first, the portio had to be colposcoped, creating a kind of illuminated looking glass in the dark inside. Samuel was second to none as far as surgical skills were concerned. It took Wirths 20 minutes to perform an operation. Samuel finished it in 5-6 minutes. The patients were given so little evipan that immediately after the last stitches, they came to again, for they had to walk from the operating table to the ward.

Samuel was helped by a German, non-Jewish photographer who was Fella's kochani (boyfriend). It sometimes took him half an hour. The women were spread out in the typical gynecological "open" position. Who else among the prisoners in Auschwitz had the opportunity to "study" girls in a warm operating room without being afraid of the SS intruding, and handling them to his heart's desire?

Dr. Wladyslaw Dering
Dr. Dering was a Polish, non-Jewish political prisoner who worked as a surgeon in the Revier (hospital). He was totally inhuman. He could be charming, but was always out only for his own benefit. He performed all the ovarectomies on the young and beautiful Greek girls for SS-physician Horst Schuman. I testified in writing at his trial.

The Inmate Personnel of Block 10

Most of the inmate personnel consisted of Slovakian Jewesses from the first Jewish transports.

Magda Hellinger
Magda was our first Blockaelteste in Block 10 for a short period of time. She was a silent, more or less good, woman.

Margit Neumann
Margit followed Magda as Blockaelteste. She and Rusenka formed one of the first lesbian couples in Block 10. Margit had a low number and had probably been through a lot. She gave the impression of not "having them all together" (as it was referred to in camp jargon), screamed at us viciously and also beat us.

Sylvia Friedmann
Sylvia occupied an important position as Professor Clauberg's nurse. All of us were afraid of her. She was assisted by Genia Lewin and Magda Hans. Genia was a small, pretty girl and a very good intriguer. Magda was ill most of the time.

Once, during our cabaret night, when I sang and danced together with Mila Potaczinska, Sylvia was enormously impressed and wanted to perform together with us. We got to know each other a little better and I had the advantage of not being chosen for any experiments.

Ria and Magda Hans

Ria and Magda were two charming sisters. The very first day, Ria lent me a needle and thread so that I could alter my dress a little. She was a prominent prisoner and I was a new arrival—a very odd combination —something that happened very rarely in Auschwitz. On the whole, we had nothing to do with each other.

Magda was ill and more or less always in bed in the Pflegestube (hospital room). She was sort of a young aristocrat, loved by everybody and cared for by Ria and the "haute volee" as the tragic and unique beauty "from all ages and countries."

Tonka Reich

Tonka worked in the dentist's station. She was a small, pretty Czechoslovakian girl with a low prison number. For that reason, she behaved as if she belonged to nobility. She was not interested in anybody except in her circle.

Ilona Vohrzykova

Ilona was a poor Slovakian person who also worked in the dental laboratory. The women in that work detail had nothing else to do but to take out the gold from the teeth that were delivered from Birkenau.

Hélène Frank

Hélène was a young, pleasant woman who worked, like myself, as part of the crew of the operating room. She came from Bruxelles and knew a lot about cooking. Once we had two potatoes and a piece of garlic and I watched her make a delicious soup out of these few ingredients. The same miracle occurred with half a head of white cabbage. How she handled with lady-like hands a huge knife, dicing minisculely fine slices and, with an onion, a bit of acid from the pharmacy and boiled water, she produced a gourmet salad.

Margot Friedman

Margot was the Pfoertnerin (gate-keeper)—a very important job. Nobody could enter the block without her permission and, of course, she could make things difficult and had to be bought to let people in.

Hélène Rosenthal

Hélène was a fantastic nurse. She was Belgian and spoke French. In my opinion, she exhibited suicidal tendencies. She had volunteered for the transport to Auschwitz. In camp she often exchanged her daily ration of bread for two cigarettes. Ironically, she came out of Auschwitz alive. I am not completely sure, but I seem to have heard that a few years afterwards she committed suicide.

Hélène was the only genuine nurse in Block 10. All the other sixteen persons were untrained. Among them were a belly dancer, office girls, a diamond polisher, a whore, schoolgirls, actresses and ordinary housewives.

Branco Van Thijn

I had seen Branco, but I hadn't spoken to her much as yet. During the hours we were forced to stand and wait on the platform before boarding the train for Auschwitz, a close bond developed between us. Bonds of friendship can be formed suddenly like this.

I had always been sheltered and spoiled at home and I felt lost through the total isolation. In that harsh environment, no one was concerned about anything except himself and his own interests. In the conversation with Branco, I felt warmth and concern, and an interest in the little "non-essential" things for the first time in months. She told me, for instance, about her father's birthday, his having received 17 plants, all different, for his greenhouse. This made not only him happy, but her as well; the happiness still radiated from her.

I thought she was absolutely lovely. She must have been about 32, ten years older than myself. She had very long, heavy, auburn hair, white skin and gray eyes. Her figure was small and compact, and she was dressed in a splendid gray corduroy trouser-suit from Liberty.

And I? I looked down on myself and this woman who had been a pharmacist in Amsterdam took me seriously and accepted me without reservation. That gave me the kick I needed to be mentally capable of coping with future horrors. Thus, a few hours of contact between individuals can establish a bond for life. Through that conversation, she pulled me out of anonymity. Something flowered, a feeling of former times. This was far removed from most of the talk then, which was about hate, politics and fear.

In Block 10, Branco was in charge of the medicine cupboard. Under her supervision, medicines were used exclusively for patients and never for exchange, as they were in every other prison camp under certain conditions. The very idea of this "organisieren" was repulsive to her. She earned a unique name for herself in this way, particularly through being able to bandage terrible wounds, predominantly boils of all sorts, beautifully and lovingly. Entirely against her own will, she had to relinquish medicines to Dr. Samuel, which he said were needed for patients, but which, of course, were exchanged for food and cigarettes.

Then Branco fell ill with an affliction of the facial nerves—trigeminus neuralgia—accompanied by insufferable pain. Dr. Samuel interceded to have an operation performed in the medical block of Auschwitz. The surgeons there were Polish gentile prisoners, but Branco was adamant. "I will not be operated on by a Pole. I won't even consider it." I argued that she couldn't last long as she was. "I'll only consent if you give the anesthetic," she finally agreed. This weighed on me, as it would be a major operation of more than an hour, but I had no alternative. And then, of all veins, I couldn't find hers! At my request, the Polish surgeon inserted the needle, naturally with the familiar arrogant look of "How stupid can you be, 'bloede Hollaendische Kuh?'" (Dutch cow!) After that, I took over the syringe and gave the anesthetic throughout the operation, which lasted more than an hour and a half. I am confident that the anesthetic during this operation, which was more serious and dangerous than an operative procedure on the cervix, was administered correctly. I am not so sure about the operation, though. To begin with, it took longer than expected, and afterward Branco was in continuous pain. That splendid, strong woman, with her beautiful, luminous skin, became old in the course of two or three weeks. After the operation, she was sent back to Block 10, where I took care of her.

The key to the medicine cupboard was temporarily handed over to Alina Brewda, the Blockaelteste, (head prisoner of a barrack) a Polish Jewish female doctor. When Branco asked me to get her an opium injection from the cupboard to alleviate the pain, which must have been excruciating, Alina answered, "Yes, I'll do it, but I'm busy at the moment and I haven't got time right now." I had to ask her three or four times. "Yes, tonight." Once Branco had gotten the injection, of course her pain was tremendously relieved. However, by the next morning the pain had become just as severe and Branco didn't get any more injections, only sleeping pills. She was in terrible pain all the time and very upset in the first place, as a result of the unsuccessful operation, and in the second place because of her anger at not receiving adequate medication. Even now the success of such an operation cannot be guaranteed.

It's remarkable that all the women who came into Block 10 after me, though they were deeply impressed by Branco's humanity, only knew her as an old woman. Gradually, the pain diminished, but the key to the medicine cupboard was withheld from her. And that too, hampered her urge to do something for others. Therefore, she approached an assistant of Dr. Clauberg's, a certain Dr. Weber, who for his laboratory experiments in Rajsko, together with Zabel, took liters of our blood, most of which they spilled. At her repeated requests, he arranged for Branco to work in Rajsko. Branco thought she would be given work in the laboratory, but she was assigned instead to the Gaertnerei (Gardening), which naturally was much too strenuous for her. She therefore asked permission to return, through little notes given to our group by the crew of the typhus laboratory, which had been moved there in the meantime. In the end, Dr. Samuel finally succeeded in finding a job for her. So, she came back to the "Pflegestube," though her strength was failing.

During the evacuation on January 18, 1945, when we had to walk for three days and almost three nights, we lost track of each other, but in Ravensbrueck I found her again in an atrocious isolation-hospital, where all who were mortally ill were brought. Branco was desperately clinging to life—her inner strength was all that kept her going. I knew the effort it took as I visited her almost every day and felt tangibly the stranglehold of death that was stalking around there. Fearing possible "selections," most of the dying didn't dare stay in bed; they walked around and their piercing eyes clung to you.

After a month we were evacuated again. "Aufstellen in fuenfer Reihen!" (Form rows of five!) We walked through the "Lagerstrasse" (main road of the camp) and there I saw Branco standing in front of the window. I saw her calling me, but naturally I couldn't hear her voice. Yet I hear it in my ears now, "Ima, don't leave me alone!"

And I'll never forget it, it will never leave me as long as I live. I owe so much to Branco. I owe her so very much.

Everyone who ever met her knew her as a torch of warmth, affection and charity, whether or not she was giving you a pill or applying a bandage or adhesive tape. That was the kind of person she was. Because of her, one can still believe that there are some good people. Your life depended on a few intense friendships. You couldn't survive alone. You felt indifferent toward all the others or you hated them.

Branco was an oasis there, although I couldn't get up in the morning without reciting, "To be or not to be," and then, "Erst kommt dass Fressen und dann kommt die Moral." (Food first and morals later.) These were my thoughts and those of many others, while all the time Branco was a sanctuary, an island where for a short time, you felt safe.

The "Rassenforschung" ("Racial" Research) Experiment

I remember very well that a "professor" came to Block 10 to look for about thirty Jewish women, as different as possible in regard to eyes, hair, height, physique, nationality, etc.

A rumor had spread that these women were going to leave camp. Thus, everybody had a look of "choose me" in their eyes. But I, having already spent one month in St. Gilles prison in Bruxelles and five months in Mechelen, tried to make myself as inconspicuous as possible and looked at my feet in order not to be chosen—because with my blue eyes and black hair there was something unusual about me. All those who were selected did indeed obtain better clothing and traveled to Germany. They were all gassed for Professor Hirt's Rassenforschung purposes in the Struthof-Natzweiler concentration camp.

The Polish Bacteriologists

The bacteriologists were Jewish "Sonderhaeftlinge" especially fetched from Lemberg University to find and develop a serum against typhus and were working in Block 10 when I arrived. I believe it was Dr. Fleck who had discovered a certain substance which could transform typhus into nothing but a bad headache. He and his wife were taken to the Rajsko laboratory to continue working on it. They were helped by the Seeman and Umschweif couples.

Both women had their children with them. Broniek Seeman was eight and Oleschu Umschweif three years old. The first had a calm and wise mother and he was a quiet boy. The other had as mother a beauty, but an intriguer. He was an impossible child, refusing to eat, etc.

About half a year later came another couple to work with them, the Meisels from Warsaw. Both were very intelligent. Mrs. Meisel was a charming person and although we had little in common, we liked each other and became friends. After the war, she visited us once in Haarlem from Poland, but she was very involved in communism. We would have liked to have learned more about it—but everything was pretty much a secret and could not be discussed.

Three-year old Peter Dattel was the third child in Block 10. His mother, Ruth, came with a transport from Berlin and was selected at the "Rampe" (railroad station). Wirths allowed her to take the child with her to the block. It was rumored that Peter resembled Wirths' small daughter. Ruth Dattel was an intelligent woman with a sense of humor, and Peter felt immediately at home among all those young women, who adored him. He became a sort of mascot of Block 10—even for the SS. He could get out of the block for a bit of fresh air and delivered secret letters from one to the other.

A few years after the liberation, mother and son (who had lost contact during the evacuation of Auschwitz) found each other again in Germany.

The Weekend Course[7]

Once, a weekend training course for nurses was held in Block 10. We prepared a cabaret night for the last evening. During that time, Alma Rosé, the famous violinist, lived in our block. She was Gustav Mahler's niece (her father was the well-known leader of the Rosé Quartet) and had been named after Mahler's wife. At the beginning of the war she had visited Holland with her "Damenorchester" and thus had been unable to get out in time. In Amsterdam, she had come to see my parents, so, when she arrived in Block 10, I recognized her at once and told the Blockaelteste that here was the wife of the renowned violinist Pzcyhoda (as famous in the Balkans as Menuhin was over here). After a few days, Alma Rosé was given a violin. She stayed in our block for about six weeks and we used to sing and dance in the evenings.

Later, Alma was transferred to Birkenau as conductor of the women's orchestra. She died about a year later, nobody knew from what. Her brain was sent to the Institute of Hygiene for research. Neumann, a Canadian journalist who wrote a book about Alma, claims she was poisoned by eating canned oysters which had been sent to her from Warsaw.[8]

For the cabaret night, Mila Potaczinska and I performed a "Damentango." We sang while dancing, pretending to love each other and kissed each other on the mouth. Immediately, Sylvia Friedmann wanted to dance with us, so somebody arranged a song for the three of us. Again that helped me not to be experimented on by Clauberg.

During that evening, one of the nurses, a Russian girl, fell in love with me and we talked till early morning. I understood a little Polish and Russian, and she made me feel quite high. I was so drunk with her enchanting words that I could not find my bed any more.

In January 1945, we were evacuated—at first to Ravensbrueck, then to Malchow and from there to Taucha in Saxony. On April 15, 1945, we escaped and hid in a wood. There was a heavy Allied bomb attack that lasted for several hours. Walking out of the forest I went right into the arms of an American elite corps. They were very kind boys who knew absolutely nothing about German concentration camps and the extermination process. I was housed in Leipzig in the Flack-Kaserne, together with Bep Jooust, Edith Goldstein, Paula Inga and Erna from the Stabsgebaeude, and was later repatriated to Holland.

In April 1946, I married Jaap Spanjaard. My husband, a psychoanalyst, had been in Westerbork only three months and he had come out as a non-Jew. After having observed how some of the Greek girls in Block 10 fasted on Yom Kippur and then at night stole bread from other prisoners, I also abandoned my religion. It made me feel free. My husband and I joined a humanist group instead.

We have three sons. The oldest, Eduard, is a conductor and pianist; the second, Lodewijk, is a bacteriologist and a cello player; and the third, Martin, is a computer expert and creative artist. There are three grandchildren. Unfortunately, my husband passed away two and one-half years ago.

I keep busy with friends, involvement in Amnesty International and a variety of hobbies, such as music, dance, gardening, reading, cooking and a houseboat.

For the last five years I have been speaking about my camp experience to school classes under the auspices of the Anne Frank House. It fulfills a double purpose—not only do children learn about Auschwitz, it also serves as therapy. It helps to evaluate one's own position, which is not a fixed one but can change with time. If only everybody could work similarly in their own circle. That would be more effective than war crimes trials.

❖

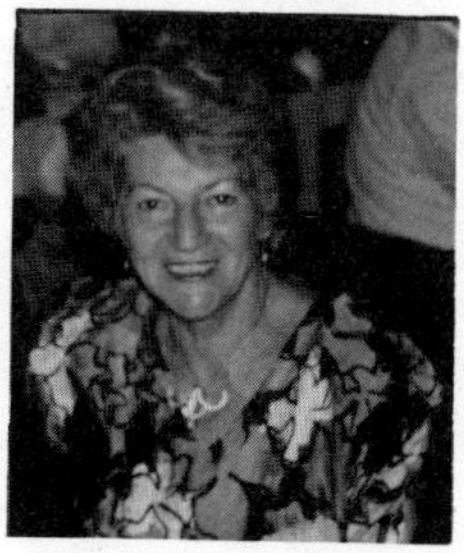

Magda Blau (née Hellinger)
Melbourne (Australia)

When I was eight years old my parents took me to the famous Hasidic Belzer Rebbe (Rabbi) to be blessed. The rabbi placed his hand on my head and said, "This child is predestined to help our people. She will save hundreds of Jewish lives." My parents could not understand the prophesy and did not tell me about it until I was deported. But from the moment I stepped off the cattle cars in Auschwitz I helped in every way possible.

I arrived in Auschwitz in the spring of 1942 and was placed in Block 9.[9] After the first few days, the SS announced that they were looking for women to work in the kitchen, sewing room, office and at other odd jobs. Most of the girls hurried to apply but I did not volunteer because I had to take care of the unfortunate few of our block who had lost their minds.

We had a German Stubenaelteste (room-elder), a political prisoner, with swollen legs. She asked me why I was not searching for a job. I told her that I was a kindergarten teacher and I hoped this kind of occupation would never be needed at Auschwitz. She stated that she was also a teacher, and so we became friends.

The next morning, when I was chosen for an outside work squad, the Stubenalteste came, slapped my face and pulled me back, saying, "You are not marching out, I need you here." She took me to her room and ordered me to help her scrub the floor. "With what will I scrub the floor?" "With your nails," she replied, and that's exactly what I did. Later, she gave me a rag. Therefore, I was able to clean the whole floor.

The following morning I wanted to march out again, but once more the Stubenaelteste prevented me from going. "I want you here inside and if you don't obey I'll kill you," she blurted out while she slapped my cheeks so hard they turned red.

I also had time to look after those girls who had initially gone crazy, but gradually were able to come to their senses again. They were very grateful and begged me to continue helping the room elder. Thus, my career as Stubendienst was launched.

I was sent to fetch the tea. The German, non-Jewish inmates had heard that the Slovakian Jewesses were all prostitutes and were there to compete with them. They refused to let us have any tea because they wanted us to die of thirst. "Anyway," they said, "you won't be able to pick up and deliver the forty liter cans." I had been excellent in sports at home and was still in pretty good shape, so I challenged one of them: "If I pick up one handle of the can and you the other and we deliver it together, will you let us have the tea?" She replied, "OK," so I grabbed one handle and she the other. After walking for some time, I shouted, "now run!" We did, and after we had arrived she developed total respect for me. Following that episode getting our tea or other supplies presented no problem.

Since the room-elder was not feeling well, I took it upon myself to see to it that the tea and other food would be delivered properly. I am a very practical person and have a good memory for faces. I made sure that nobody came twice for tea and food, and also that the bread, margarine, etc., would be evenly divided. Nobody would go without food. I held this position until the women's camp was transferred from Auschwitz to Birkenau, which was approximately during August 1942.

Birkenau was awful. There was total chaos. All the room-elders were housed in the same block. I believe it was Block 2 or 3, which was close to the kitchen. By this time, I was already a full-fledged room-elder myself under block-elder Katja Singer, also a Slovakian, because the Germans had already changed the system. They now also put the Jewish girls in powerful positions. It suited them nicely—I found out later—to place the responsibility and culpability on the Jewesses. "Whom do you remember?" the Germans theorized. "Of course. The block-elder and the room-elder who give you food and drink—none of the others. Once the war is over they can let out their pent-up anger at these Jewish girls."

Birkenau was a tremendous change from Auschwitz. There were open ditches all over the camp and there was no water. Only one single well existed. Imagine—so many women depending on that sole well. A lot of girls who wanted to get to the water so badly fell into the well and drowned. Water was so restricted that women could not wash their hands or faces or even drink a little bit.

Despair grew. Among our group of room-elders there was one youngster called Surka. She was blond and blue-eyed and her younger sister became a Laeuferin (messenger). Surka came to me and asked, "Tell me, tell me are we going to survive in this camp? Do you think we'll once again be free?" I assured here that we would because I firmly believed in our survival.

Of course, you could only survive if you instilled hope in each other, because there was no way to survive Birkenau without supportive friendship. I tried to give Surka strength and by giving her strength I helped myself. "Yes, we will survive. We will be together. We will help and protect each other as much as possible." Surka was very young and kept on asking, "How do you know?" "Look," I said. "Remember Noah's Ark in the Bible? There the people and animals survived. It will be the same for us. We shall be the ones who will survive if we believe in it and if we work toward it by helping each other." She survived, her sister survived, I survived and Katja Singer survived, too.

Friendship and solidarity were very important, especially in cases of illness. Here is an example: Katja Singer, my first block-elder in Birkenau, became Rapportschreiberin and a German, non-Jewish prisoner replaced her as the new block-elder. Just about this time I fell ill with typhus and typhoid fever. I had a very high fever, my tongue was as dry and rough as a chicken's stomach turned inside out and I had horrible diarrhea. I could not eat. The only thing I was craving for were tomatoes. Imagine, tomatoes in Birkenau! But by certain connections and through solidarity and friendship, the girls from Rajsko brought me some tomatoes. I was also asking for soda water and lemonade and there was a girl who worked for the SS canteen and somehow she smuggled out a bottle so that I could drink.

I was so weak that I could not even stand up and whomever SS-Blockfuehrer Stiewitz found in bed he took to the gas chamber right away. So, one of the girls said, "You pretend to belong to the night shift so that you can sleep during the day—we'll do your work for you." So again, there was solidarity and friendship, and the commitment to help each other.

Ruzenka, whom I took along to Block 10 later on, was a very good organizer. She asked the girls from the peeling kommando (who were peeling vegetables) for the kitchen to roll a few potatoes and onions behind the fence. At night, Ruzenka would run out of the block, collect the potatoes and onions and do a little cooking for me. She also knew how to sew very well and she told the block-elder, "I'll sew and cook for you if you'll let Magda stay in the block," since the block-elder had tried several times to send me away. She was scared of covering up for me for such a long time. "But if Magda goes, I go and you won't have any cooked meals any more, and nothing will be sewn for you. I will ask one of the girls to do the night shift for Magda and clean the wheelbarrows of human excrement."

A day check was carried out by Stiewitz. Many young, beautiful girls from Slovakia, who were lying near me were sent away by him. In spite of my fever, I quickly jumped up and told him in perfect German that I was on the night shift. He said, "Halt Deine Schnauze!" (shut up!) and my life was spared.

When I recovered a little I could neither walk, hear or see. Again the girls were very helpful, teaching me, like a baby, to walk. A few days later, approximately in December 1942, there occurred one of the largest selections Birkenau had ever encountered.[10] Everybody was sent out of camp to a huge frozen field and there we stayed until the evening. The strongest girls put me in the middle of a row of five and carried me by the elbows. They kept very close together so that nobody could see how I was dangling from their arms like a puppet. They put me on a big rock in the field and changed my position from time to time so that I would not freeze. Somehow, they had organized some tea from which I could take a sip occasionally. Many girls froze to death in this field, but my friends miraculously managed to carry me back to the camp after having smuggled me through the scrupulous selection process.

Following my recovery, I resumed working as room-elder but my function and the jobs changed continuously. Once I was room-elder, then I was ["verfuegbar"] (available temporarily without a permanent job). Again I became room-elder somewhere else, and later deputy. Finally, I was chosen to be block-elder in

Block 13. The prisoners I was in charge of were all Polish Christians. I don't believe that other Jewish block-elders had exclusively non-Jewish prisoners as their charges. However, Rapportschreiberin Katja Singer had known me for a long time and knew how I handled people. She always said, "If they are difficult, let Magda take them." The Polish women did not object at all to this situation because I looked after them very well. For example, epidemics were raging in the block. Typhus, typhoid fever, cholera, malaria, dysentery and others—all attacked the helpless prisoners. It was absolutely impossible to be on the top row of the bunks while suffering from diarrhea. The inmates used the bowls intended for soup to relieve themselves and the contents they then spilled through the broken windows. Naturally, it made matters worse. I tried to change the situation. At first, we organized a few latrines and put them into the block. Then I found out that there was clay in the back of the camp—the type similar to adobe which peasants use to build their huts. I approached a male prisoner driver of a horse-drawn carriage who usually delivered goods to the Lagerfuehrerin (SS-woman in charge of the women's camp) and asked him to bring me some clay and two barrels of whitewash. It was dangerous to attempt to obtain it, but we got the stuff. I picked the strongest Polish women and explained to them what we were going to do. We organized buckets, sticks and rags, and when it was dark in camp, one group applied the mud outside our block, the other group covered the window frames and walls with the whitewash to avoid further spreading of the disease.

The following morning, Katja Singer cam running to me exclaiming, "What did you do? The Lagerfuehrerin and the rest are going to hang you. They say you did it on purpose so that pilots can single out the camp."

I explained to the Blockfuehrer that sanitary conditions in camp were dreadful. Somebody had to do something about it, otherwise the diseases would attack not only the prisoners, but others as well. He concurred, stating that a large number of SS-men had died of typhus. Then he went to the camp commandant to clarify the situation. They called me "nach vorn" (to the gate) and I was put in charge of the project to see to it that other blocks would follow suit with the same program.

Once there was Blocksperre (nobody was allowed to leave the block) while I was helping to pull girls out of the ditches into which they had fallen. SS-man Stiewitz arrived and took all the girls from the ditches on the truck, destined for the gas chamber. He made me climb in together with the weak Muselmaenner (skeletons) and I just said to myself, "Goodbye, cruel world!" and thought my life was finished. But just then a German, non-Jewish kapo passed by. She was the woman with whom I had carried the tea during my first week in camp and who had considered us all prostitutes. She was a lesbian and had become very fond of me, but I had convinced her that this lifestyle was not for me. We had not seen each other for a long time, but when she caught a glimpse of me on the truck, she immediately pulled me off, screaming, "I need you in my kommando," and slapped my face hard. She talked briefly to the SS-man, but he did not object, and so she saved my life.

The Polish non-Jewish women prisoners of my block showed their appreciation by similarly rescuing me.

It was customary that those prisoners who were "verfuegbar" (available) were frequently taken in rows of five to Block 30 for sterilization and irradiation. Indeed, the next time I was available they marched me to Dr. Schumann's block. But I already had a very good reputation at that time and the Polish male non-Jewish prisoners who knew that I handled people in a very humane way, committed sabotage on my account. It was a very cold day. The water in the pipes was frozen and, consequently, there was no electricity. The Polish inmates managed not to repair anything all day long so that the sterilization experiments had to be cancelled for that day. Nevertheless, I was advised to disappear for some time. The Polish Christian women whose block-elder I had once been hid me in their block and provided me with food and blankets.

In January 1943, the only transport of French non-Jewish political prisoners arrived in Birkenau. They came from prison and most of them were professionals, i.e., scientists, doctors, lawyers, journalists, etc. They marched into the camp escorted on both sides by SS and sang the "Marseillaise." They were considered dangerous, and the SS was afraid that they would start a revolution—so all other prisoners had to turn their backs while they passed by. I was available at that time and Katja approached me,[11] saying, "Magda, you take the French women." I remonstrated, "I don't speak French. What do you want from me?" "Do you want some brutal girl to get them? They are too valuable," Katja replied. Thus, I became the block-elder of the French women, who appreciated me. They had an opportunity to reciprocate in kind exactly two years later.

After the evacuation of Auschwitz in January 1945, we were sent to Ravensbrueck, where the non-Jewish French women had already been transferred several weeks earlier. When they found out that I had arrived, they invited me to their block. They all had their own beds while our group was sleeping in tents without any covering in the bitter cold. They bathed, nursed, fed and looked after me. I spent each day with them, joining my group only for roll calls and recuperated a little from the tremendously trying death march.

As a matter of fact, I am still in contact with two of them, Dr. Hautval, who worked at one point as a physician in Block 10, and a scientist by the name of Marie-Elisa, who is a friend of Dr. Hautval.

I don't know of anyone else who was in charge of inmates of as many nationalities as I was. Later, I became block-elder of Czech non-Jewish women. Some of them were relatives of Eduard Benes, who later became President of Czechoslovakia. I was also block-elder of "Aryan," wives of mixed marriages and once I was personally chosen as block-elder by Commandant Hoess of the "Russian village." There were small children and pregnant women among these Russian inmates and rumors were circulating that they might be exchanged for German generals. I had been selected because of my background as a kindergarten teacher.

I told them, "If you want me to be in charge, you have to grant me the following: no roll calls for these women and children. I want them to be able to go to the sauna daily so they can wash freely with plenty of water. I want them to receive food similar in quality to the SS food, and I need some Russian women to help me." To my astonishment he said, "All right, you will get everything you asked for." I did everything possible for them. The Russians repaid me, just as the Polish and French women did, in the following way:

The final days in captivity were spent in a satellite camp of Ravensbrueck called Malchow. It was toward the end of April or beginning of May 1945 that the Germans pushed us on the road again in a futile attempt to evade the approaching Russian Army. While we were marching I suddenly noticed a group of Russian partisan women who had been in my barracks when I was block elder of the "Russian village" in Birkenau. They recognized me too and realized that as a camp functionary prisoner, I would be considered to have been a collaborator and was in danger of being hung or shot. They knew me well, since the entire village had been under my supervision and, out of comradeship, felt it necessary to hide me. They took me with them and I asked whether I could bring a few of the girls along. They explained that it would be very hard to build a shelter in the woods for many persons. We bargained, and finally, they agreed that I could take three of my comrades. The Russian women built the shelter out of twigs, provided us with food and waited for the Red Army. When the Soviets arrived, they established themselves in a flour mill. The partisan girls went to see their compatriots and explained the situation, especially clarifying who I was. After two days they came to fetch me, and I became a celebrity. They placed me at the head of the table and were extremely nice to me.

Because I was so capable and efficient, I encountered a lot of intrigue and jealousy. Stenya, the sadistic Polish block-elder, as well as Maria Mandel, the chief of the SS-women, wanted me out of the way and succeeded in transferring me to Block 10 as block-elder, approximately in the spring of 1943. I asked for twelve girls to accompany me as room-elders. The request was approved.[12]

Block 10 was located in the men's camp of Auschwitz. All windows had been barricaded with wooden planks tilted outward at the top, with meshed wire—so only a very little bit of light seeped through. We were locked in all the time. Every morning an SS-woman opened up the door and then locked it right away. The food was brought to us from the men's kitchen only up to the door, from where the room-elder girls carried it inside.

When we arrived, Haupsturmfuehrer Dr. Wirths, whose brainchild the experimental Block 10 was, waited for us. We talked for a while and Dr. Wirths stated that I surely could not be Jewish because of my very blond, wavy hair. He insisted that a mistake had been made in my case.

I quickly thought, "Why not use his idea for the benefit of my comrades?" So I said to him politely, "If you want to have a hospital here, then we'll need sheets, blankets, soap, towels and nighties." It sounded incredible, but Dr. Wirths assured me that I would get whatever I asked for. Slowly, we received the supplies.

The nighties came in bundles. Each of the unfortunate women who had been chosen for experiments received a nightie. I had the idea of brightening their lives up a bit by arranging a fashion parade. Since a tall woman occasionally received a short nightie and a short woman a long one, it created quite a bit of amusement. That gave me the idea to organize entertainment once a week. I recruited some talented women and a theater was established.

Of course, this did not prevent the SS physicians from performing their experiments on these women. Often, after they had been operated on, they were of no further use. They would then be returned to Birkenau, where most of them perished. New women would arrive. All of them were Jewish, but of many different nationalities—Belgian, French, Polish, Greek, Dutch and others.

I received permission from Dr. Wirths for the women to march out of camp to the surrounding meadows and woods to enjoy nature a little. At one point, a herbalist male prisoner went with them and the women collected different herbs for the SS-kitchen.

Adjacent to Block 10 was the "Black Wall," where executions took place. Once, when I peeked through the slits in our barricade windows, I saw Dr. Weber, the chief of the Bacteriological Institute, cut out pieces of flesh from the thigh part of executed prisoners. It was rumored that it was used in his laboratory as a culture medium in which bacteria were grown.

Our group also included the wives of famous Polish Jewish scientists. Their husbands were working in Dr. Weber's Institute of Hygiene as researchers and the women were in Block 10. Two of them even had children. Thus, two small Jewish boys lived in the midst of the main camp of Auschwitz while hundred of thousands of Jewish children were being gassed.

After the evacuation of Auschwitz, Karol, one of the little boys, was in Malchow with his mother, Natalie Umschweif. She was very ill and asked the physician, Ena Weiss, a Slovakian Jewish prisoner, to take care of her son in case she should die. Ena kept her promise and took care of the boy after the liberation. He emigrated to Israel, is a grandfather by now and is still in touch with Ena, who lives in Australia and whom he considers to be his second mother.

In Block 10 there was a Slovakian Jewish girl from Hungary named Ria Hans.[13] She worked as a nurse and always admonished us to use our eyes and ears to memorize everything that was going on, since we were not allowed to put anything on paper. She said that if we should ever get out of this hell alive it would be important to bear witness to the fiendish crimes committed here.

After the war, Ria Hans lived in Israel and was accused of war crimes. She was thrown in jail, although she was pregnant at that time. My husband, Bela Blau, who had also been a prisoner in Auschwitz, appeared as a defense witness for her. He testified that during the incident in question on a beautiful late summer morning in 1944, Ria did not hit or knife anyone as claimed by some of her accusers. She only screamed at the women from Block 10 who were intermingling with male prisoners who belonged to a large work squad of 1300, of whom my husband was kommando secretary. Of course, speaking with these men was prohibited. Bela told the judge what happened and thanks to his testimony, Ria was acquitted. Those girls who accused her had absolutely no idea of what was going on. They could not even recollect whether it was summer or winter when the incident occurred. Ria Hans left Israel afterward and is supposedly living somewhere in Brazil.

I remember quite vividly the mask experiment which was carried out in the summer of 1943.[14] A certain number of women were chosen and subsequently the experimenter made masks of their faces. It was said that they wanted to prove that the Jewish "race" was different from and inferior to all other races. I escorted these women to a block in the men's revier (hospital) where these masks were made. Being curious myself, I requested that a mask of my head be made as well. The researcher complied but did not pick me for the experiment because I was a protege of Dr. Wirths.

All women who were chosen for this experiment were later locked up in a room whose key was entrusted to me. They were supposed to leave by train at 12:00 o'clock.. According to the researcher who had made the masks, they would be transported to his sanatorium near Strassburg. Of course, we did not believe the sanatorium story. Later, when I passed by the locked room, two of the girls begged me to let them out, which I did. One of them was Mila Potashinsky, a Polish Jewess from Belgium, who once was an actress and who later worked as a nurse in Block 10. She now lives in Melbourne and we are very friendly because she knows if I had not let her out, she would not be alive. I also permitted a Greek girl to leave the room. When I lived in Israel, she visited me with her husband and sister and thanked me for saving her life.

When the women were taken to the train it was discovered that two were missing. I had had the key, was accused of sabotage, and an SS-woman, Irma Greese, came to take me back to Birkenau to spend seven days in the Stehbunker for punishment.

A Stehbunker is a tiny booth measuring approximately one cubic meter. There was only room to stand—not to sit down or crouch. There were four of us who were forced to spend each night in the Stehbunker—of course, sleep was impossible.

In the morning, after roll call, I had to clean the toilets. I was very lucky that the male prisoners who worked in the women's camp found out that I was being punished for having saved two women. They instructed me, "You lie down and rest till the evening roll call, because you won't survive working all day and standing up all night. We are going to clean the toilets for you!"

After seven days, Blockfuehrer Taube came and took me to a wooden barrack which contained mostly non-Jewish women who had office jobs. Thus, from toilet cleaning I had been promoted to block-elder once more.

Afterwards, I also worked for some time in the Schreibstube (office) of Birkenau together with Zippy Tichauer. In the spring of 1944, when the Hungarian transports started to arrive, they were looking for a Lageraelteste (camp elder). I was picked by Maria Mandel, the SS-chief of the women and her deputy, SS-woman Drechsler. When I heard about it, I immediately went to Drechsler and told her naively, "Forgive me please, but I can't be Lageraelteste. I have never been one and I would not know how to perform this function." She started to laugh (she had very protruding teeth, almost like a horse) and replied, "Of course you don't know. Who has ever been in a concentration camp before? But here you'll be Lageraelteste."[15]

Then I implored Katja Singer, who was still Rapportschreiberin. "Please, don't let me become Lageraelteste, because it is very hard. You have to handle many thousands of people without proper supplies and facilities. You can't help everybody. After we'll be free, just the ones you were unable to help will point a finger at you and accuse you."

But Katja countered, "Do you want Stenya,[16] this Polish anti-Semite, to be there in your stead? You will at least try to do your best and help whenever you are able."

So, I became Lageraelteste in the C camp of Birkenau.[17] Soon Commandant Kramer came to see me. He was a giant of a man, about 6 feet 5 inches, with enormously big hands and was capable of taking a man by the neck, squeezing him, crushing him and dropping him like a doll. At that time, the camp consisted of empty barracks with beds, i.e., the wooden planks with nothing covering them. We also did not have any bowls. There were 31 barracks and they were expecting about 30,000 women. I told him, "Herr Lagerkommandant, how do you expect people to exist here? There is nothing here for them. You might just as well take them directly to the gas chamber. How long can they survive here without a mattress, without straw, without a blanket, without a bowl from which to eat, without a spoon, without anything?"

He turned around. "Why do you care so much what happens to them? Is that your business?"

I don't know how I dared, but I replied, "If tables were turned and you were in a concentration camp and would have the function of Lageraelteste, if you would not do anything for your comrades I would call you a coward."

He looked at me and the girls near me froze, because they were convinced that at that moment he would grab me by the neck, squeeze me and drop me like a doll. To everybody's amazement he said, "You are right. By tomorrow, you'll have blankets, bowls and spoons for everyone." I received these supplies, but I cannot recall whether they delivered the straw or the mattresses.

There were many of us girls who attempted to stand up to the mighty SS, because we told ourselves, "One only goes up the chimney once, so at least if I can help, I will help." By standing up to Kramer, I earned his respect. Therefore, the few other times I demanded something from him, he gave it to me. Via these means I was able to save lives, and, in retrospect, I believe that Katja was right.

However, I paid dearly for it. After the liberation I had a few unpleasant episodes. Former inmates accused me—but for each person who spoke against me there were always ten who pleaded for my case.[18]

When I was living in Israel I was denounced by one of the Hungarian girls whose life I actually had saved when I was Lageraelteste in the C-Lager in Birkenau. She denounced me and I appeared in front of a judge in Tel-Aviv. The story was the following:

There was a despicable SS physician in Auschwitz, named Dr. Klein. He came from Transylvania and spoke Hungarian. He approached the first arrivals, young, naive Hungarian women and said, "Oh, you are so young and pretty and strong. Why should you stay here in such an ugly, dirty camp? I have a beautiful sanatorium and I'll take you there if you volunteer." I knew he was recruiting for the gas chambers, but the young Hungarian girls had no idea what was going on. They gathered around him and one after the other started to volunteer. I could tell that I did not have much more time, so I just went and slapped the women, one after the other, saying, "You are not going to go to the sanatorium. You are going to work here together with me. If I have to stay here, you should too."

Suddenly, to my surprise, Dr. Klein just left. He could have sent me to the crematorium straight away, but he did not and I was able to rescue the girls from the gas chamber.

One of these girls pressed charges at my trial, declaring, "I know she saved my life but I don't forgive her for the slap." When the judge heard this, he dismissed the case stating, "If she had not slapped you, you would not be alive today." He then said to me, "It is odd, but these women did not deserve you. You saved their lives and instead of being grateful, they have made life miserable for you. Go home and tell your children they can be proud of their mother."

Our main purpose in camp was to fight the Germans and to save as many lives as possible. I would like to give another example of our modus operandi:

When I was Lageraelteste in the C-Lager, I separated the young girls and put them in Block 8. I approached a gymnastic teacher and told her to do exercises with them during the day because it was very important for the morale of the kids. One day, SS physician Dr. Mengele came to the C-Lager. He could not stand the sight of these young, beautiful girls and put them in Barrack 3, which, unfortunately, had just been emptied because all the prisoners had been sent to the gas chamber. They were to stay there overnight and the next morning the crematorium truck would pick them up. An SS-man was put in front of the door to guard them.

I deliberated with Gilda, my deputy, about what we would do to save the girls, and decided to approach the guard. Through small talk, I discovered that he was unhappy because the next day they were sending him to the Russian front. I returned to Gilda and told her, "Listen! He is very upset. We have a chance. We have to make him drunk."

There was always Schnaps in camp. We took some to the SS-man. "Here—have a little. You are going to the front tomorrow. Who knows what will happen to you? Have a little drink. Be a little merry." And so, once I visited, once she visited, and we always offered him a little more, until finally we gave him the whole bottle, which he finished. When he fell asleep, we quietly entered and removed thirty girls at a time and took them to a block. We told the block-elder to distribute them among her inmates. Thus, very slowly, we emptied the entire block. We left the guard sleeping there and went to bed ourselves. It seems as though our good deed was never discovered. No one ever came to ask us how the girls had disappeared. In this instance, we saved eight hundred young women.

Whenever there were selections in C-Lager, I had to be present with Dr. Mengele. When the selection was over and they did not come right away to pick up those who had been selected, I tried to conceal some of them. I could not save them all, but I did my utmost to divide them into groups and to distribute them in different barracks, sometimes 200-300 persons. Nobody knew about it and no one should have known, because it was dangerous. Only now am I able to talk about it.

During my time in camp, I was moved around quite a bit. I could be in one place for two or three weeks and in another place for two or three weeks, in addition to being block-elder of the French communists and the Polish political prisoners, the non-Jewish Czech women, the non-Jewish Russian women and the "mixed marriages." I also had Dutch and Belgian inmates under me in my block.

I forgot to mention that I was camp-elder in C-Lager with one interruption. There was a short period of time during which the camp was empty. The Hungarian transports had stopped and the inmates had either been transferred to other camps or, unfortunately, sent to the gas chambers. Kramer personally took me to Birkenau—a gesture which was unheard of. He wanted me to become kitchen kapo. I knew that the present kitchen kapo was a German, non-Jewish prisoner who was good friends with the camp-elder. I did not want to make the mistake of depriving a woman of her position, so I just sat around and told the SS-guard in charge of the kitchen, Aufseherin Franz, I would rather be assigned to the food warehouse. My task would be to count out the rations for the entire prison population. The job suited me well, and I also requested to have another girl who had just lost her position as assistant. The request was granted and I took Regina along. We attempted to enlarge the prisoner portions to almost double their initial size. Inmates did not know why they suddenly had a little bit more to eat than before.

After a while, Kramer personally took me back to the C-Lager in his car. He jokingly said that since I had done everything possible in the best interest of the inmates, he would install me once more as camp-elder in the C-Lager.

I would like to add something which I think is very important and which has never been mentioned. When they took us to the concentration camp we were young girls who had no idea where we were going. We were not prepared, nor had we any idea of what was in store for us. After the war, we were asked, "How did you survive? What did you do that you survived and others didn't?"

The question mainly concerned those who had been functionaries in Birkenau and Auschwitz. Moreover, no one asked, "Did you volunteer for it?" or "Was it a steady position you had?" They did not know that the Sword of Damocles was hanging over our heads every second. Today you might be in and tomorrow you might be out. I emphatically declare that nobody ever volunteered to be a functionary. No one desired to be in a prominent position—the Germans wanted us to occupy them. They just happened to choose us.

Naturally, when a girl was placed in charge of thousands of hungry, sick, thirsty, desperate women, she herself was in despair. She was young and had never been in a similar situation. She did not have even an inkling about how to handle such a crowd of people. The roll call had to balance. The food and drink had to be delivered. The bread had to be distributed. The sick had to be separated. How could a girl of sixteen or seventeen cope with these problems? If something went wrong, for example, if the roll call did not look too good, she herself could be selected together with the others and sent to the crematorium.

It is very sad that nobody ever posed this question after the war—a question of how a young girl, suddenly thrown into a position of power and authority, could survive without any help or encouragement.

I don't know why I was chosen by fate to have so many functions. Not that I wanted them—believe me, I always protested against them. It was unbelievable that they chose me to be Lageraelteste. But I occupied this position in the C-Lager from approximately spring 1944 until the evacuation of Auschwitz in January 1945 (with one short interruption). I knew I could not please everybody, since I was in charge of 30,000 women (there were 30 barracks and they were filled to capacity during the mass arrivals of the Hungarian transports). But I always attempted to do as much good as I could.[19]

❖

CHAPTER THREE
Human Guinea Pigs

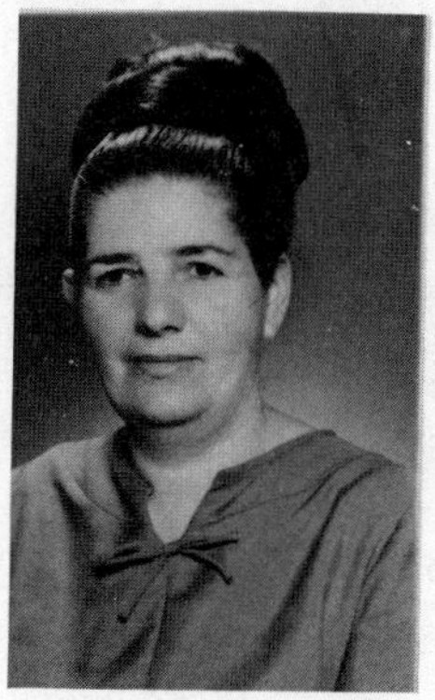

Aliza Barouch (née Zarfati)
Hod Ha-Sharon (Israel)

In 1939, when the war broke out, I was 11 years old. I was born in Saloniki on May 10, 1928, not far from the sea. On April 9, 1941, the Germans came into town and my childhood was over. The school closed down and community members were arrested.

Jewish streets got Greek names. Diseases started spreading, there was a shortage of food. My father was fired from the docks. Special Jewish laws were enacted and we were beaten. We were given numbers and taken to Forced Labor Camps.

At night, someone went through town with a bullhorn telling us to prepare packages. They said we were going to Poland to start a new life.

Our Rabbi, Dr. Zvi Koretz,[1] promised that it would be okay and everyone believed it. He told us to hand in our jewelry and money and in return we were going to receive certificates entitling us to plots of land in Cracow.

We took a few personal belongings, such as warm clothes, and started walking to the "Baron Hirsh." Baron Hirsh was the Ghetto, an old dark quarter. It remained as it was. A big wooden wall with barbed wire on top surrounded the Ghetto. The Germans guarded the gates and rudely pushed the ones entering.

Thousands were cramped together here. They slept in the toilets and on the side walls. Tens died every day. Boys and girls were married fictitiously in order not to be separated. I married a young boy in a "mariage blanc" ceremony. I was 15 at that time.

We stayed in the Ghetto about a week. One day they told us we were leaving tomorrow morning. Each family got a money order of 600 zloty. Those who took gold or jewelry were endangering their own lives. We were forbidden to take suitcases and we were not allowed to take more than 20 kilo. We were given blue certificates with which we would be able to purchase land in Cracow. We did not doubt it for a minute.

The Germans pushed us. Those who were slow were beaten. People were screaming, sighing and crying and fighting to be the first on the trains.

Children were separated from their parents, wives from their husbands. The railroad cars used to transport horses; 8-10 horses per car. And here we were 80-100 persons penned into one car.

We believed that the suffering was worth it. In a few days we would reach our destination and start a new life. The railroad cars moved along slowly; 2,800 persons were stuffed into them, touching each other.

I was with my "groom," my parents and my brother. If somebody wanted to stretch one's legs all the others around had to get up. There was no air. The windows were narrow and barbed; the doors locked. There was a small pail to be used as a toilet.

We had a few loaves of bread and olives, but people did not eat. We thought we would soon arrive and eat like humans, but the journey stretched longer and longer. We did not want to eat, so that we would not have to use the "bathroom" in front of all those people.

It was hot. We took off clothes. People fainted, people died. I was sitting there, picturing the reunion with friends that had gone before me. They would probably wait for us with flowers. I believed we would manage all right in the new country. We would be able to speak Spanish, and we would have a great time.

We travelled for eight days and arrived on April 17, 1943, on Shabbat-ha-Gadol (the Great Sabbath.) The train stopped, the doors opened. We were in shock. Germans were standing there with dogs, shouting and hitting. Down below (on the ramp) were people in striped clothes. The poor things, I laughed. They were probably crazy. Why did they bring us to a nut house?!

The smell of a kitchen came to me. Good, there is food. Smoke was coming from the chimney. How much food are they preparing there?

They got us out of the cars screaming "Raus, schnell," hitting us, dogs biting our legs—and I was expecting my friends to greet me with flowers. "That's not nice," I said. "No one came!"

They separated us. Men to the right, women and children to the left. They took my "husband" from me. Mother stayed with me. When she saw that they were putting father on a truck, she left me and got on the woman's truck. All the money orders and documents we had received from the Germans were with her. She wanted to be with father, so that she could prepare the house and arrange all that had to be arranged before we came.

She asked me to go with her, but I refused. I wanted to walk all the way, so that I would get to know the area, so that I would know how to return when my friends from Saloniki would arrive with a later transport. I wanted to welcome them with flowers—not the way I had been greeted.

Father was already sitting on the truck. My brother saw that I was not joining Mother and was angry. He shook his fist at me, saying I should not be silly and go with Mother. Mother begged, but I was stubborn. "If something should happen to you," she said, "don't blame anyone."

She gave me her scarf and asked that I cover my head so that they should not shave my hair.

Morning dawned. One hundred of us, aged 15-20, were selected at the ramp. They took us young girls with knee socks and fur hats on a long march. We were told we were registering for school and would then go home. I was excited—until I passed through the gate—until we went into the barrack—until we smelled the fire—.

There were big showers in the barrack. We had to strip naked. Our hair was shaved and we were taken to Block 10. There were already about 15-20 girls from Greece. "This is it," the girls said. "This is where life ends. You won't see your mother or father any more. They are gone." I did not want to believe it. "You want to say that the chimney is not from the kitchen?"

One hundred girls sitting and crying—what a welcome!

The Great Sabbath in Saloniki was a festive day—New clothes, joy. And what has God arranged for us here?! Death to our parents. Shaved heads!

I was not called Aliza anymore. They had tattooed on my flesh my new name: 41544. Sometimes I would dream of coming to the train to greet my friends, but on the way I would not see anyone.

Gradually we found out that Block 10 was an experimental block and that we women were to be used as guinea pigs. Two of the main experimenters were Clauberg and Schumann. Professor Clauberg was a short ugly man who appeared in civilian clothes and always wore a Tyrolean type of hat with a long feather. Dr. Schumann was a handsome, tall blond man who had a big scar on his face and a preference for very young Greek Jewesses to be used as subjects. He considered them "good stuff." Both Clauberg and Schumann conducted experiments. Both of them tortured the girls: they removed their virginity, irradiated and sterilized them, removed their ovaries and contaminated them with cancer. They violated and disfigured their bodies and transformed them into female eunuchs. Mentally and physically crippled, the victims would then be sent to the gas chambers.

In the beginning, I wept all the time in Block 10. Dora Gershon was there with her mother and she treated me like her second daughter. I did not want to have anything to do with strangers and associated only with Greeks.

One of the girls in our circle was Allegra. She had arrived with my transport and was later chosen as a specimen for Professor Hirt's skeleton collection at Strassburg University. She was gassed for this purpose, together with 29 other women in the concentration camp of Struthof-Nazweiler.

It was dark in Block 10. The windows were shut and blocked with boards to prevent us from looking out at the Black Wall, the death wall, located between our block and Block 11, the Bunker. There executions took place.

We peeked through the cracks and saw all. When we heard a truck unloading gravel, we knew that today the killing would take place. They executed once or twice a week. The condemned sang songs. Then they took them out naked, placed them against the wall and shot them in the back of the neck. They fell on the gravel, row upon row, until the trucks came to cart off the bodies.

Food was no problem in Block 10. The male prisoners were standing outside and we were at the windows. And if you gave your number or name you received packages when the cauldrons were delivered from the kitchen. We received a lot.

The first time they took a group of us Greek girls to Birkenau to irradiate our ovaries was in May/June 1943. They put us into a dark, locked and sealed room. We thought they were killing us. You could smell medicine in the air. Very soon the gas would come through. We stood in the corner, holding each other, and then SS Dr. Horst Schumann arrived. He took one, Forforca (who now lives in Spain) and closed the door. The minutes were like eternity. What are they doing in there? Will she cry, will she scream? It was very frightening.

I, at 15 the youngest of our group, looked through the key hole. I saw only legs. Fifteen to twenty minutes later she came out. Then Bella went in, then I. Schumann stood behind a glass divider. On my abdomen (front and back), he put a wooden board with many wires. Then I had to stand naked between two x-ray apparatuses. After 20 minutes, he let me go. It did not hurt.

When Forforca came out she was snow-white and she felt like vomiting. The same with Bella. I thought, maybe they are poisoning us in there.

It lasted a long time, until all 20 women had received their dosage of x-rays and were ready. We felt so miserable that it took us twice as long to walk back to Block 10 in Auschwitz since we had to vomit continuously. Afterward, we stayed in bed for 18 days.

A little later, we lost all our hair and after the second irradiation experiment, our entire body was burnt and turned black and we had blood in the stool. All the other girls underwent radiation only twice, but Dora Gershon and I had to endure it three times. Dora does not want to talk about it, I am the only one who speaks out.

Incidentally, of the twenty girls, only four are alive now: Forforca Bachar, Germaine Pichon, Dora Gershon and myself. Forforca, Germaine and I were lucky that Dr. Samuel performed the subsequent ovariectomies, ordered by Schumann. He cheated and, consequently, all three of us were able to have children after the war (Forforca had 4, Germaine 1 and I, 2). But Dora, whose oopherectomy was done by Polish prison physician Dr. Dering (whose notorious trial occurred in London in 1964), remained childless.

One morning, they said: "Go down. We have to open up your stomach."

"Why," I asked. "I don't have a baby."

They called my number, but I did not answer. They called again and I did not go. I got hysterical, I turned into an animal. I hid behind beds and screamed. Dr. Schumann came with a woman doctor and pulled out a gun and screamed: "You either go down or I shoot. Crawl like a dog and come down." I had no choice.

When I awoke from the operation, I saw Dr. Samuel standing by me. He stood there and stroked my head. "If you live, remember me," he said.

One week later they took out the stitches. Because of the radiation, the skin did not grow together and there were suppurations. The abdomen opened and pus came pouring out. They put toilet paper instead of a bandage and closed the skin with a safety pin. I saw the Angel of Death—my body was boiling.

I lay there for 11 months in excruciating pain and terribly high fever. I did not drink water. I did not know what they had done to me.

The ones who survived the operations were sent to Birkenau to the crematoria. I hid and when a new transport arrived, I got back into bed. No one noticed.

Meanwhile, the Germans found out that Dr. Samuel did not do what he was supposed to do. For instance, in my case he removed only one ovary and one half of the uterus instead of everything. He agreed to work in Auschwitz as a doctor in order to save the lives of his wife and daughter, but when he found out they were killed, he decided to take revenge on the Germans. When he was ordered to operate on Jewish prisoners, he tried to minimize the damage as much as possible.

When this was found out, the German doctors searched for all Jewish prisoners of Block 10 in order to operate again.

It was my luck that I was sent just at that time to Birkenau and thus saved from a second operation. However, Dr. Samuel was sent to the gas chamber. Germaine Pichon named one of her sons "Schmuel" in his memory and I am working very hard to see that he will be honored by Yad Vashem.

In Birkenau, I had to do hard labor. Only the ones who worked stayed alive. I could barely move, my abdomen hurt so much.

Every now and then Dr. Mengele would come and perform selections. We stood in line. One by one we stepped out and walked in front of him. The ones who had lost a lot of weight were sent to the crematorium. The ones who had undergone operations were sent to Auschwitz to continue the experiments. I walked up to Mengele naked, hiding my scar with my skirt. Luckily he did not notice and, once again, I was saved from the experiments. For about two weeks, I worked in an outside kommando. Then, a part of the group of women who had been transferred from Block 10 was sent to work in an ammunition factory. My job was to sort out bombs. It was here that I met my future husband.

One day a male prisoner, who also worked for the Weichsel Union Factory, was beaten. They whipped him with a lash of leather and metal. After each lash, they made him leap like a frog, and the others stood around him laughing. Suddenly, he fell down and called out "Oj Madre." From his accent I knew he was Greek. When nobody looked, I came closer and asked if he was from Greece. "Yes," he answered, "and you?" His name was Ovadia. Only our eyes spoke, we kept silent.

I was present when the four girls who had smuggled explosives out of the Union factory were hanged. We returned from the night shift and we had no idea what was going on. We tried to sleep, but it was so noisy that we could not. We asked, "What's happening?" They replied, "There is going to be a concert." The SS ordered us out. I was always the first one. "Du, Kleine, come listen to the concert." The SS wanted us to see. Suddenly, we noticed that there was no concert, but gallows on the podium instead. Two girls were hanged for the nightshift to watch and two for the dayshift.

In January 1945, the Russians advanced and the Germans retreated. They took us, the tortured prisoners, skeletons in rags, with them. We went on the death march with no food and no water—rows and rows of skeletons. Whoever slipped or fell in the snow was shot.

After the death march, we came first to Ravensbrueck and later to Malchow. On May 1, 1945, Malchow was evacuated and the following day we were liberated by American troops. The American Red Cross gave my four Greek friends and me a food parcel.

A few days later, the Russians arrived in Neustadt, where we were staying. Then we, the five Greek girls from Block 10, took trains and went wherever the train was going, all over Europe, hoping to get home fast. However, we did not arrive in Greece until September 1945.

Ovadia had returned to Saloniki[2] much earlier. One day, he saw my name on the list of survivors.

When I arrived, he wanted to get married immediately. I said, "No way. I know you lost a very large family and you know what they did to me in Block 10. I regret I will not be able to provide you with happiness in life. I will not be able to bear children."

But Ovadia told me that he loved me very much. He wanted me, not children. And finally, in November 1945, we got married. However, I had to make myself a year older because one had to be 18 in order to obtain a marriage license in Greece.

In 1946, we emigrated to Israel and rented a barn in Magdiel for two Lira per month.

My stomach was swollen and I was afraid I had caught some intestinal disease. My neighbor always invited me to come to her to make peepee, etc. (our barn/stable did not have a toilet. I told my husband, "I believe I have the same disease as my neighbor." She had a waterbelly (ascites). "I got infected. I am not going to go to her anymore." My belly grew larger and larger, but I did not consult a physician. I knew I could not have any children. Finally, the public health nurse sent me with an interpreter (at that time I did not yet speak Hebrew) to the hospital.

At Belinson Hospital, they found out that I was pregnant. The doctors heard my story and could not believe it. But, I recalled Dr. Samuel, "If you live, remember me!" Dr. Samuel was killed, but on the second day of Rosh-ha-Shanah 1946, I gave birth to Jacob. It was a difficult delivery, but the boy was a healthy baby and weighed 2 kilos and 700 grams. For a whole month, I stayed in the hospital and I was told that for eight years I should not have another child, and preferably, I should refrain from sexual intercourse altogether.

I had a lot of milk, and my son grew and developed well. When he was 6 months old he already weighed 12 kilograms. Today, he is a tall, handsome man. I have a good daughter-in-law and I am also a good mother. They are living close by here in Ra'anana.

I did not obey the doctors' advice. I wanted to show the world that the Germans had not won. One after the other, I had four children. They all died 2-3 days after being born. In 1960, I tried again, and two times I did lie in bed during almost the entire nine months of my pregnancy, with my feet elevated and my head down so that the embryo would be better positioned. I gave birth to a healthy baby girl. The doctors said it was a miracle. But, I was very sick.

In 1962, during an operation, they found I had only half a womb, one ovary and a cancerous growth as large as a grapefruit. In 1983, I had blood in my stool, and a second operation was performed during which polyps were found. Most of the Greek women who had been irradiated by Dr. Schumann in Auschwitz and who survived camp developed cancer. Many of them had to undergo colostomies and were living with a "sakit" (plastic bag for feces).

Three of them died in spite of their "sakit:" Rigreta Azi-Aaron, Auschwitz prison number 38968; Eleonora Malali, #41579 and Bella Riva-Nifusi. Two are still alive, but very gravely ill: Dora Cohen-Nachman, #38782 (with "sakit") and Dora Varsano-Gershon, #41624 who had, in addition, one kidney removed.

Unfortunately, I am again hemorrhaging. But, I don't want to undergo another operation. I want to die without a "sakit."[3]

In the spring of 1987, together with seven other Greek Holocaust survivors, I returned to Auschwitz on a pilgrimage. The trip had been organized by

Galei Zahal (a radio station), the Israel Ministry of Education, Yad Vashem, and the World Jewish Congress.

Each of us was accompanied by one offspring. I took Jacob along whom the Germans had not wanted to be born. He was forty years old, a proud sabra, tall and husky. I wanted to show the world that the Germans did not win.

❖

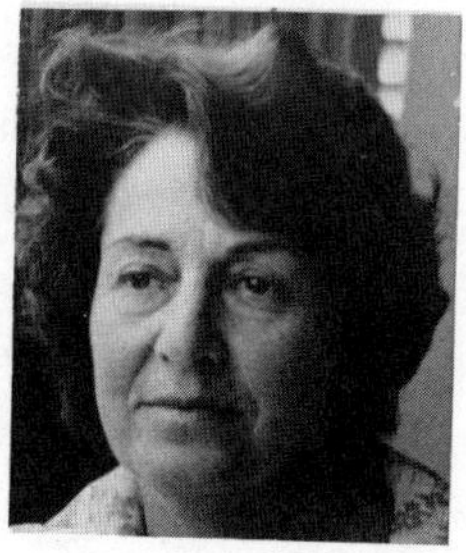

Renée Duering
Daly City (USA)

I was living in Amsterdam, Holland when the Germans invaded that country during their Blitzkrieg in 1940. The round-up of our fellow Jews began immediately, but we were not taken at first.

We were allowed to stay because we were employed by the Dutch government. In a matter of months, however, the Germans lifted that provision and all Jews throughout Holland were considered to be fair game for capture and imprisonment.

I married Fritz Kramer in 1942, and shortly afterwards my parents as well as my husband and I were sent to the holding camp of Westerbork. Fritz, who had a beautiful deep voice was selected to be a telephone operator for the camp. That meant he got to have a private room, but we were separated. I was living in a giant barrack with hundreds of other women and was not allowed to see my husband until our first wedding anniversary.

A few weeks later, the names of Fritz and myself were chosen for a list of thousands who were to board the jammed freight trains for Auschwitz. We knew we were going to Auschwitz but we did not know it was a death camp at the time. Fritz thought we would simply be forced to work very hard for the Nazis.

When the wheels ground to a halt and the freight car doors parted, we jumped out of the train and some SS man told us to drop all our belongings where we stood. Fritz turned to me and said, "We will never see each other again, Renée, goodbye." He said he could tell this would be the end for us.

An SS guard then separated us taking Fritz with the large group of men. I was hurried into a gathering of women where the young married women were then separated from the young unmarrieds.

They marched us to a building and ordered us to remove all clothing. We were given shabby dark gowns with red crosses painted on the backs. Then they herded us before men who cut every bit of hair from our bodies (see Illustration 1). We were each bald from head to toe dressed in these strange gowns and terribly frightened. We did not know what was going to happen to us.

We were marched five abreast to a nearby red brick building. I was placed upstairs with about 500 others. A bed was ordinary straw covered in burlap. Two shared one mattress. Our meals, as we were soon to learn, consisted of a small portion of bread, a cup of tea from leaves and a cup of soup each day.

Soon after our arrival, a man came into the big room and began tattooing numbers into the flesh of each woman's lower left arm. When he came to me, I asked why I had to have my arm marked. He told me to be glad I was getting a number because that meant I was going to live (see Illustration 2).

The following day was a Thursday, when we were exposed for the first time to the shootings that occurred each Thursday at the Black Wall between Blocks 10 and 11. That's why all the windows of our block were boarded up and we did not get much fresh air (see Illustration 6).

A day or so later, a man came to us and announced to all new arrivals that we had a choice of signing up for "certain physical examinations" or being killed (see Illustration 3).

Almost all of us signed the piece of paper. Some women who lived through it say today that they never signed anything for the Nazis, but they did, everybody who remained in Block 10 and was used as a guinea pig did if they wanted to stay alive.

The only one I remember who refused to sign the declaration was Gerda Mueller. She was transferred to Birkenau and miraculously survived the war. I met her in the summer of 1945 in Amsterdam at the Joodsche Invalide, the former Jewish Hospital for the Elderly, where many survivors were sent for recuperation.

I soon discovered the so-called physical examinations were actually part of the notorious Nazi human experiments at Auschwitz (see Illustration 4).

First they took our blood for the Nazi soldiers. Our blood was good enough to save them, but we were like animals to the Third Reich, not human beings (see Illustration 9).[4]

The first experiment they did on me was a series of injections into my back. I don't know what they were shooting into me, but there were about 42 places where they stuck me (see Illustration 7).

One morning I was summoned along with ten other women to the operating room downstairs. There I met a man in a white coat and he explained he would be performing an experiment with me (I later found out his name was Goebel). I was laid on an x-ray table and my right ovary was injected with an unknown serum (see Illustration 8).

I was also subjected to numerous radiation exposures on my female organs.

When he finished with me, there was a terrible pain on my right side. It lasted for about three days. All the women who were experimented on said they had these pains afterwards.

I was called to the operating table three times during my confinement at Auschwitz. Two of those times, the experiments were carried out. The third time I was lucky.

They had destroyed the ovary on my right side and had me scheduled to do the left side, which would have made me sterile. There were seven of us standing outside the room waiting for the experimenter. When he arrived, he became angry because there were not ten women as he had requested. He said he would not operate if there were not ten and he stormed off. We were taken back upstairs.

I, along with groups of other women, was used for assorted work behind the barbed wire. For a long time, I gathered leaves from which they made the tea we were given to drink (see Illustration 11). I lost weight and became like a skeleton. I would reach with my hands completely beneath my rib cage. The only flesh left on my body was in the calves of my legs.

On January 18, 1945, Auschwitz was evacuated (see Illustration 21). We were marched from camp to camp. Many died of starvation and exhaustion or were shot on these marches. I was imprisoned in four other concentration camps after leaving Auschwitz (see Illustrations 25 and 26).

I remember one night shortly before I escaped, when I was lying with ten women who were all trying to huddle beneath one blanket. It was very cold and the concrete beneath us was wet. I was shivering beneath one edge of the cover when a male voice called out to me.

He asked if I wanted to cross over this wire fence and sleep on that side under a blanket by myself. I asked him what else he had in mind and he assured me—nothing. So, I crawled over that fence and he made a place for me to sleep between a stack of boxes (see Illustration 27).

I recall lying there covered by that wool blanket, looking up at a clear sky with all those beautiful stars. I could remember Fritz's warm smile, my mother and father and when I had been a little girl, growing up in my home town of Cologne, Germany. For the first time in almost two years, I felt a sense of tranquility (see Illustration 28).

A few days later, we marched through a small German town and I noticed an open courtyard gate just ahead. I manuevered myself to the outside of the column and positioned myself.

I knew there would be only one chance, and I was ready to risk it. Glancing back over my shoulder, I saw the SS guard turn his head to bark an order. At that instant, I leapt from the crowd and behind the courtyard gate, pushing it closed as the columns continued marching past (see Illustration 29).

I hesitated momentarily, resting my head against the wooden door. Did the guard see me? Would he follow and shoot me down? Was I actually free?

The shuffling feet continued. No one followed. I was once again a free person (see Illustrations 30 and 31).

▼

After the war, a doctor informed me that I could have a baby through certain methods. He said although one ovary had been destroyed in the experiments, one remained intact.

I remarried a Jewish man and we lived in Israel. A daughter, Naomi, was born there in 1954.

My second marriage failed after seven years. Naomi and I came to San Francisco in 1958, and five years later we became American citizens.

Even now, after almost 45 years of freedom, I still frequently awake suddenly from a sound sleep. I dream the same dream: that I am trying desperately to scale a massive stone wall. Soldiers with guns are trying to stop me with shots and screams. I am stretching and straining with all my might to climb that wall...

▼

In the small vignettes and illustrations that follow this text (pp. 106-136), I have attempted to represent some aspects of my camp experiences.

My First Wedding Anniversary in Westerbork

I was 17 and Fritz was 19 when we first met. We waited for four years until we married on August 12, 1942. The only place Jews could get married anymore in Amsterdam was at the Zoo, which was an hour's walk. Jews were not allowed to use streetcars and all bicycles had long been confiscated. So we walked with our parents, sisters and witnesses.

On August 12, 1943, our first wedding anniversary, we were already in Westerbork, where men and women lived in separate quarters. Fritz had arranged with his five room-mates to let him use their room during one hour in the early afternoon. I was working the night shift in the tailor shop. For one special day, I had to sacrifice my sleep, and when Fritz came to pick me up we walked to his place. He was hugging me when there was a knock at the door. Fritz jumped up and looked from the window. "It's your mother," he said.

She had made us a cake, with the ingredients available; it consisted of old bread and some raisins.

Fritz had managed to get one carnation for me which stood on the little table. He had also given me a silver broach with my initials: RK. It had been made by a jeweler from a silver Gulden. The pin was a simple safety pin, and I succeeded in smuggling it into Auschwitz in my shoes. However, there I lost it or it was stolen.

Fritz had been so glad that he would be alone with me for one hour and now my mother sat there. He had thanked her politely at the door when she dropped off the cake, but she sat down and we did not know what to do. Then Fritz said to her, "Would you kindly leave now, I would like to be alone with my wife." She got up and started to cry, she was speechless and left. I did not enjoy that last part of the hour at all.

A few weeks later we were deported to Auschwitz.

Margit Neumann

When we arrived in Block 10, Margit, the block elder, introduced herself. She stood in front of us straddle-legged, her head resembling a Beethoven mask with natural curls sticking out on all sides, a stern expression and high front, speaking to us in German with a strong Slovakian accent.

"I have been in camp a long time. When we arrived we were wading in the mud. I saw the construction of Birkenau and am still alive. I have been appointed to be your block-elder and I want to do my job conscientiously and honestly. To accomplish this, I need your help. I want Block 10 to be an exemplary block and I want you to know that this is going to be tough on you and me. I'll punish you if anything does not go smoothly. I haven't been asked to come into this camp, neither have you; but I want to survive this war and I'll do anything to accomplish this goal. Please keep this in mind. You'll have to obey every order, otherwise you force me to be strict. So, it will depend on you how things will be here in the block." Then she disappeared.

We looked at each other silently and everybody felt that this reception did not bode well. The Dutch girls started to develop a dislike for Margit—and Margit considered us all as Dutch because we had come with a transport from Holland.

One day, during our first week, Margit discovered some dirty plates on the table. She asked who had left them and nobody stepped forward.

"If the culprit does not have the guts to come forward, is there at least somebody willing to wash the plates?"

I had a clean conscience and volunteered to clean the dishes. When I passed Margit, she hit me viciously in the face. I stood still and just stared at her. Probably, nobody had ever looked at her so accusingly and so frightened. Everybody always tried to avoid her glances. Then I washed the plates downstairs. There was still silence when I returned to our dormitory.

From then on, Margit glanced sideways whenever she saw me. She never raised her hand to me again.

We were already in the new block when I talked to Lien about the rumors concerning Margit and Margot. Lien was a seamstress working for the SS women. She was a nice person and had a workroom to herself.

It was already late. I saw light through a chink in the door, knocked and Lien was happy with my visit. She continued to sew while we talked.

I discovered that there was a small room behind Lien's studio without any outside door to the hallway.

"Is there anybody in this room? Can anybody listen to our conversation?" I asked.

"No," Lien answered. "Margit and Margot often meet in this room, you know..."

I pretended to be surprised. "Tell me Lien. You must know more. Is it really true?"

Lien looked at me for a second and laughed. "You are still doubting? Don't you remember how the two often sat arm in arm in front of the stove in the old block at night when everybody was asleep?"

I did remember.

"I would prefer to run away when Margit passes my room because I know that Margot will follow soon. I always ask Margit if I should leave, but she tells me to stay and continue my work."

"What is in that room?" I asked.

"Just a bed," Lien replied.

▼

After the war, I lived in den Haag and went to see Lien who had been reunited with her family in Scheveningen. She was an excellent cook and kept me for lunch.

"Do you remember, Renée, when you came to see me in the sewing room? I forgot to tell you something." Lien seemed to hesitate.

"Why don't you finish the story."

"Don't laugh, Renée, but I can't forget the sounds coming from that room. They were horrible!"

Dr. Samuel

One day shortly after my arrival in Block 10, Dr. Samuel entered our dormitory. He was a tall man. My mother had often mentioned him. "He has a beard, but he is a handsome man," she always used to say. She always referred to him as "King of women." There, in Auschwitz, he did not have a beard anymore, but he carried himself very erect.

He had been my mother's obstetrician and had delivered me. On January 7, 1921, he was called to the house my parents had just bought in November 1920. There were no paved streets yet. My father paced back and forth in the bedroom while my mother was in agony. Dr. Samuel motioned him to come outside. He had to talk to him. The situation was very serious and my father should choose whether to save the mother or the baby. He opted for his wife, Esther. As luck would have it, we both made it and lived happily ever after until Hitler came to power.

I had the courage to talk to Dr. Samuel in Block 10. He must have noticed a family resemblance and immediately addressed me by my mother's name as Esther Duering.

"Please, tell me, Dr. Samuel. Are you going to also use me as a guinea pig?" I asked.

He stared at the farthest corner of the wall—my question must have been very unpleasant for him. "I don't think so," he said briefly and hurriedly left the dormitory.

Dr. Samuel did hysterectomies for Dr. Wirths in Block 10. It was rumored that he was in cancer research and writing a book. Once I was present when he let an SS Obersturmbannfuehrer glance through the colposcope. The SS man was not very interested. The not so young woman on the table was Samuel's show piece.

After Dr. Samuel had completed his studies, he was dragged away, still in his white coat, to be shot.

Mrs. Levi, the Gate-Keeper

Everybody knew her, not only the inmates of Block 10, but anybody who entered the block, because she was the gate keeper.

She sat near the door from early morning when the SS women arrived until after the evening's roll-call when we were locked in. It was not difficult to guess why she had been chosen for this job. She was like a police dog.

Her eyes were as sharp as pointed knives, here nose was too prominent for the small head, her mouth was large but she had very thin lips. She had arrived with a transport from Belgium long before me, was not a youngster anymore and occupied a third tier corner bed in my dormitory going toward the road, from where she probably could watch the gate even at night.

One day, shortly after my arrival I was introduced to Mrs. Levi. "Well this is Renée," she said. "Come a little closer. How old are you?"

"I am 22," I replied.

She smiled, and I could see her ugly yellow teeth, turned to a woman next to her and remarked, "Look how beautiful she is." (see Illustration 5.)

Nobody had ever told me that I was pretty—nor did I think so myself. Either this woman is a liar or a flatterer, I thought and went back to my quarters.

From that moment on, Mrs. Levi always greeted me quite cordially whenever we met.

Diphtheria

I had diphtheria and was in the Revier (sick bay). On my left lay a Dutch woman suffering from the same disease. Her throat was full of pus and she had great difficulty breathing. The stench of the pus poisoned the air.

She was so weak that she could not go to the potty herself. Since the nurses were scared of infections, I had to help her although I was quite sick myself.

She was fully conscious, but could not speak and attempted in vain to gasp for air. I asked the nurses to fetch the physician. It was after midnight when Dr. Brewda just showed her head at the door without entering.

"Are you going to operate in order to relieve her?" I asked.

"No," she answered shortly and closed the door.

The patient now lay quietly in her cot, foam bubbles and mucus slowly dripping from her lips. At dawn she died. I do not recall her name, but I remember her face very well (see Illustration 10).

Margot Meier

Although Margot, originally from Berlin, had lived in Amsterdam, she did not belong to my transport. When I saw her the first time, she was standing at the window trying to communicate through gestures with her husband who was in a block across the road.

She told me how she had landed in Auschwitz. Her husband and she had tried to smuggle themselves from Holland to Switzerland in a lift. In Cologne, the lift was inspected, the two were arrested, sent to Berlin and from there to Auschwitz.

Soon Margot got the news that her husband had not been able to evade a selection—a few times, previously, he had successfully hidden himself in the toilet. Margot cried a lot, none of us could comfort her. We all had suffered a similar fate.

When I was in the Revier with diphtheria, Margot was one of the nurses and we befriended each other. She even dared to talk to the physician on my account. After two weeks, I was supposed to be discharged although I was still ill. Margot mentioned me to Dr. Brewda, who took the trouble to examine my throat and simply said, "She has to stay."

After the death march, Margot and I met again in Ravensbrueck. While we exchanged experiences, I mentioned that my underpants which I had hung close to the stove had been stolen.

"What are you wearing now?" she asked.

"Nothing," I said.

Margot got up, took off a panty she was wearing and gave it to me. "Here, take this. I can live without it."

I was speechless and very happy, and did not have to be afraid of catching a fourth bladder infection (see Illustration 23).

In the early sixties, Margot visited me in California. I told her that I had never forgotten how she had generously let me have one of her panties when I was without any during the severe winter of January 1945 in Ravensbrueck.

"Did you believe I had only two pairs of panties?" she asked.

"Of course!"

"No Renée, I had three pairs at that time."

"All these years I was under the impression that you just ran around with one pair."

We both laughed.

Martha and Erna Heimann

These two sisters had married two brothers and had arrived with a transport from Holland. During our first conversation, I noticed that they had a Rhineland accent. It turned out that they were from Cologne, Wetticher Strasse. They both had children my age who were hiding in the Netherlands.

I went to see them regularly and found out that they had played as children together with my mother. In Block 10, they knitted diligently. Every day they completed a pair of gloves or a pair of socks together.

One day, when we had returned from a walk to our block, sugar beets were unloaded. The male prisoners were clumsy on purpose and quite a number of beets rolled on the street. I marched on the other side of the column and they were beyond my reach, but many women stooped and collected them. So did, for example Margit, she quickly ran with her apron full of beets to the block-elder room and then came outside again.

The SS woman on duty had observed this incident. She gave an order to Mrs. Levi, the gate keeper, and when we entered Mrs. Levi checked every inmate. Whoever had a beet had to step aside.

Erna Heimann, the younger of the two sisters, was also among the culprits. Margit came upstairs to our dormitory with a list to punish the guilty ones. Each received 25 whip lashes. Some women did not utter a sound, but Erna screamed pitifully. She returned weeping and Martha had to help her climb up on the bed. Both sisters were crushed by the occurrence. Erna only got up for the roll-call. For soup distribution, Martha presented her plates and Pola, the room elder, gave her two portions. Erna's screams were still in everybody's ears (see Illustration 15).

The two sisters were almost always together. From time to time they were separated when one of them was again used for an experiment. Usually, the absence lasted between two hours and two days. But this time, I had not seen Martha for a long while. I visited her in the Revier and found her skinny, weak and dejected. I tried to encourage her, but she only shook her head. Martha probably had typhus which had to be kept secret. Even Dr. Brewda, our inmate physician, described these diseases as nothing but colds or slight indispositions during SS inspections.

After the war, I met quite a few of the women of Block 10 in Holland. I inquired after Martha and Erna. Both of them still had to endure a lot, but they did not live to see the end of the war.

I was told that the surviving son of one of them had refused to speak to any person who had known his mother in camp.

Marushka

Marushka came from Cracow in Poland. One day, she approached me timidly and said, in broken German, "Are you Renée about whom Tonka told me?"

I answered in the affirmative. Previously, I had given a full massage to Tonka and received many compliments and a piece of bread. Marushka wanted a facial. I was very happy about the proposal because it meant an extra portion of soup.

Erna and Martha Heimann let me use their upper cot. I had once received a little vaseline from the pharmacy which I had saved.

At first, I did not want to ask Marushka what type of work she did downstairs since she had come to me to relax. She used to see me twice a week, and I was always looking forward to our session. Marushka was very pleased and grateful.

But, one day I could not refrain from asking her what she was doing as a dental technician in our block because from time to time I saw a ton full of dentures, gold teeth and partials in the hallway.

"Please excuse my question, Marushka, but I am very curious to know what type of work you are doing here?" I asked.

Marushka swallowed hard and answered, "All day long I sit at a table and sort gold teeth. Then they have to be fastened on cards. In Cracow, I was a dental technician, that's why I was chosen for this work. Believe me, it is not a pleasant occupation."

The Red Shoes

I had bought the shoes in 1938, in Maas Street in Amsterdam when I still worked at Tante Lina's. They were dark red sport shoes with leather laces, which one day would save my life.

When we arrived in Block 10, the shoes were the only possession I was allowed to keep. I used to wear them daily and was very indebted to Martha Heimann, who once took them to the shoemaker shop to have them outfitted with black rubber soles.

I was also grateful to Margit because she ordered Gutya, the room elder, to return the shoes to me. This happened when I was in the Kraeuterkommando (herbal detail). I was entitled to wear a pair of wooden boots which, mostly, I did not do—only on rare occasion to preserve my own shoes, since I was aware of their tremendous value.

While I was outside working, an inspection of the block took place and all burlap mattresses were searched as they were the common hiding place for every inmate. My shoes were found and confiscated, and the room elder wore them for two weeks until I gathered enough courage to tell Margit about it. It was the only time that I talked to her. At first, Gutya did not want to give back the shoes but, in the end, she had no choice and obeyed. Feeling my own shoes on my feet once more, it was as if I had received a new lease on life.

During the evacuation of Auschwitz, on the so-called death march, my friend, Lucie Heidemann, was heavily hanging on my arm because, with her wooden shoes, she had great difficulty walking on the slippery snow. After two days, we rested in a barn, and I carefully removed the shoes to examine my feet, which had been numb for many hours. I discovered a few red spots and quickly put the shoes on again so that they would not be stolen while I was asleep.

A week later, I had an opportunity in Ravensbrueck to look at my feet again (see Illustration 22). By then, the spots had turned black and the big toe was frozen. I kept this discovery a secret, because I did not want to have my toe amputated, and only told Manya, who had been a nurse in Belgium, about it. She massaged the toe and slowly the numbness subsided (see Illustration 24).

Shortly after my escape in April 1945, I was spending one night in Radebeul on the Elbe in the house of the stationmaster's daughter. In the morning, she brought me some fresh water and said, "My dear woman, please tell me honestly, what have you been through? I can tell from your shoes that it must have been something dreadful."

Absentmindedly, I had put the shoes in front of my door in the evening, as if I had spent the night in a hotel and expected somebody to clean them the following day.

"Unfortunately, I can't tell you, I replied. "Thank you very much for your hospitality, but don't ask me. I can talk only after the war."

When the woman removed the water, she again murmured something about frightful events. The water was so dirty, that it was a disgrace. However, I did not have any time to bother with such trifles. I had to get to Dresden.

The shoes carried me still to Frau Gerber's fourth floor flat in the Scheufussstrasse. While I was asleep, Frau Gerber took the shoes away and burnt them in the kitchen stove. She gave me a pair of black worn-out women's shoes which were much too large for me. On top of it all, I had to thank her, but I was quite sad (see Illustration 19).

Bathing in the Sola

As usual, thirty women were standing in front of the block ready to march out to collect herbs.[5] It was a beautiful summer day. The sky was blue and there was no breeze.

Today the SS man decided to collect peppermint. We crossed the bridge outside the camp, turned toward the right and walked along the river bank. There were a few bushes and we collected herbs.

The women who had been in camp longer started to tell us events that had occurred before our arrival.

"Do you see the Sola? It leads to freedom as well as to death. When we passed by here about a year ago, the SS women allowed us to take a bath. There was also an SS man who sat a little further away. One of the women, who spoke French, was a good swimmer. She tried to swim away and the SS man shot her. Auf der Flucht erschossen (shot while trying to escape)."

That was the reason that, until now, we had avoided the Sola on our walks, they did not want to run the risk. But gradually, we marched there again. The peppermint season was over, now we collected blackberry leaves. These bushes did not grow directly on the banks but also were not far from the Sola.

On our way home we sang, mostly Dutch hiking songs. The marching went better, and we did not feel the pangs of hunger so much. In the meantime, we had become a nice cohesive group. Suddenly, we fell silent. One could see the chimneys in the distance. Never had we seen the flames shooting so high skyward. We continued to march at the same pace, but nobody uttered a word. The SS man marched at the end of the group. He advanced and commanded, "Sing!"

He repeated, "Sing! I told you to sing." When nobody started to sing, he delivered a speech.

"You mean the fire. I saw it long before you. You have every reason to sing because you are still alive. Sing!"

We were still waiting. He continued, "I saw my comrades fall next to me, and I had to bury them with my own hand and had to continue to fight. Sing! Do you understand, "Sing."

And we sang, softly. He screamed, "Louder, louder!" and we sang a little louder, but we were all broken. We came to the block and did not speak.

Once, during the dandelion season, we were on the left bank of the Sola. The weather was still beautiful (see Illustration 12). We rested not far from the bank. Whoever had a piece of bread from the previous evening ate it, the others stretched out and rested.

I disappeared unnoticed, and went down to the Sola. There was a tiny sheltered bay, not deep enough for swimming. I undressed and went into the river, lying on my back. From far, I heard the women's voices. After about ten minutes, I dressed and went back to the resting place.

The reception was not as easy as I had imagined. The group had been counted and they had noticed that one was missing. Nobody knew who. When I arrived from behind the bushes, they asked me, "Where were you?" I pointed in the direction from which I had emerged and said simply, "Down below."

The SS man said, "In the future if you have to relieve yourself, you have to tell me so. If it happens again, you will not be allowed to march out with us any more."

I did not tell anybody that I had taken a bath in the Sola (see Illustration 13).

Peter Dattel

Peter was the mascot of Block 10. He would goose-step in front of us women at roll-call, imitating the SS. He was six years old and was blond and blue-eyed and Dr. Joseph Mengele had decided to let him stay alive when he arrived in Auschwitz. He and his mother, Ruth Dattel, had arrived with a transport from Berlin and were sent to Block 10 right from the ramp. Both survived (see Illustration 14).

I met the two of them in Cologne in 1957, when I was waiting for my papers to emigrate to the USA. Ruth had remarried but did not have any more children. Peter was 18 years old and had to decide whether or not to enter the German Army.

Stefan Dziwlik

As punishment on the occasion of the attempt on Hitler's life in July 1944, our outside walk had been cancelled. A high SS officer had ordered that we could only be in the fresh air a short while in the morning between Block 10 and 9. The area had been cordoned off with heavy ropes.

I stood next to the wall because the sun was shining and had my eyes closed. Beside me were three giggling Greek girls. They spoke Ladino and I could not understand. I opened my eyes and saw a male prisoner crossing the cordon. He handed me a note as well as a bottle of soda water before he stepped back. I shared the bottle with the Greek girls and was very surprised to have received the gift.

Cautiously, I read the note which said, "Please let me have your name and number. I have been observing you for the last four months. I want to help you. My name is Stefan and I am Polish. I want to share the packages which I receive from home with you. I deliver the soup in Block 10 on a daily basis, be close to the staircase and hand me a small note at that time because we cannot speak to each other."

The next day, when the soup detail arrived, I went downstairs and unobtrusively handed Stefan a note and he pressed an envelope into my hand. The note said, "My name is Renée Kramer and my number is 62,501. I come from Holland. Thanks for your nice words. Please write more about yourself. Why are you allowed to receive packages?" The envelope contained sugar which I shared with Lotte and Henny.

Thus Stefan became my "kochany." From now on a new era started. The days were passing faster because across from me in Block 9 there was a man who was thinking of me. We could not talk to each other, but we communicated in sign language. The women in the dormitory respected me more. All of a sudden, I had only friends in the block. Even Margit did not say anything and turned the other way when Stefan and I exchanged notes while he delivered the soup.

I learned that Stefan was a political prisoner and had a wife and five children in Cracow. He had studied law in Marseille (France) and spoke five languages, including Esperanto. He gave me his address in Cracow, which I learned by heart, and assured me that his wife would welcome me there like a daughter. A few times we managed to see each other when I went to the dental block to get some fillings. Stefan also promised to find out what happened to my husband.

A few days after we had moved from Block 10 in the men's camp to Block 1 in the newly constructed camp enlargement (see Illustration 16),[6] I received Stefan's last letter: "Dear Renée, when you are reading these lines, I am probably not in Auschwitz any more, but on my way to Buchenwald. Here is the news about your husband. Be strong. He died on December 20, 1943. I know how you feel and I am very sorry that I have to be the one to transmit the bad news. Please do not forget my home address and stay in touch."

I never saw Stefan again, but I wrote to him after the war. For years, we have been sending each other New Year's Cards. He also sent me a photo and wrote that he had become a grandfather. After the war, he was deputy mayor of Cracow—a post he held for four years. A few years ago, he passed away.

Otto Gerber

When we moved from Block 10 to the new camp, less and less experiments were carried out, but still the fear was hovering over us at all times.

Sewing machines were brought in, and the large room was used not only as a dining room but as a work room as well. There was a stage with a grand piano meant for performances and entertainment.

One day, a German Kapo with a green triangle (signifying incarceration for criminal reasons) came to install a large stage curtain. He asked some of the women to help him sew on the rings. I was the only one who volunteered.

The Kapo, whose name was Otto and who was also in charge of the artists, asked me if I played an instrument. I did play the piano a little. One night I had sneaked downstairs and played a piece from "Die Weise Dame" on the grand piano and many of the women had been surprised. Nevertheless, I told Otto right away that I was not good enough for the orchestra (see Illustration 17).

"Will you be able to copy music?"

"Sure," I said.

So I was recruited for the orchestra detail together with Ima van Esso who was a flutist.

On January 18, 1945, the day Auschwitz was evacuated, I was waiting for hours near the piano. Finally, he arrived, handed me a small card and said, "If you should be in the vicinity of Dresden, try to escape, bring regards to my mother and tell her that I'll come later." (see Illustration 18.)

I followed his advice. On April, 15, 1945, I escaped in Risa/Elbe and went to his mother's house in Dresden. She took me in until she found a small apartment for me near her place. Otto returned home only 7 weeks later.

The Hanging

They walked tall toward the double gallows. We stood in a mass of prisoners head to head everywhere filling the large space of the courtyard. The shorter one of the two seemed to shy away a little at the sight of the hangman's noose. Her taller friend walked without visible emotions. They both walked briskly in step, side by side as if synchronized, taking great strides, as if to say, "Let's get it over with."

There was one SS woman who wanted to hide among us prisoners, but another SS woman held her by the arm and told her, "You should be ashamed of yourself. Look at all these inmates." She put her behind our lines so that she could barely see what was going on.

Before the two women were hanged, an SS officer made an announcement. He screamed his written speech and his voice was twisting at moments. He said it was to be a warning for us not to do what those four girls had done, never to play with fire and end up this way. The order to hang them by the neck for sabotage had come from above. In the line of duty, it was his job to carry out the order for the fatherland—Heil Hitler!

He gave a sign to Bunker Jacob, the hangman, who was in charge of Block 11. The ropes had already been around the neck of the two girls and their hands and feet were also tied. The smaller one used her bound feet to struggle with death by pushing herself against the pole she reached on one side. We watched silently until they both did not move any longer. Jacob took them down and we marched away (see Illustration 20).[7]

❖

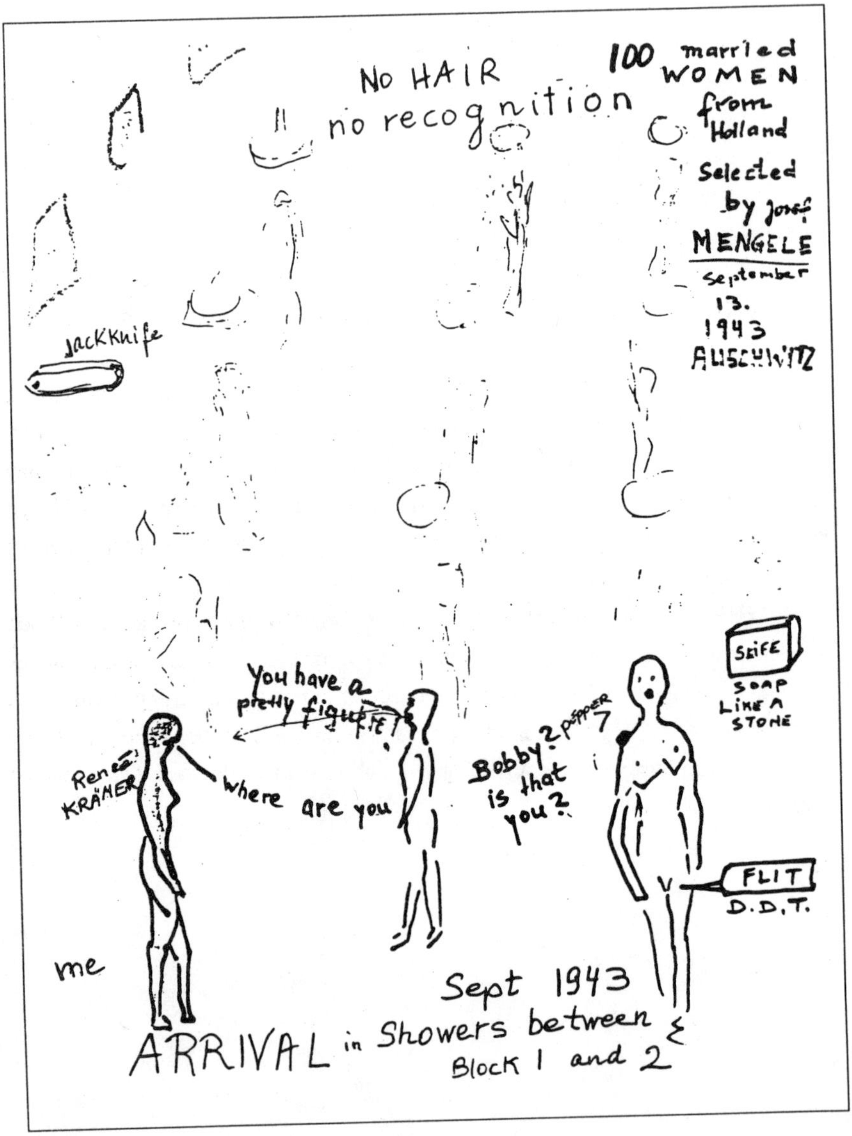
No HAIR
no recognition
100 married WOMEN from Holland
Selected by Josef MENGELE
September 13. 1943
AUSCHWITZ
JACKKNIFE
SEIFE
SOAP LIKE A STONE
You have a pretty figure!
Where are you
Bobby? is that you?
FLIT
D.D.T.
me
Sept 1943
ARRIVAL in Showers between Block 1 and 2

1. *No Hair*

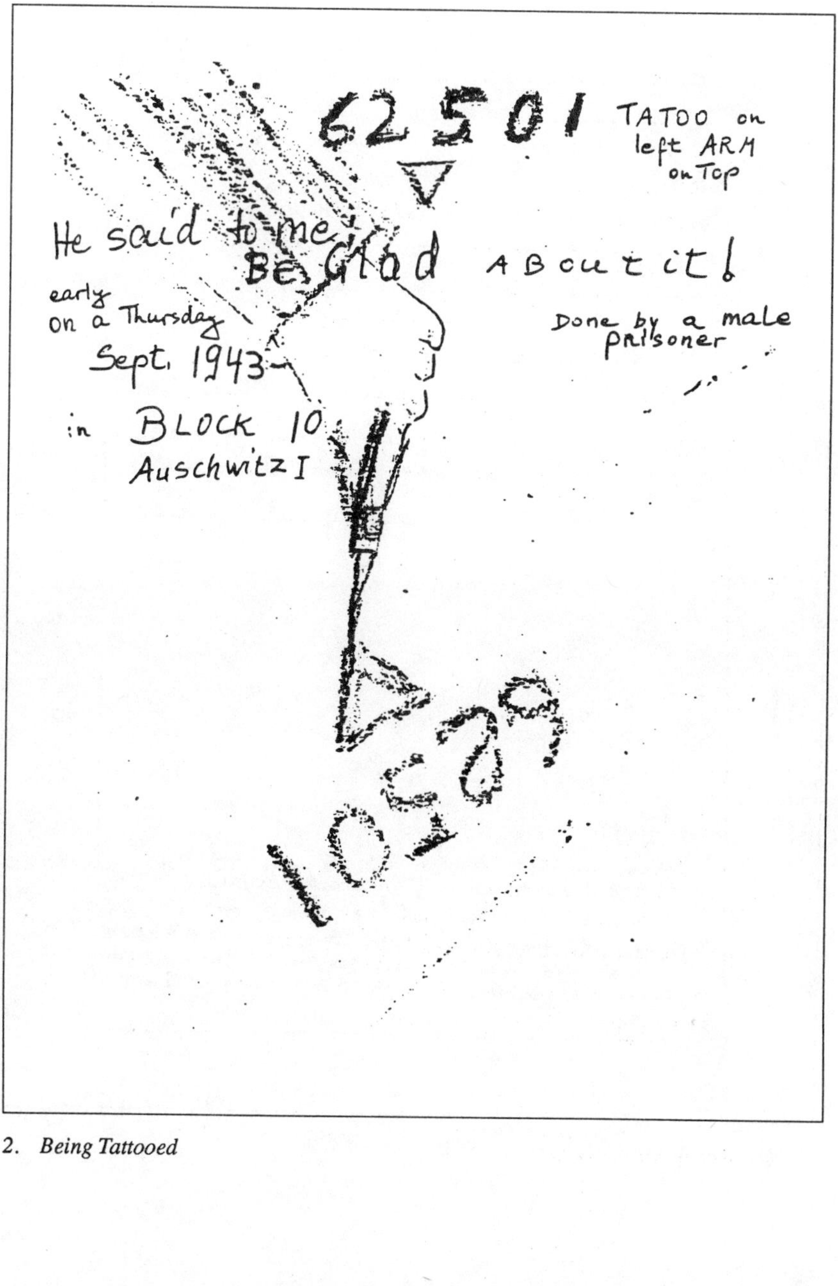

2. *Being Tattooed*

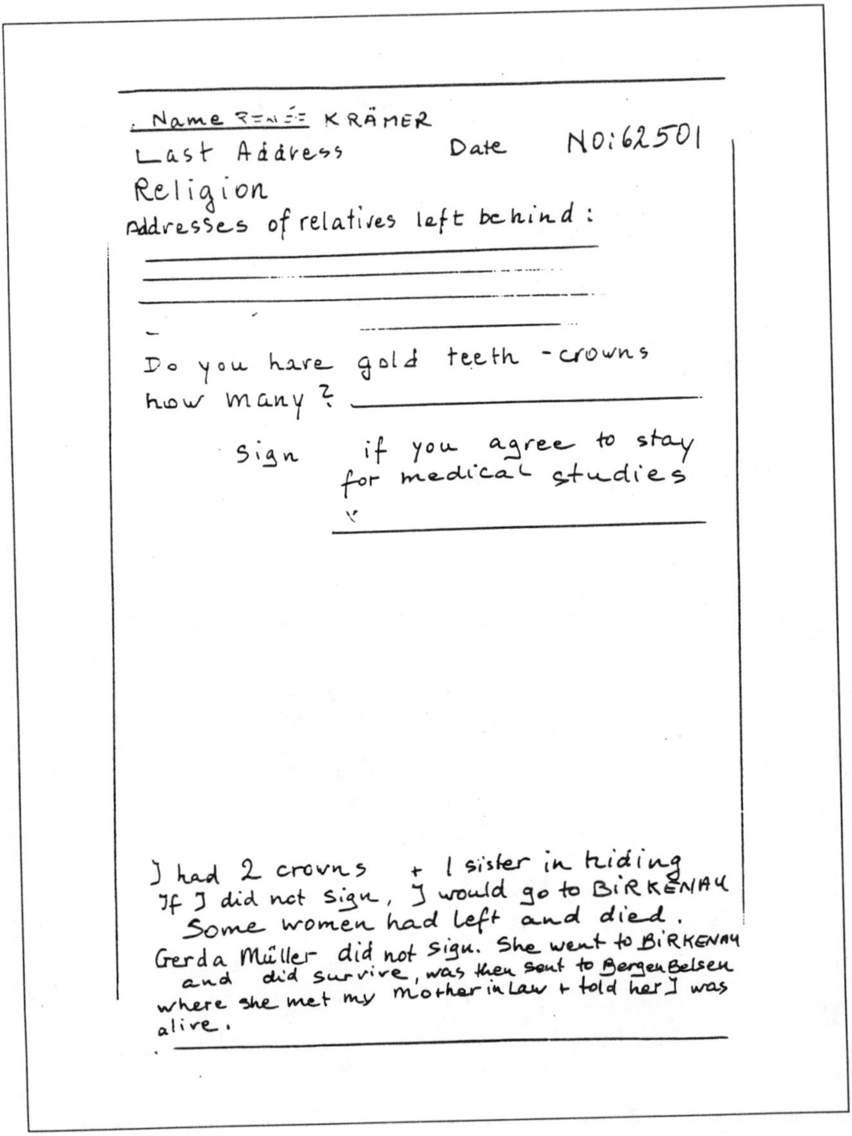

Name RENÉE KRÄMER
Last Address Date NO:62501
Religion
Addresses of relatives left behind:

Do you have gold teeth - crowns
how many?

Sign if you agree to stay for medical studies

I had 2 crowns + 1 sister in hiding
If I did not sign, I would go to BIRKENAU
Some women had left and died.
Gerda Müller did not sign. She went to BIRKENAU and did survive, was then sent to Bergen Belsen where she met my mother in Law + told her I was alive.

3. *Consent for Medical Experiments*

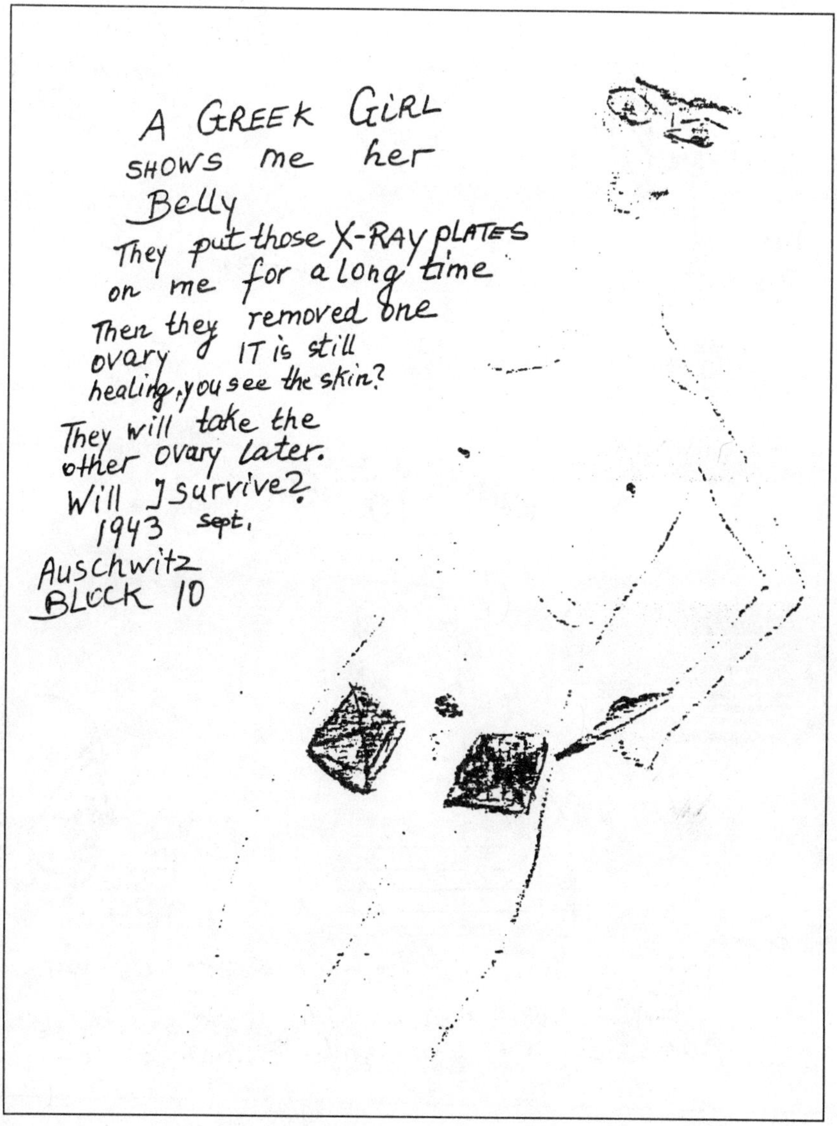

4. *Greek Girl with Irradiated Ovaries*

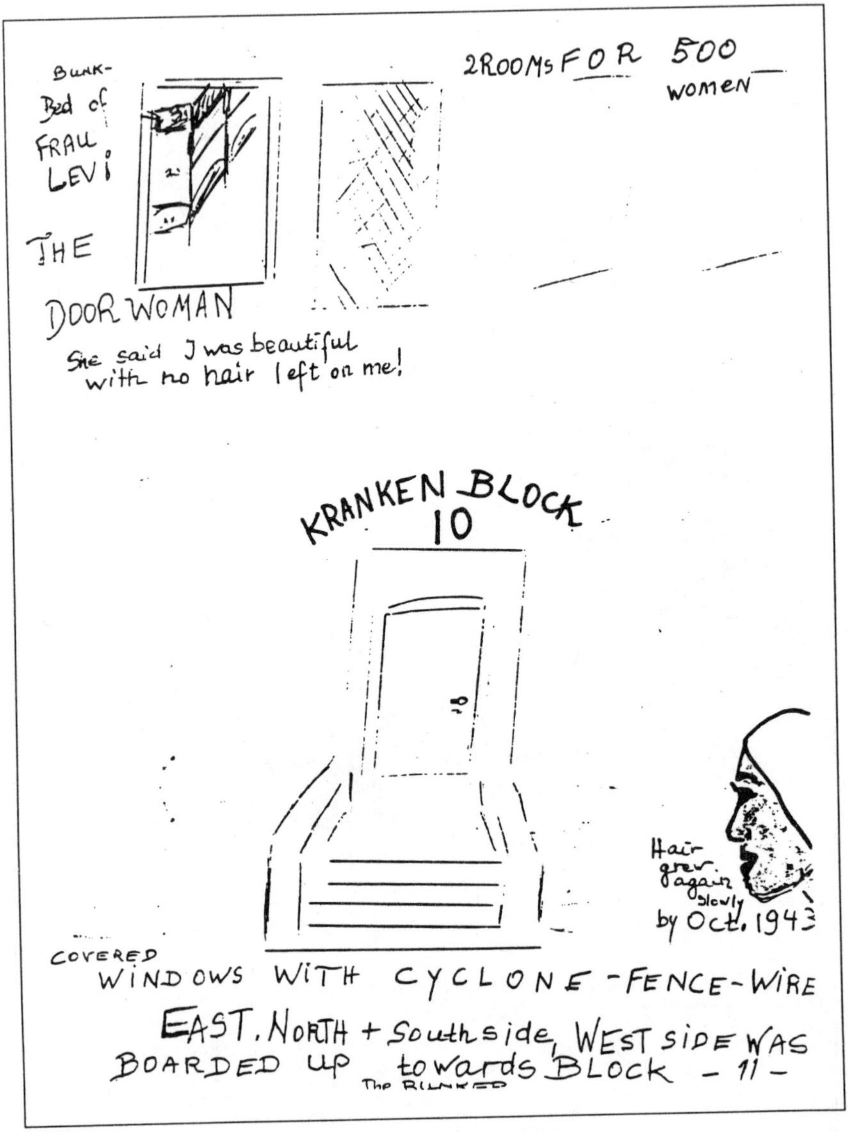

BUNK-
Bed of
FRAU
LEVI
THE
DOOR WOMAN
She said I was beautiful
with no hair left on me!
2ROOMS FOR 500
WOMEN
KRANKEN BLOCK
10
Hair
grew
again
slowly
by Oct. 1943
COVERED
WINDOWS WITH CYCLONE-FENCE-WIRE
EAST. NORTH + Southside, WEST SIDE WAS
BOARDED UP towards BLOCK -11-

5. *Frau Levi*

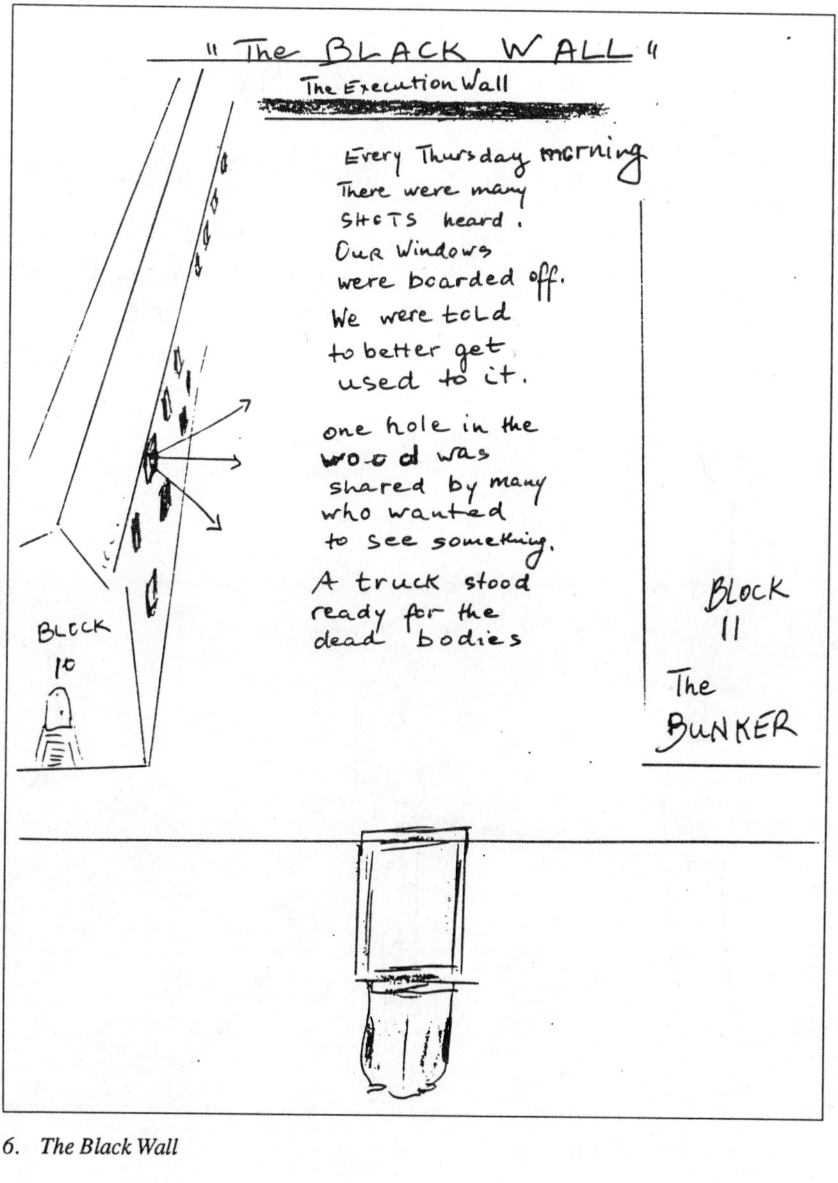

6. *The Black Wall*

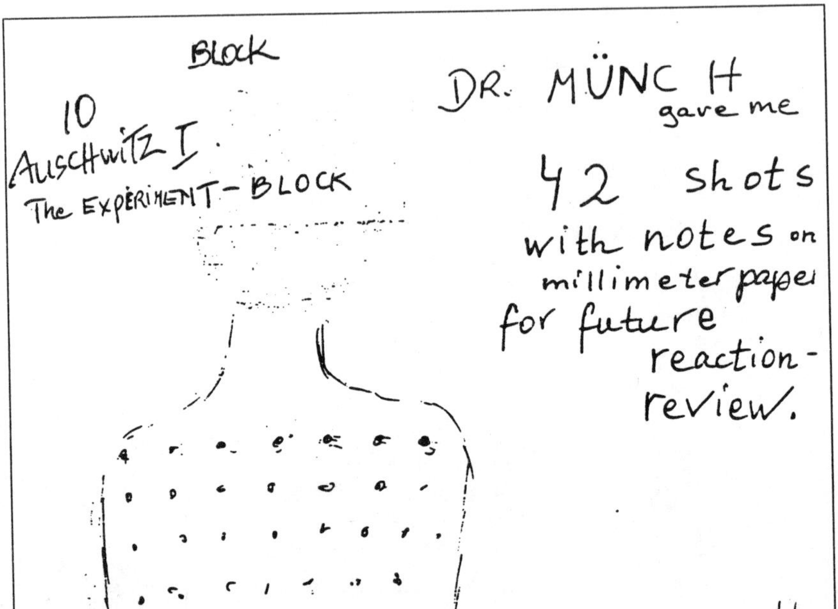

7. *Dr. Muench's 42 Shots*

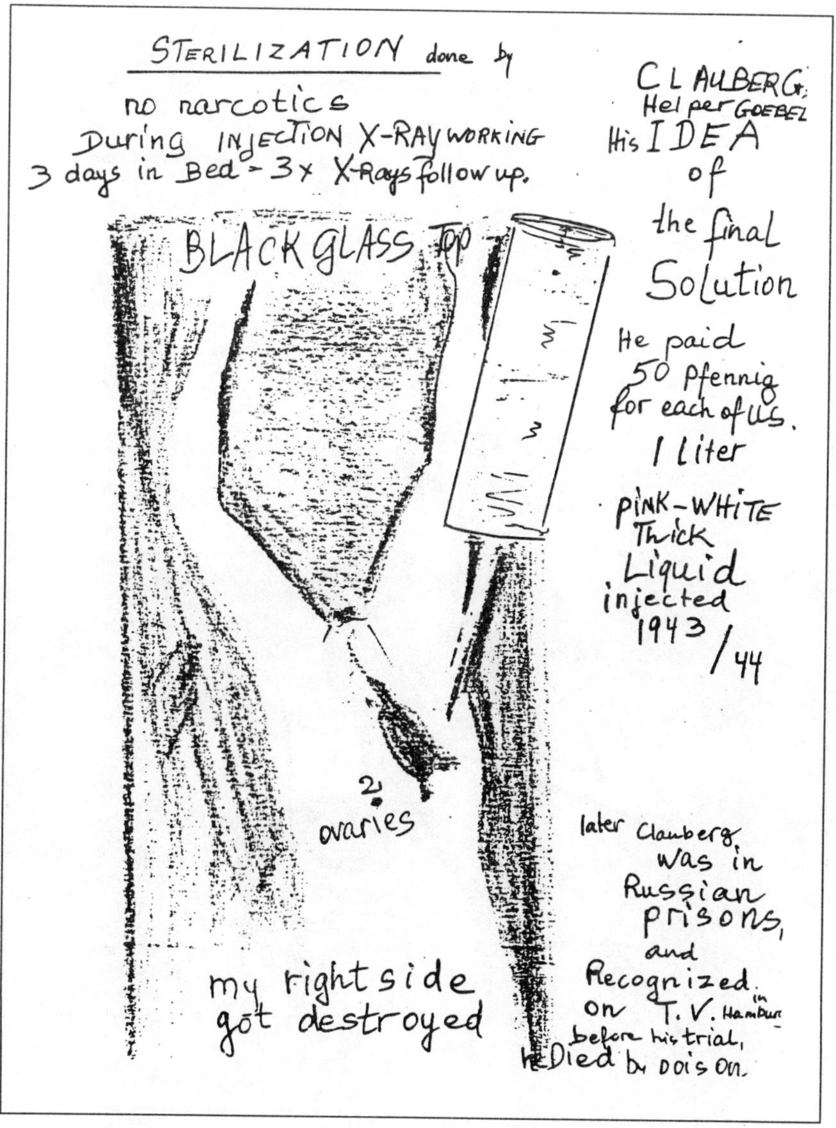

8. *Dr. Goebel's "Spritze"*

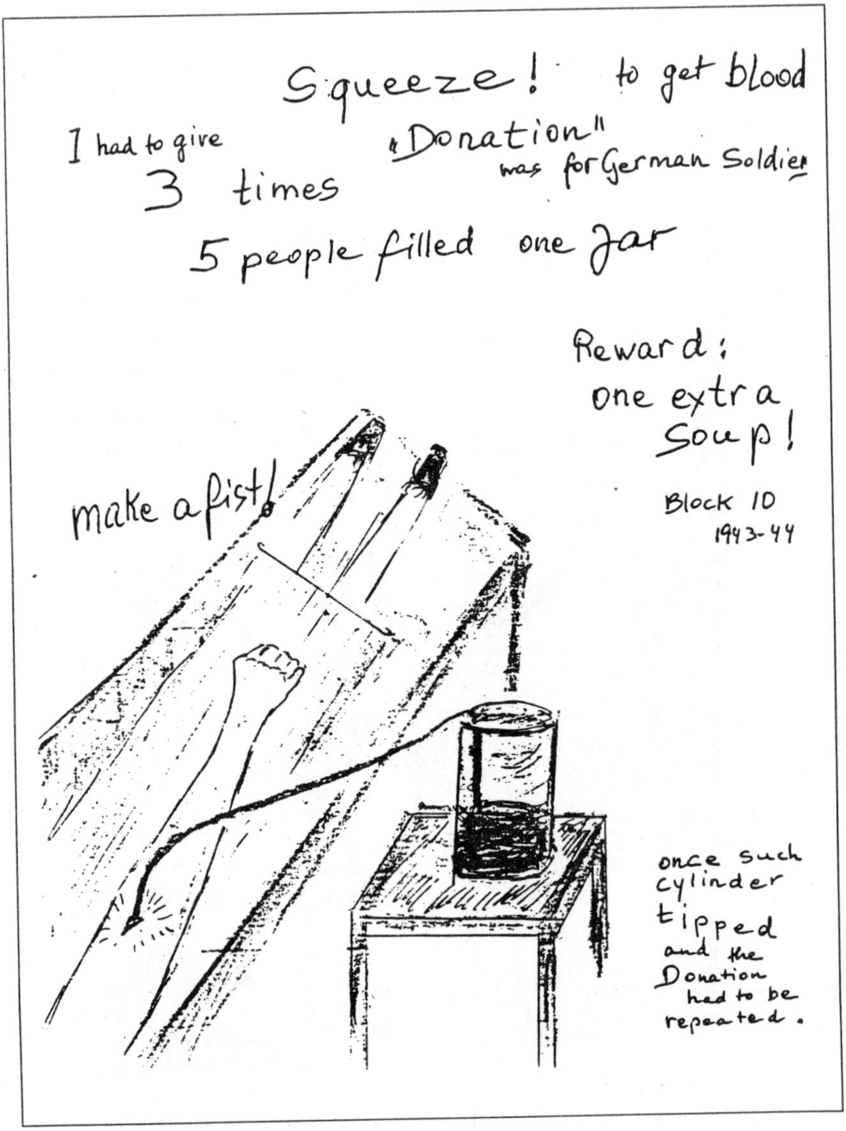

9. *"Donating" Blood*

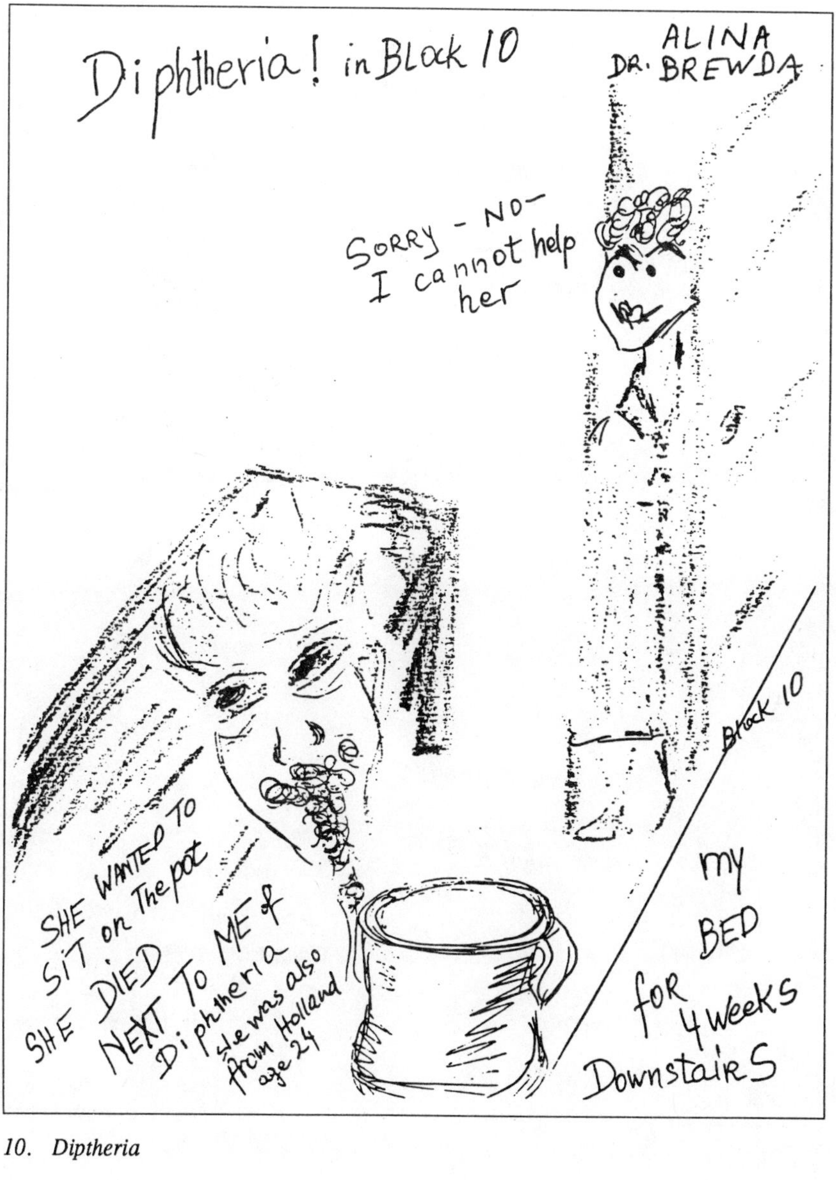
Diphtheria! in BLock 10
ALINA
DR. BREWDA
SORRY - NO -
I cannot help
her
Block 10
SHE WANTED TO
SIT on The pot
SHE DIED
NEXT TO ME of
Diphtheria
she was also
from Holland
age 24
my
BED
for
4 weeks
DownstairS

10. Diptheria

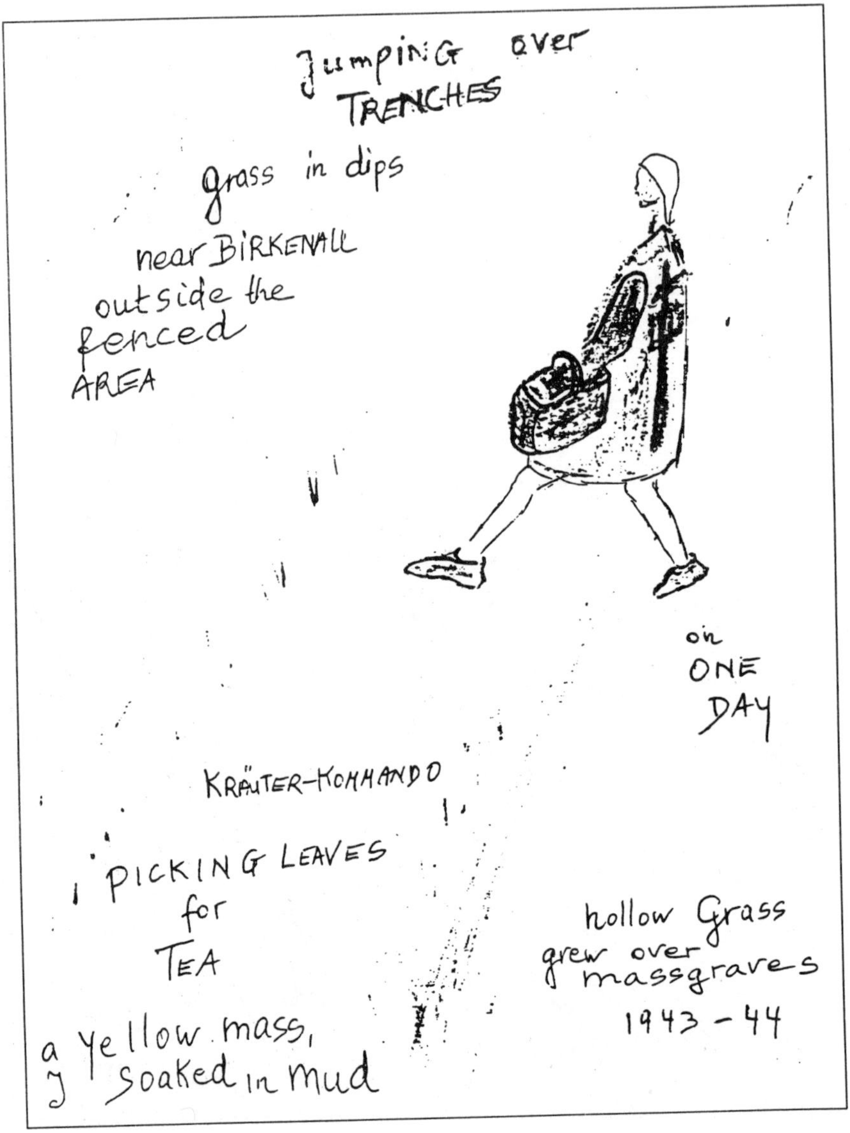

11 Kraeuter-Kommando

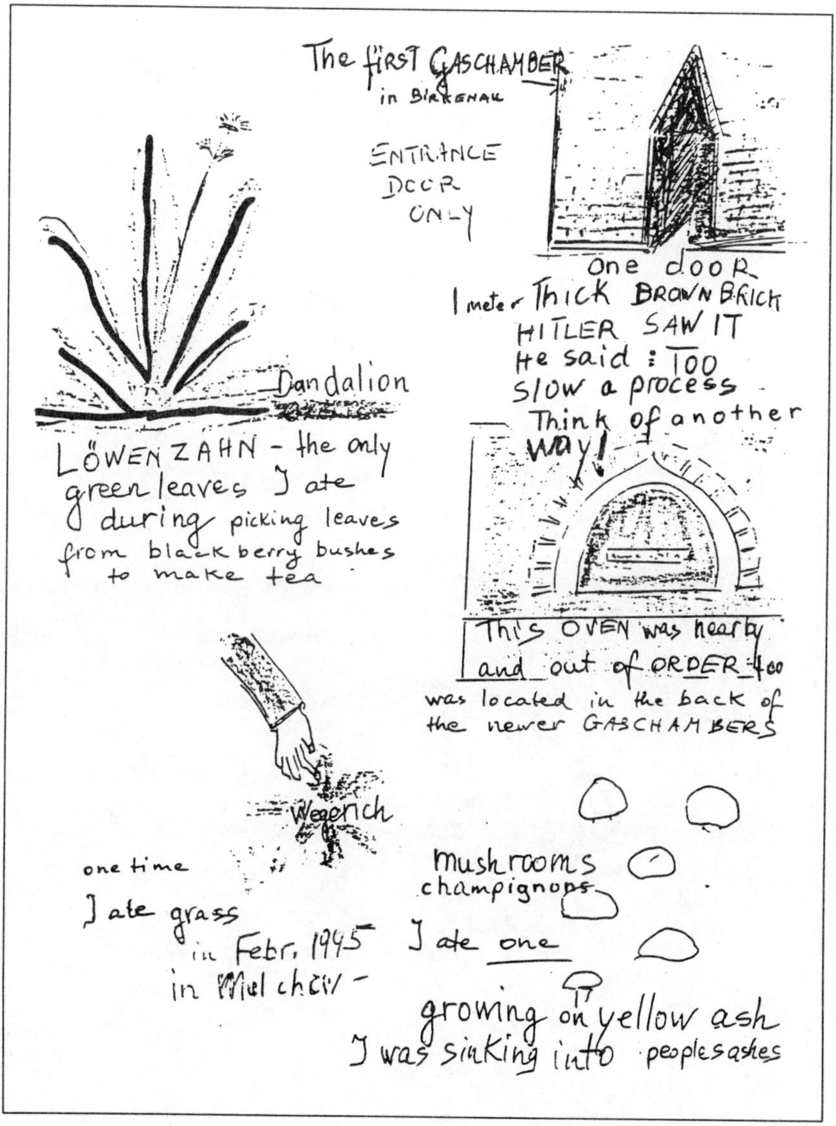

12. Picking Dandelions

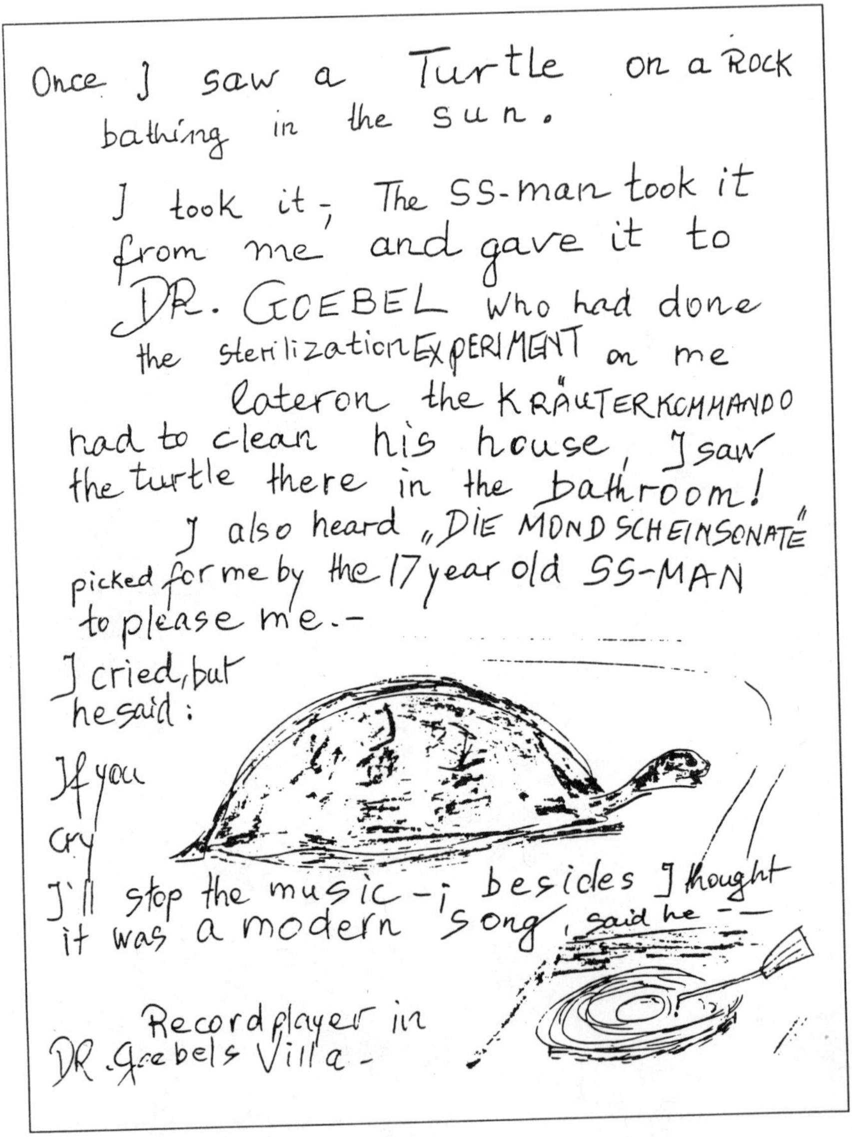

13. *The Turtle*

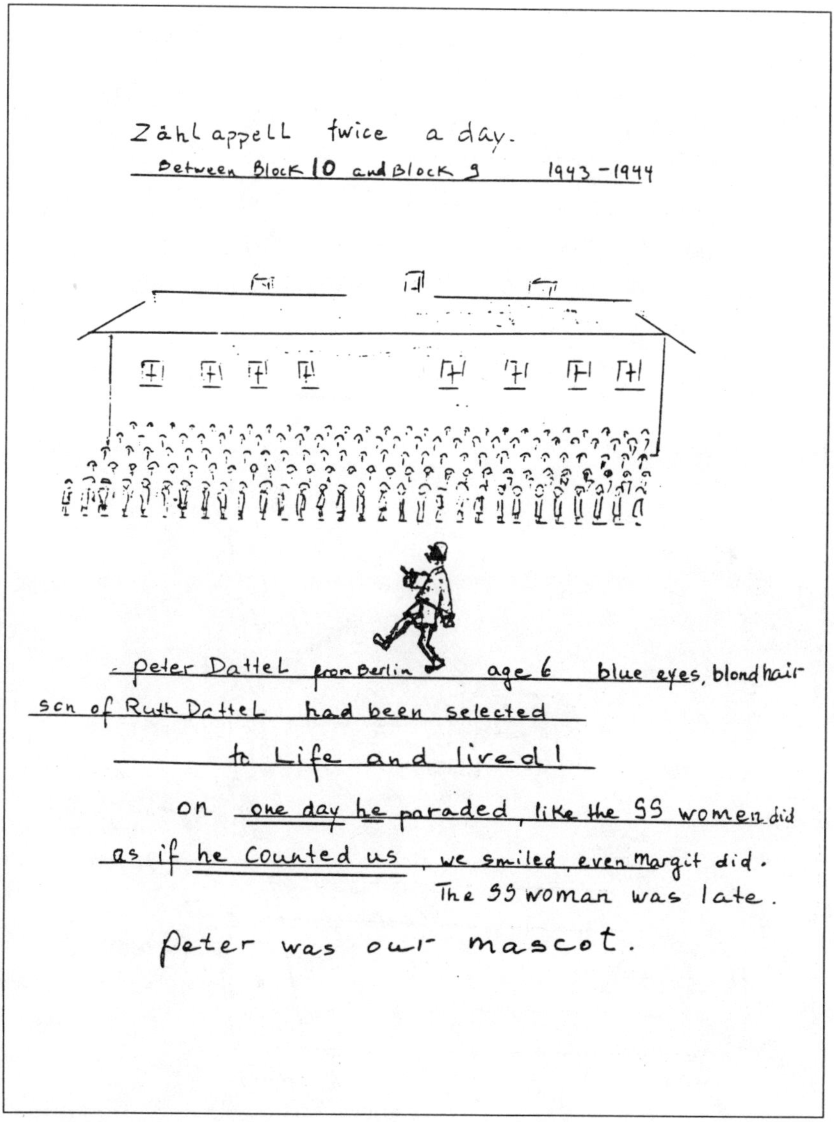

14. *Peter Dattel During Roll Call*

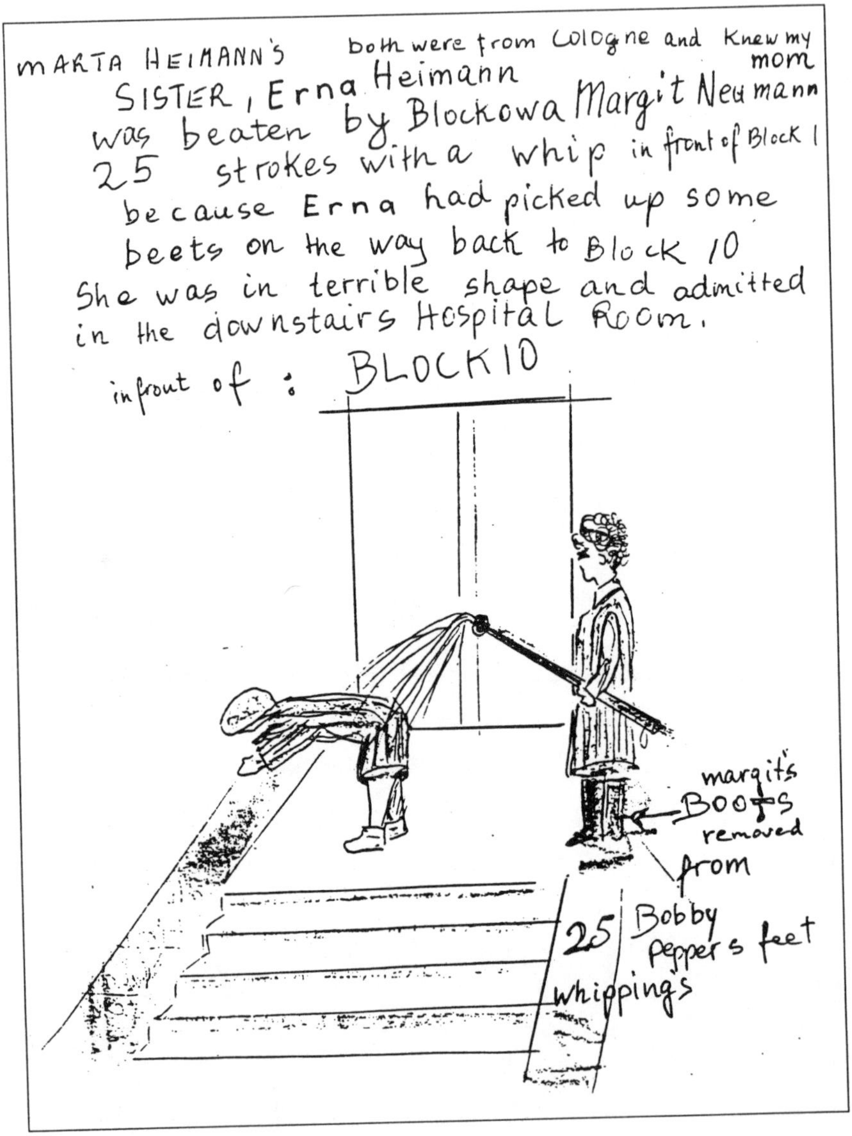
MARTA HEIMANN'S
both were from Cologne and Knew my mom
SISTER, Erna Heimann
was beaten by Blockowa Margit Neumann
25 strokes with a whip in front of Block 1
because Erna had picked up some
beets on the way back to Block 10
She was in terrible shape and admitted
in the downstairs Hospital Room.
infront of : BLOCK10
margit's Boots removed from Bobby pepper's feet
25 whippings

15. Erna Heimann Receiving "25"

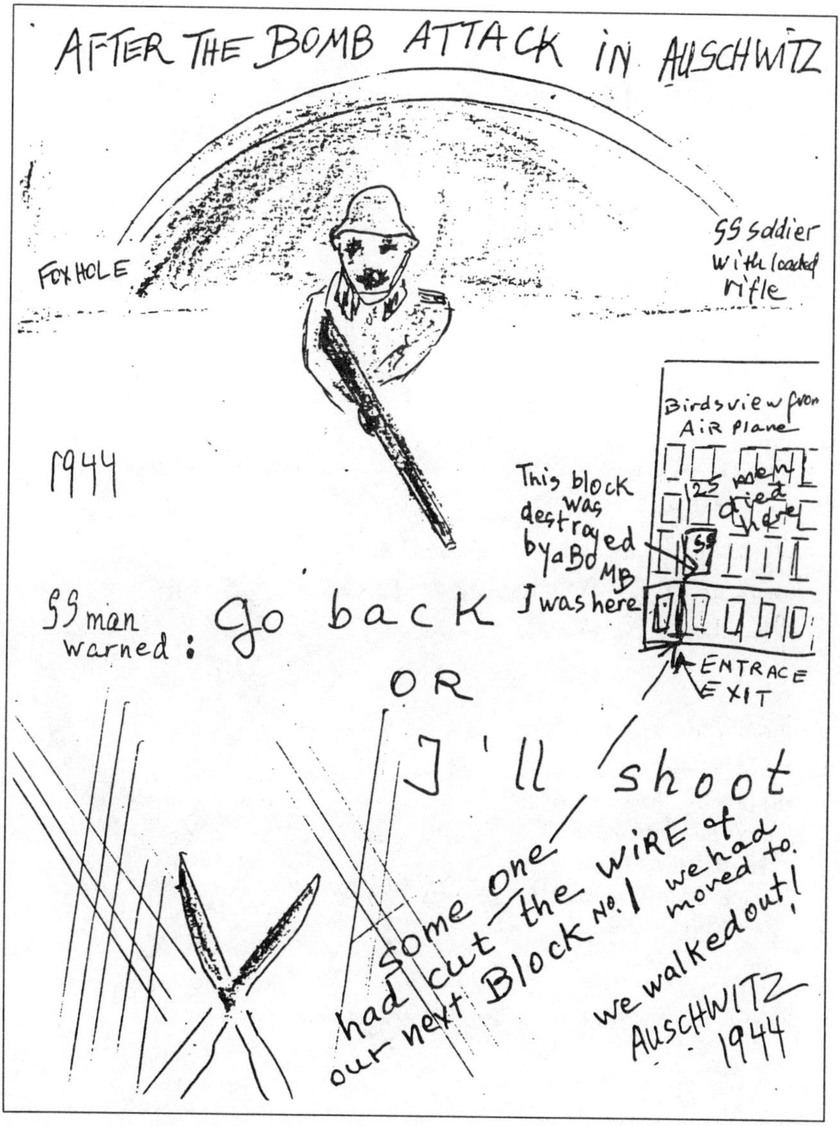

16. *After the Bomb Attack*

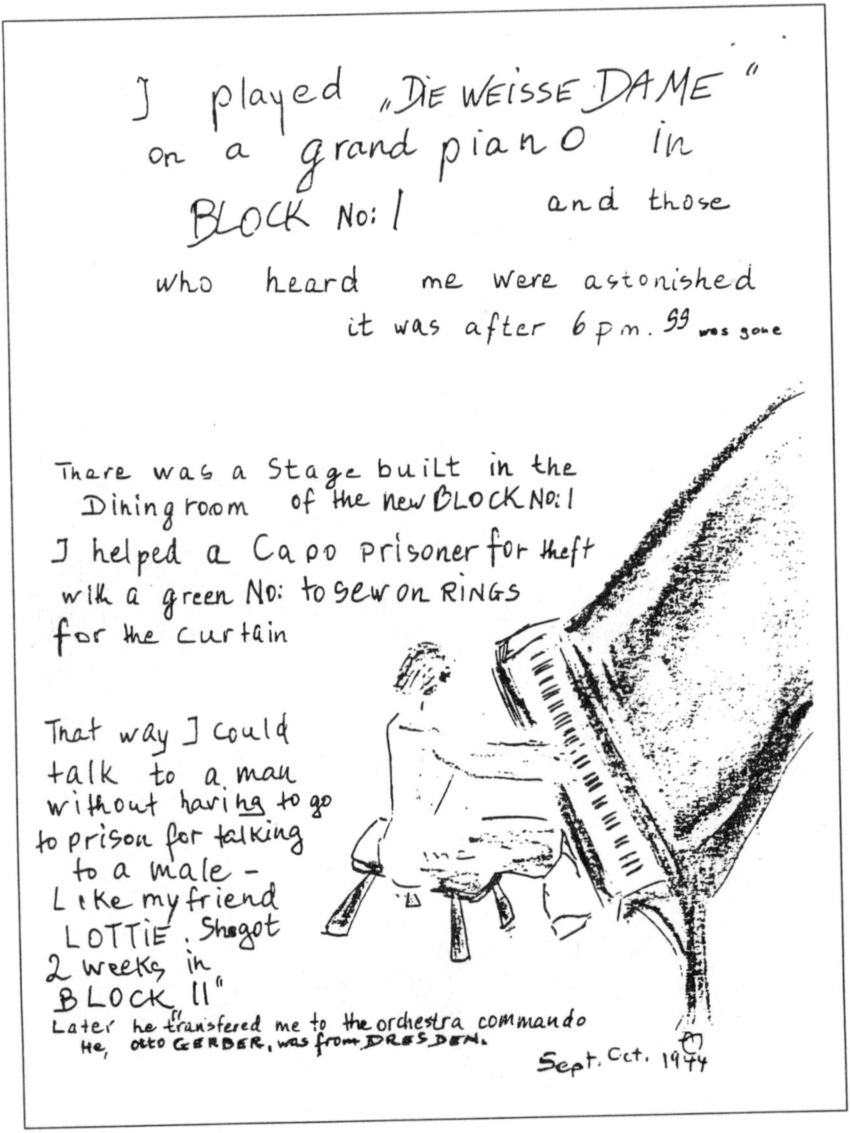

17. Playing "Die Weisse Dame"

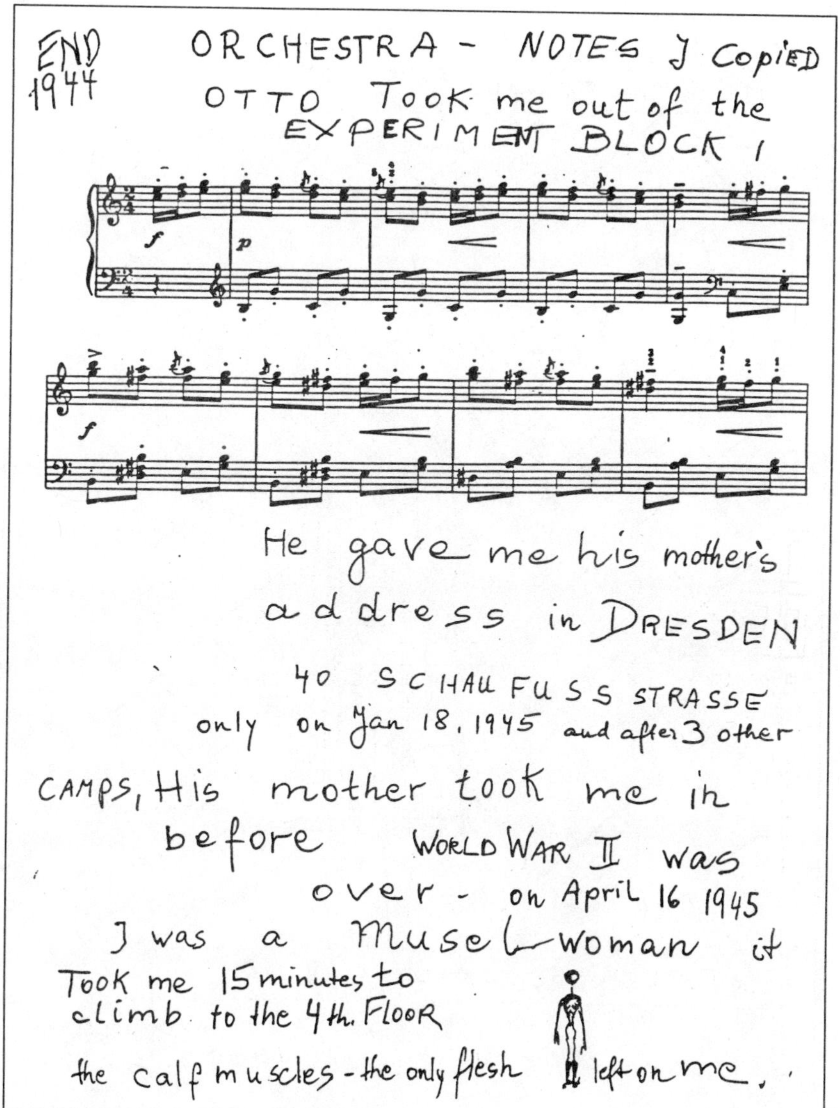
END 1944
ORCHESTRA - NOTES I COPIED
OTTO TOOK me out of the EXPERIMENT BLOCK I
He gave me his mother's address in DRESDEN
40 SCHAUFUSS STRASSE
only on Jan 18, 1945 and after 3 other CAMPS, His mother took me in before WORLD WAR II was over - on April 16 1945
I was a Musel-woman it Took me 15 minutes to climb to the 4th. FLOOR
the calf muscles - the only flesh left on me.

18. *Note Copying and Mrs. Gerber's Address*

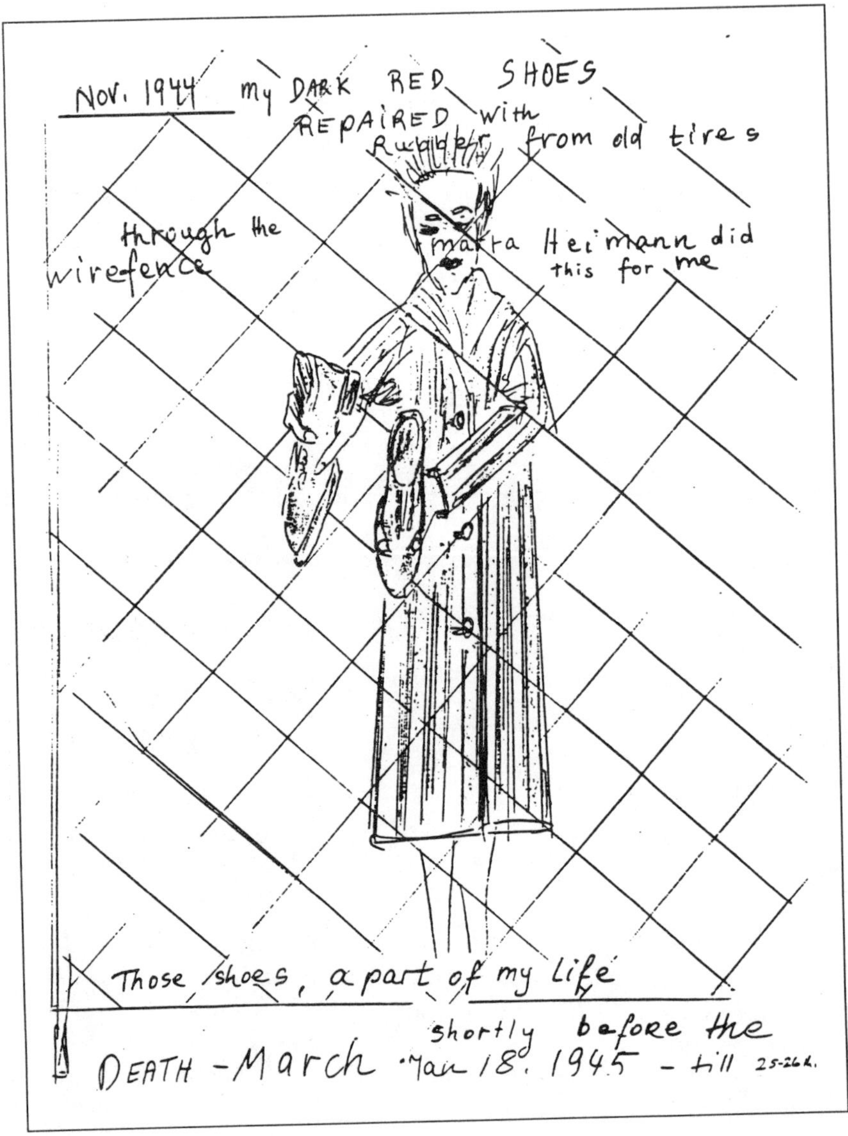

19. The Red Shoes

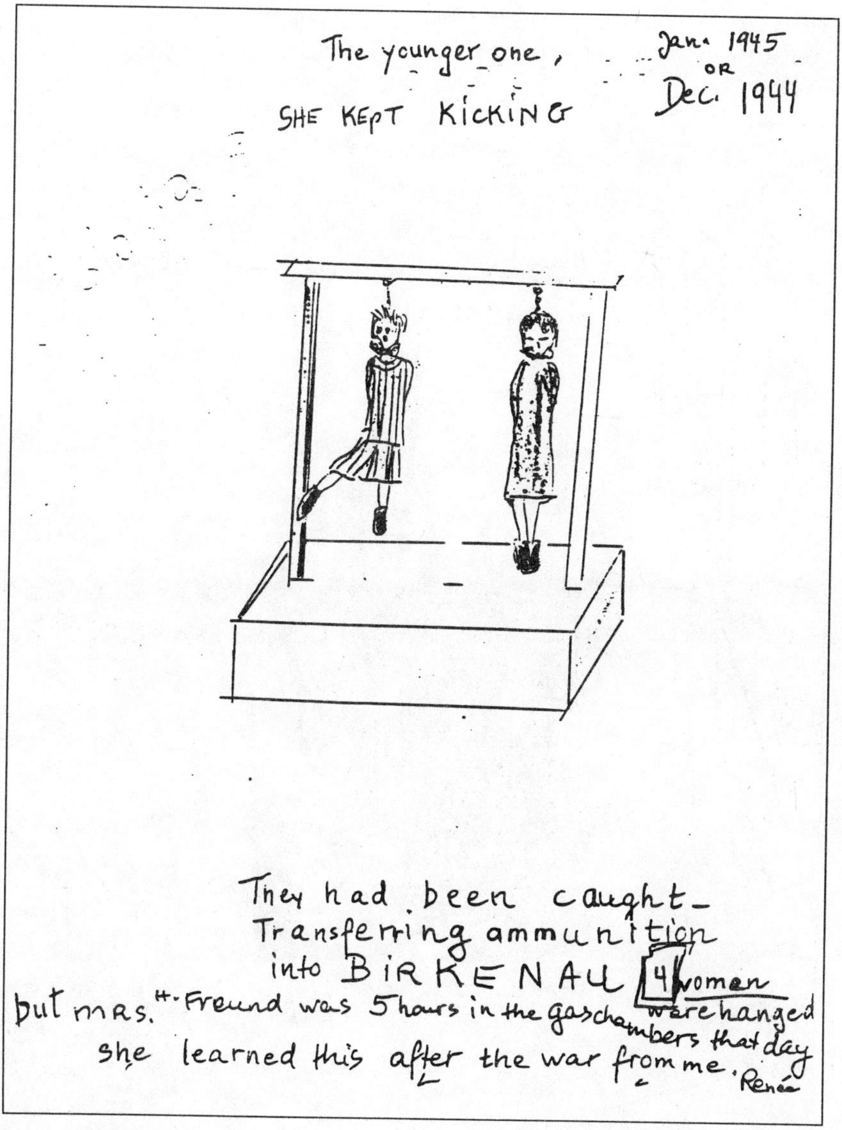

20. *The Hanging*

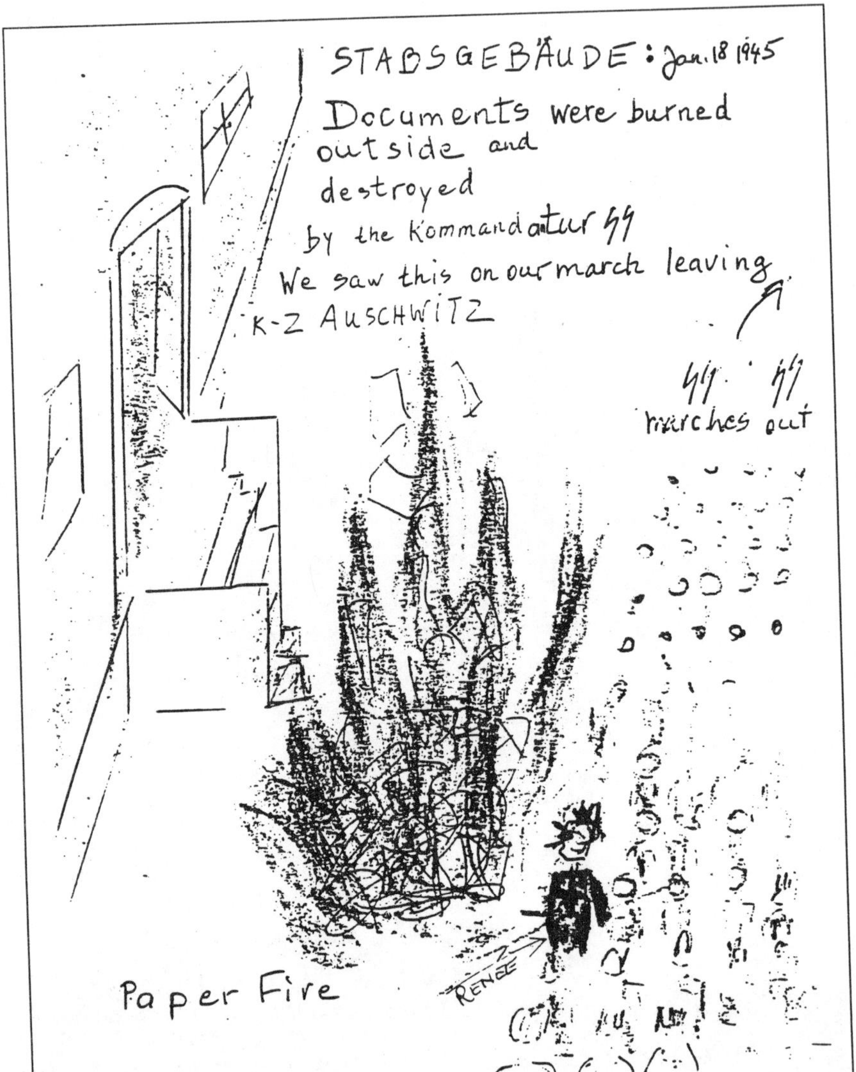

21. *Document Burning Before Evacuation*

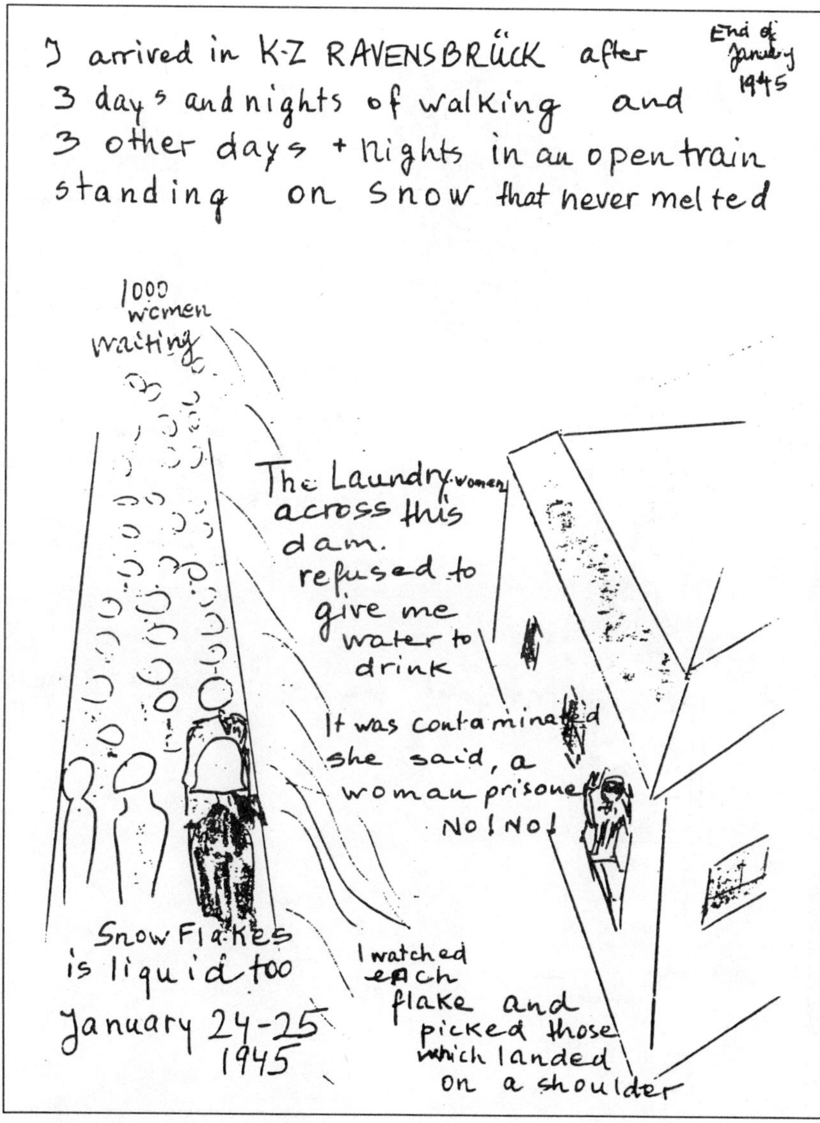
I arrived in K-Z RAVENSBRÜCK after
3 days and nights of walking and
3 other days + nights in an open train
standing on snow that never melted
End of January 1945
1000 women waiting
The Laundry women across this dam. refused to give me water to drink
It was contaminated she said, a woman prisoner NO! NO!
Snow Flakes is liquid too
January 24-25 1945
I watched each flake and picked those which landed on a shoulder

22. *Eating Snow in Ravensbrueck*

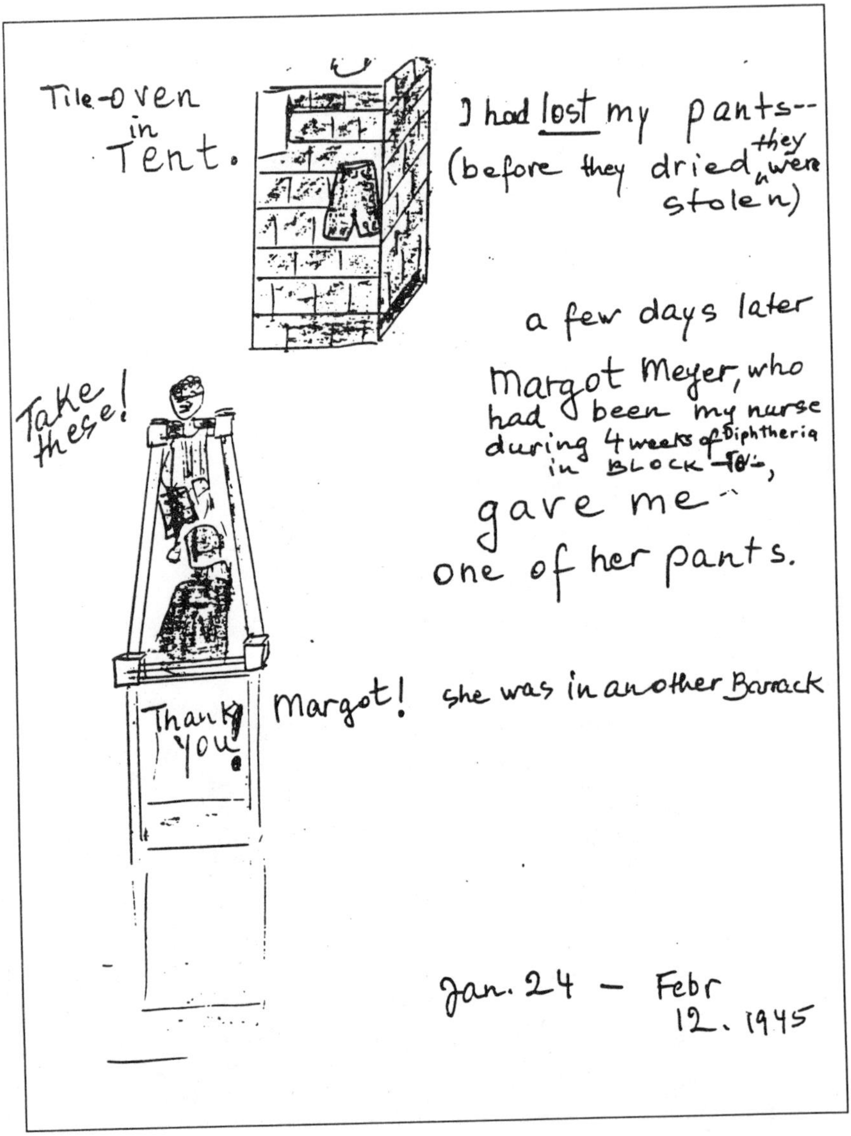

23. *Margot Gives Me a Pair of Panties*

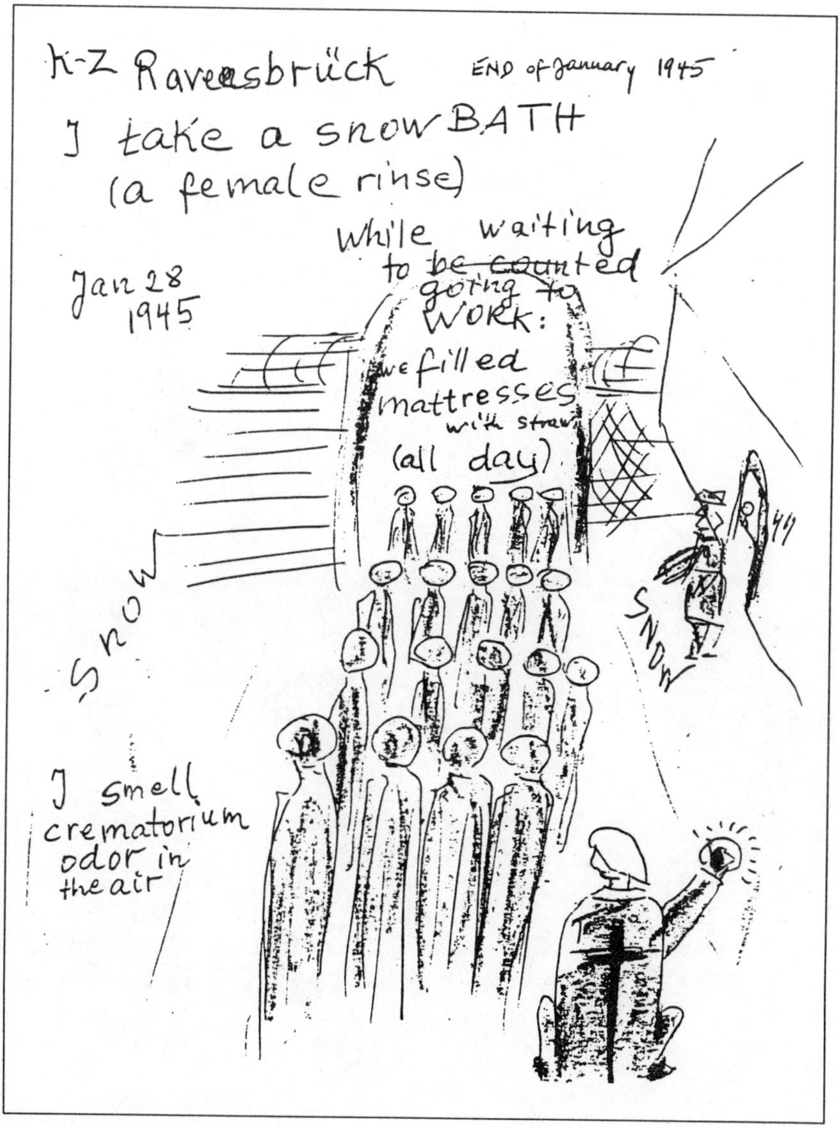
K-Z Ravensbrück
END of January 1945
I take a snow BATH
(a female rinse)
while waiting
to be counted
going to
WORK:
we filled
mattresses
with straw
(all day)
Jan 28
1945
SNOW
SNOW
I smell
crematorium
odor in
the air

24. *Snow Bath in Ravensbrueck*

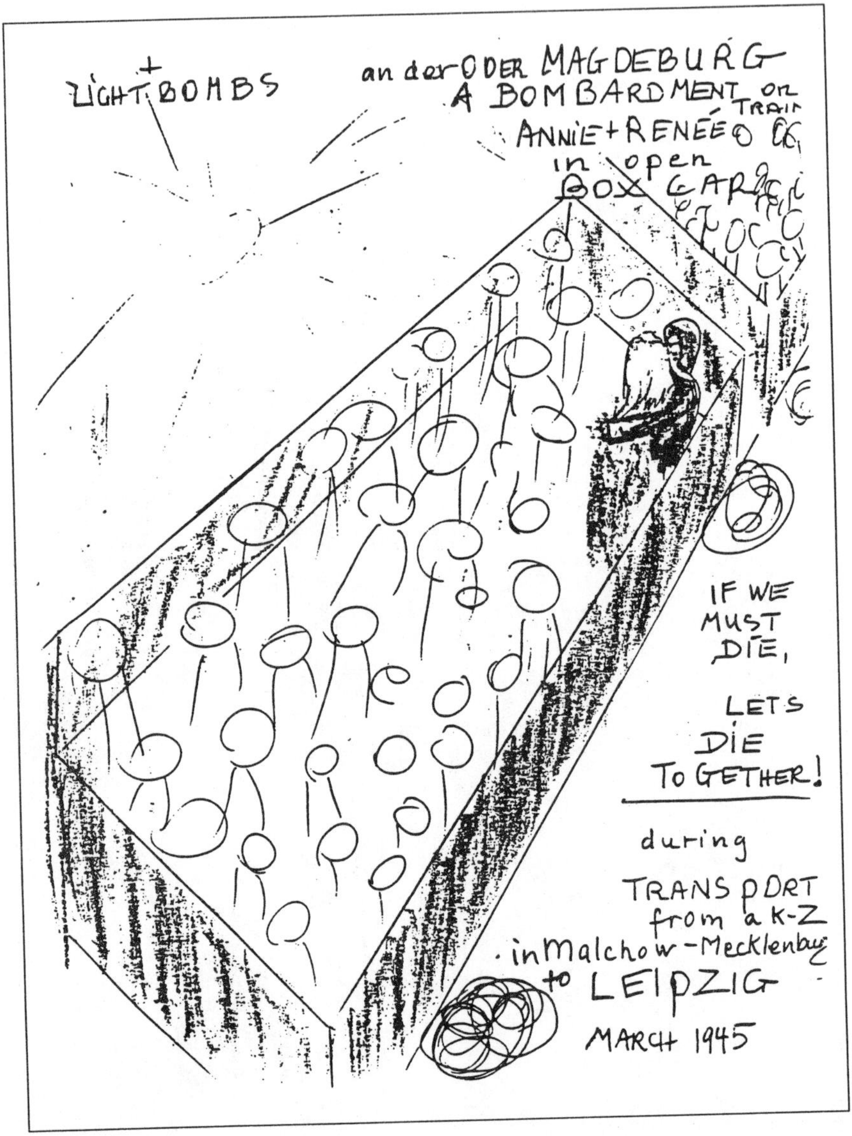
LIGHT + BOMBS
an der ODER MAGDEBURG
A BOMBARDMENT on TRAIN
ANNIE + RENÉE
in open BOX CAR
IF WE MUST DIE, LETS DIE TOGETHER!
during TRANSPORT from a K-Z
in Malchow-Mecklenburg
to LEIPZIG
MARCH 1945

25. *Air Raid on Train in Magdeburg*

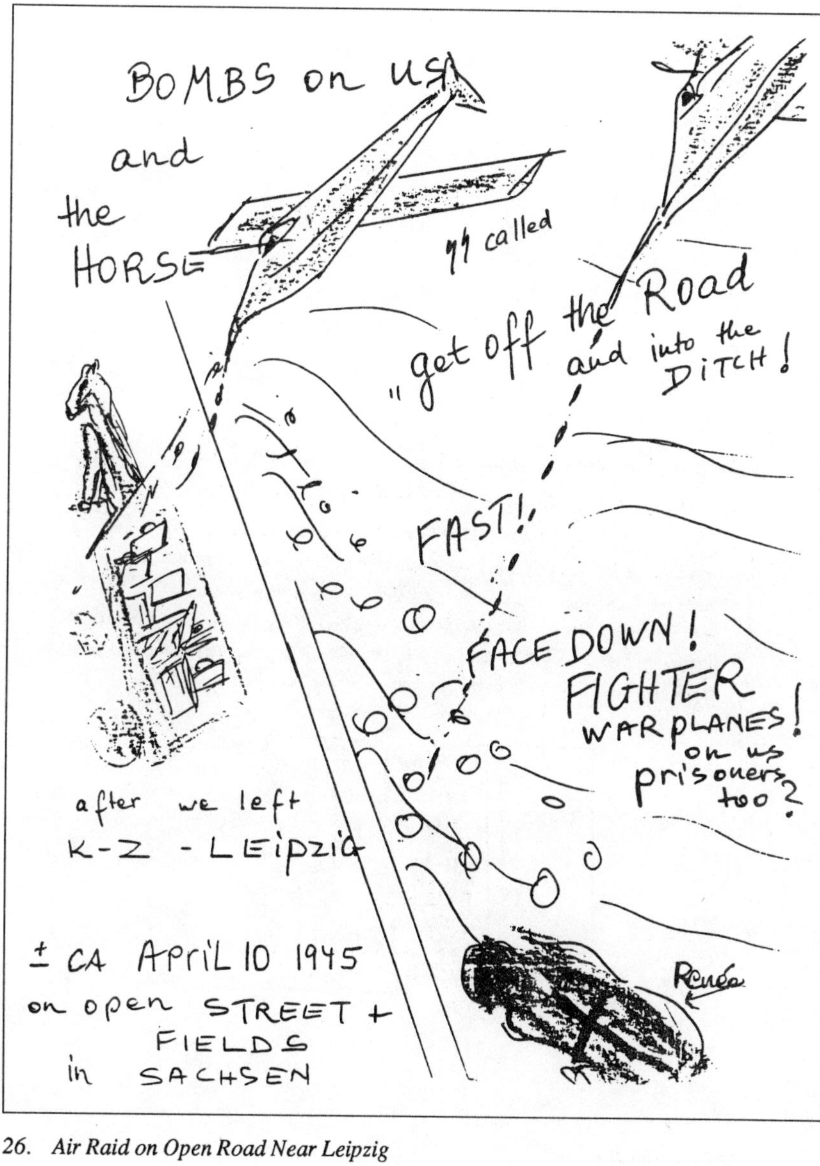

26. *Air Raid on Open Road Near Leipzig*

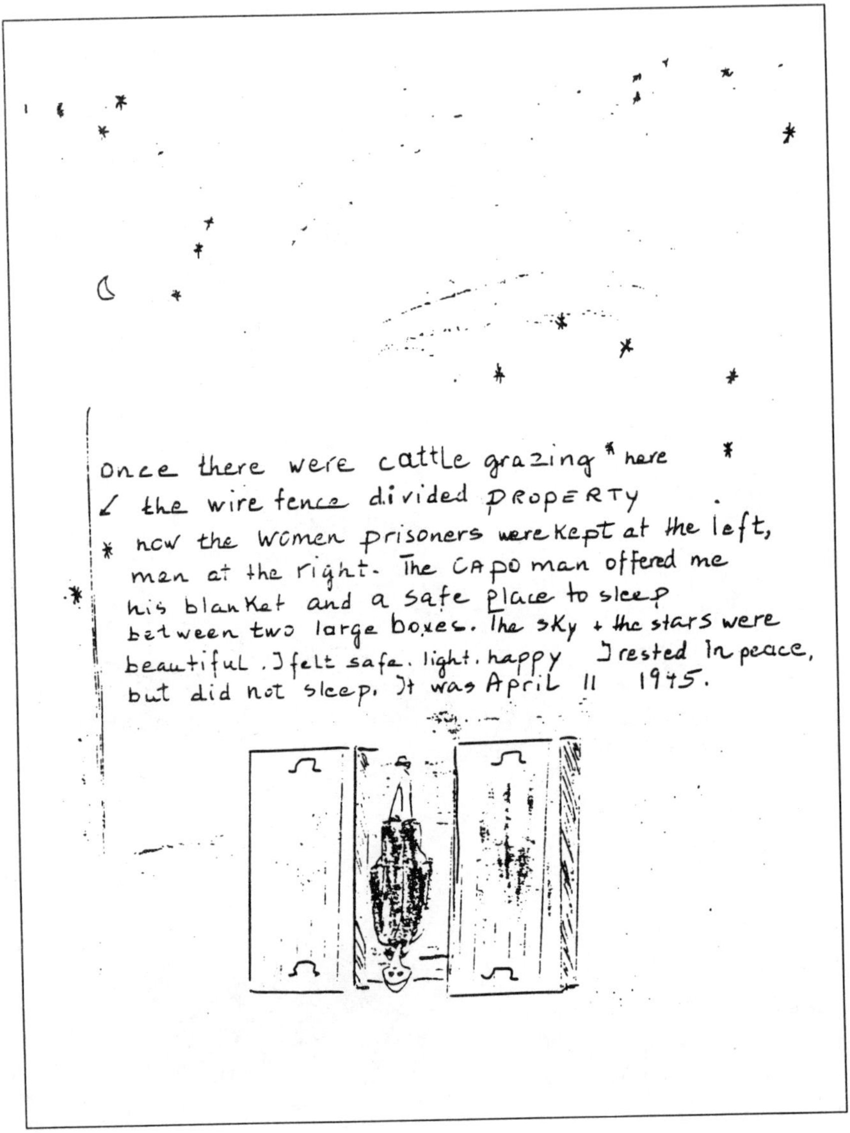

27. *Sleeping Under the Stars*

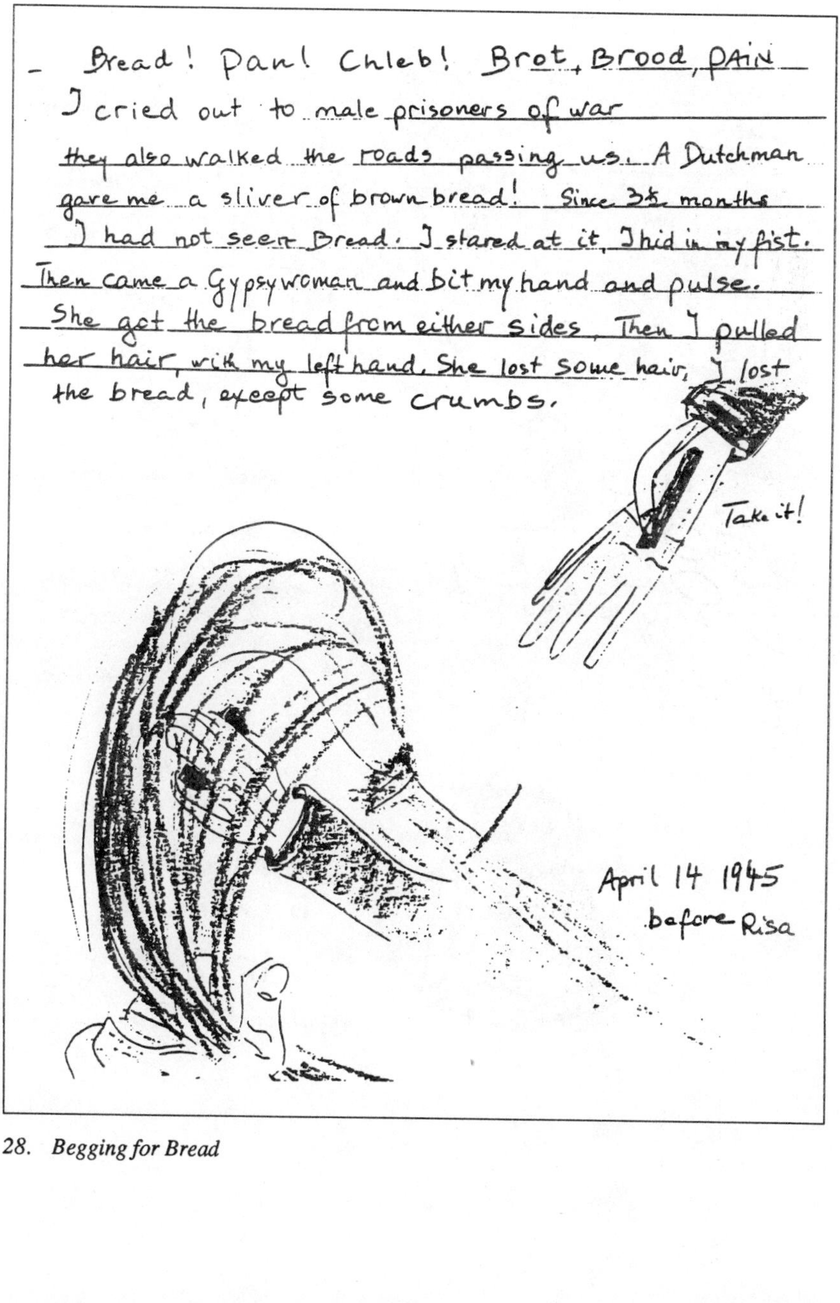

28. *Begging for Bread*

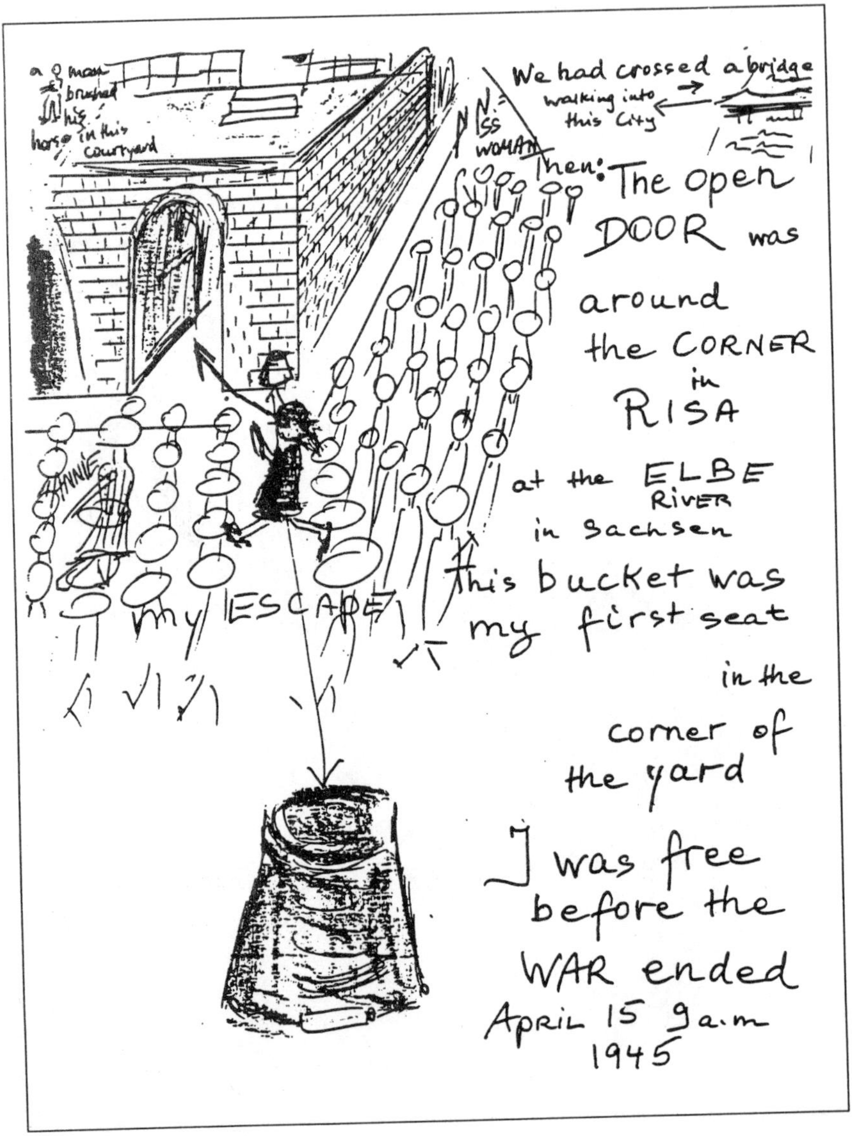
a man brushed his horse in this courtyard
We had crossed a bridge
walking into this City
SS WOMAN
Then: The open DOOR was around the CORNER in RISA at the ELBE RIVER in Sachsen
ANNIE
my ESCAPE
This bucket was my first seat in the corner of the yard
I was free before the WAR ended
April 15 9 a.m 1945

29. *Escape in Risa*

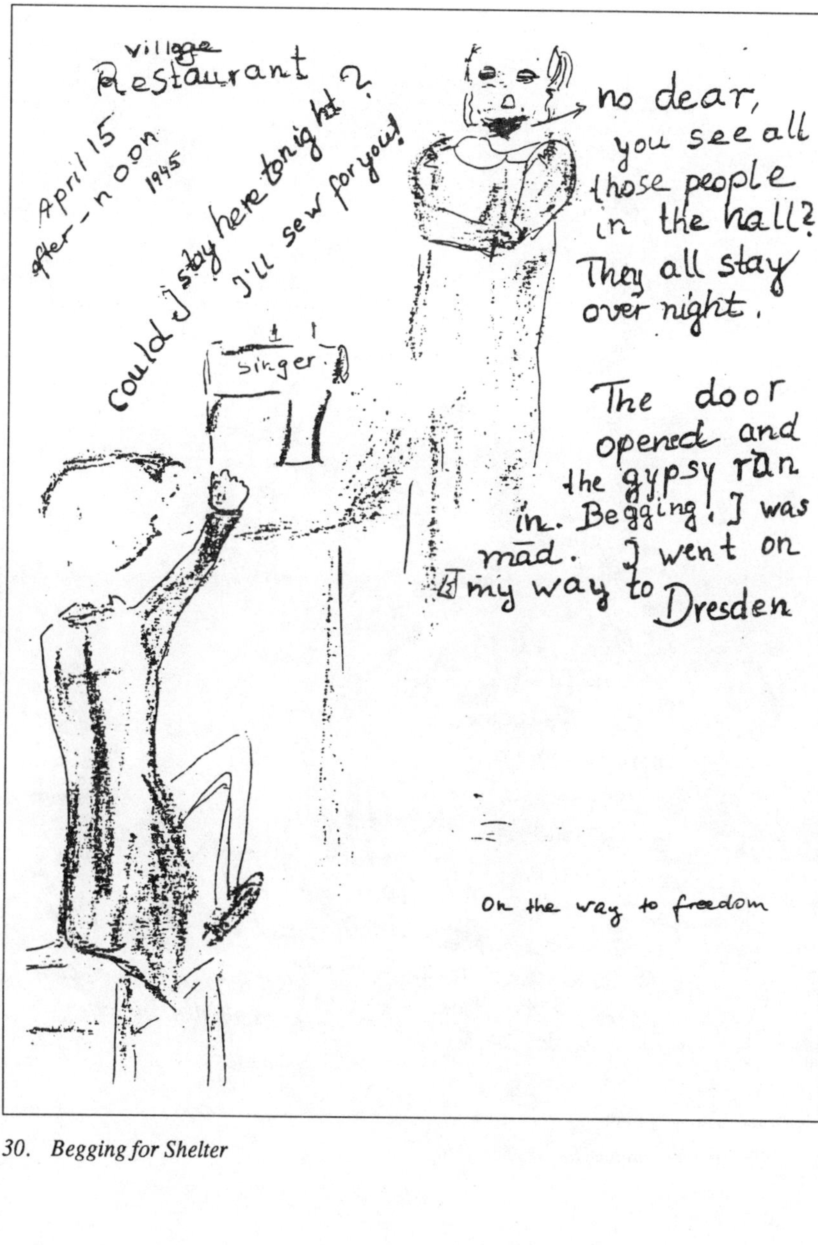

30. *Begging for Shelter*

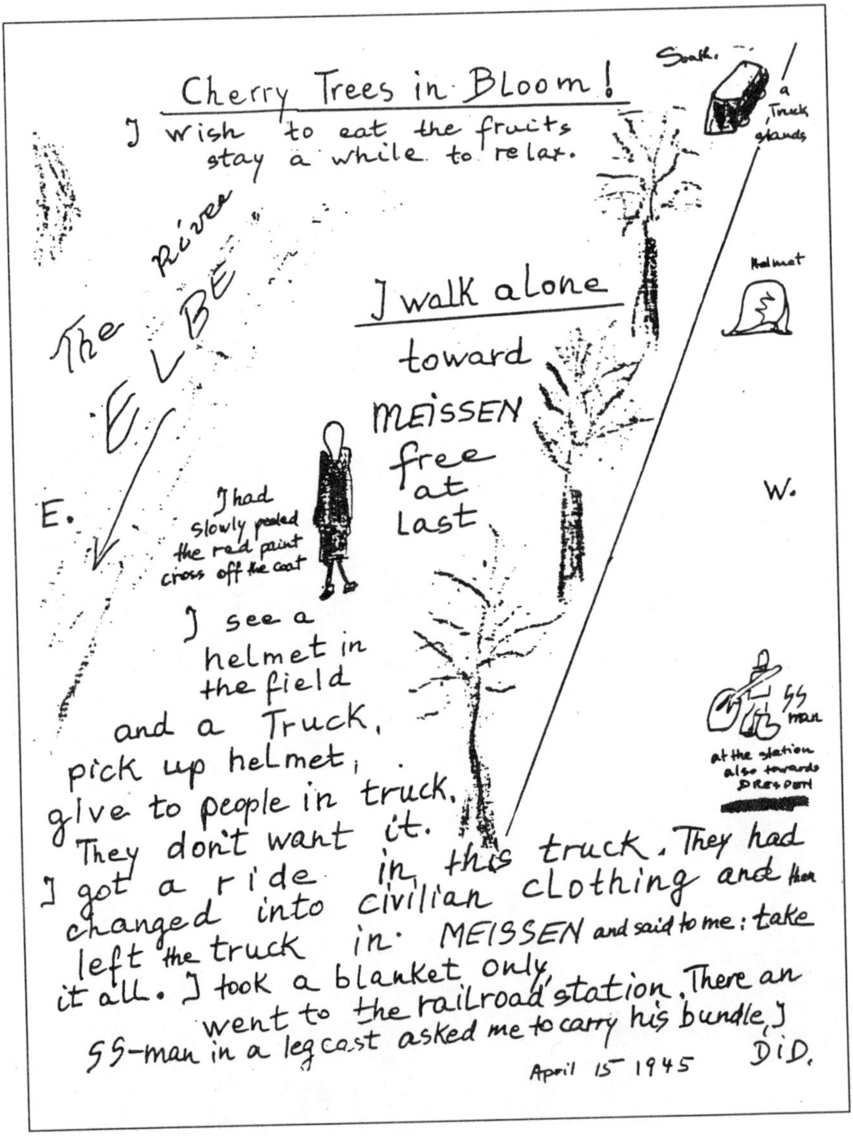

31. In Freedom on the Road to Meissen

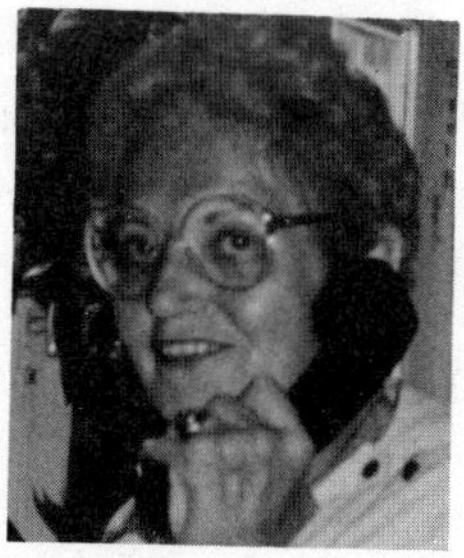

Trees Soetendorp
Amsterdam (Holland)

When I got married in March 1942, we had to move into the Jewish quarter of Amsterdam because outside there were no apartments available. We immediately tried to obtain a "Sperre," i.e., to be put on a list to delay deportation for plausible cause. For example, there existed a diamond—"Sperre," the Barneveld-"Sperre," etc. Most of these "Sperren" cost a lot of money and could be terminated from one day to the next. We were told we would be able to obtain a "Sperre" if we would have a Jewish business. Thus, my husband started a wholesale perfumery.

In May 1943, all "Sperren" were rescinded and everybody was informed to report for deportation. The only way to stay in Amsterdam was to go "underground." I was pregnant, but it would have been impossible for me to deliver a baby while in hiding so I had to undergo an abortion. Strangers accepted us into their house and were extremely helpful. They provided us with food rationing cards and other essentials for daily living. There was another man in the same hiding place. This person was not sufficiently cautious, went into the street and endangered everybody. The couple who gave us shelter was very angry and told all of us to get out. However, my husband and I were given to understand that our expulsion was only pro-forma and that we could stay—they had to act this way because of the other family. One of the other inhabitants of the house must have betrayed us. Very soon, two German officials and two Dutch SD men (Security

Service) came to pick us up. They rang the bell and knew exactly where the hiding place of the people with the "J" (Jewish) documents was, which was known only to the initiated. On September 7, 1943, we were transported to the "Hollandsche Schouwburg"—a theater that the Germans used as a collection-center for Jews who were to be "transported" (meaning to be sent on to camps). With 24 others, we were put into a military "attack-truck" and brought to this theater.

None of the 24 people I shared the truck with survived. I am the only one left.

We spent 10 days in that place. There was no possibility of escape. After the 10 days, we were sent to Westerbork, a transit camp for Auschwitz.

We were only in Westerbork until September 21, 1943, 4 days altogether. When we left Westerbork, people still believed that at their point of destination they would be re-united with their family members. In order to take along as much clothing as possible, we put on a multitude of apparel. I wore 4 pairs of panties, 4 shirts and a pair of slacks. For three days, we traveled in a cattle car, sitting on our rucksacks. There was a bucket so that men, women and children could relieve themselves. One of the cars was marked with an "S" for "Strafgefangene" (penal prisoners). In Westerbork, these persons had also been identified by an "S." But in the train every differential treatment stopped. The "S" sign had only served to scare people.

On September 23, 1943, we arrived in Auschwitz. The madness had started.

The men were separated from the women. The men's hair was shaved. My husband's hair had already been shorn in Westerbork because as "underground" man he belonged to the "Strafgefangenen" (penal group). We saw how the men marched in prison uniforms to their blocks. One woman of my group went mad at that sight.

Needless to write about the undressing, the bald-shaving of our heads, the disinfection and the tattooing of numbers; those events are already well known.

When I arrived in Block 10, I met an acquaintance who said, "How lucky you are; here you're only operated on!"

I was 22 years old at that time and quite healthy and my shocked reaction was, "I don't need an operation, I am as healthy as can be!"

She then explained that we were in a so-called "experimentation-block."

When my number was called the next day, I was terror-stricken, but it appeared that a mistake had been made with the number-tattoos. My number should have been 63229 and not 62229. With "deutscher Gruendlichkeit" the decision was made to correct the mistake.

In Block 10, a variety of experiments was performed on girls. There were very young 17 year old Greek girls who were being "treated" by a doctor Schumann. These girls' ovaries were x-rayed until terrible wounds appeared. The screams and cries of these girls petrified us; we lived on the floor above them. Most of the girls succumbed, but only after terrible suffering.

There were also operations on the uterus. Probably pieces of the neck of the uterus were cut away, after which the wound was sutured. This was done so "expertly" (sic), that during a follow-up examination the sutures had to be removed again. A Jewish physician—a prisoner, of course—was forced to take part in the experiments. He assured the women that it was all "harmless" and that they would be able to have children later.

Was he betrayed by somebody? It is certain that he suddenly disappeared and that he consequently was shot by the Germans. The last two arriving transports "belonged" to a professor Clauberg—a well-known German gynecologist.

It is also beyond my comprehension how a physician could sink so low as to what he did.

The first few months nothing happened. Then they asked who would volunteer for injections into the uterus for Clauberg. Those who did not volunteer were sent to Birkenau to be gassed. Of course, I "volunteered," similar to most of the other women. The injections were not administered by a physician but by a chemist, Dr. Goebel. His assistant was a hairdresser or a butcher. When he gave the shots, they were even more painful than usual.

We were, of course, not informed as to the meaning of the experiments, but our thoughts went to sterilization and, as some of us feared, a cancer-provoking process.

After "spritzen" (injections), we had terrible abdominal pains. It felt as if we were on fire. We got a high fever and we vomited. I underwent three of those "spritzen."

I avoided thinking of the possible consequences. As I did so often in Auschwitz, I "pulled up a curtain." Shutting out the cruel reality was for me the only way to try to survive. Besides being "spritzed" we were also, at regular intervals, called in to donate blood. (For whom...?)

There was also a period during which we received injections in breast and arms. Some of us got bad infections in the spots where the shots were given.

I did not show any effect. Was this a good sign, or maybe just the opposite, a bad one?

A few days after the "Clauberg-spritzen" we were x-rayed. The "doctors" were delighted with the results.

After all those years, I still panic when I have to enter an x-ray room.

After these experiments, they left us alone.

The younger women, to which I belonged, were put into a "Kraeuter-kommando." This meant that very early in the morning, and with very empty stomachs, we had to search for herbs in the area surrounding the camp,i.e., black-berry-leaves.

We returned to our Block around 3 or 3:30 in the afternoon.

The block elder, secretary, assistant of Professor Clauberg and the other cleaning and nursing personnel were all Jewesses, mostly Slovakian, Polish and Greek women. Unfortunately, these Jewish girls also hit us inmates, sometimes they were worse than the Germans. I once received a horrible beating because I had spilled a drop of water, another time I was hit so violently that my eyeglasses broke, because my bed was not straight enough.

And so we plodded on until the 18th of January 1945, at which date Auschwitz was evacuated. It was then that we began our so-called "death march."

We stayed together as much as we could. We, that is ten Dutch women. I believe that the ten of us managed to survive simply because we were so young.

Many around us succumbed.

On April 26, 1945, we were liberated near Naunhof, close to Leipzig. We had left behind Ravensbrueck, Malchow, Taucha and a seventeen day "walk."

For me, the result of the experiments is that I remained childless.

I think sometimes, "Thanks to Block 10, I'm still alive," but the experience has changed my life thoroughly. My husband was murdered in Auschwitz.

In 1949, I remarried, out of loneliness. When, during an argument, my 2nd husband blurted out, "Why did I marry you anyway, you can't even have children," I left. I divorced him and never married again; I was not taking a chance of hearing those words again!

For a little over 26 years I have lived with a woman-friend who, lucky for me, also had terrible camp experiences.

After the remark made by my second husband and when rheumatism struck me, I needed professional—psychological—help to keep going.

❖

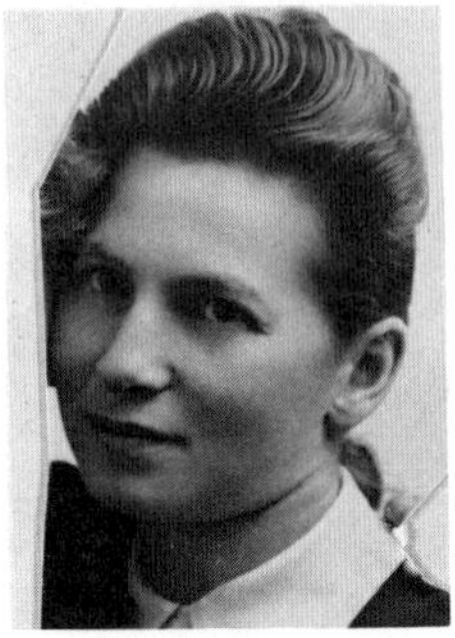

Eva Golgevit
Paris (France)

I was born on June 16, 1912 in Lodz, Poland. In 1933, I left Poland with my parents and settled in Belgium. I lived in Paris with my husband from 1936. In 1937 our son was born, and in 1939 my husband voluntarily entered the French Army for the duration of the war. He was taken prisoner in 1940. I remained alone with my son. In July 1942, the big razzia at the Velodrome d'Hiver occurred. I sent my son to French friends in the countryside, left my house and started to work for the Resistance.

On July 3, 1943 I was arrested and deported from Drancy on July 31, 1943 in a sealed cattle car. I arrived in Auschwitz on August 2, with a transport of one thousand prisoners. During the selection process, I was chosen with 55 other women for Block 10, the experimental block in Auschwitz. We alighted from the train in a sinister dawn which foreshadowed death that always followed us and has accompanied us every minute of our lives.

The memory is forever present in my mind: the shaved hair, the beatings, the screaming, the dirty and lice infested rags replacing our clothes, the threats, the infernal apocalyptic atmosphere, this inhuman universe into which I had been thrust. Everything gave the impression of having fallen into a demented world.

At first we went to the bath; the famous "Sauna," the purgatory before entering Block 10.

I looked at my old friends from Paris whom I knew quite well. They were transformed, unrecognizable. Their hair was shaved to the skin and some of them vaguely resembled their sons.

I remember the tattooing process. "I felt as if my heart was being tattooed," our Polish friend said. That was the same for all the women.

Going up to the Polish prisoner whose duty it was to tattoo us, I said furiously and indignantly, "They are raising henchmen!" Surprised, I heard his answer in a barely audible voice: "For themselves."

And then I was pushed into Block 10, the famous block of the so-called "medical" experiments.

On one side of Block 10 was the Bunker, where patriots were executed after having been atrociously tortured, on the other side was the "Krankenbau," the men's hospital from where the sick were being sent to the crematorium.

In Block 10, I found women with extinguished eyes, with dumb and desperate expressions, as if they were afraid to utter a single word, as if they had not encountered "normal" people for a very long time.

In whispers they, nevertheless, tried to make us understand where we were.

And, suddenly I had the feeling of having fallen into a worse trap than the one of my arrest in Paris when the two policemen grasped me with their paws while uttering with a sarcastic smile, "C'est fini." ("It's all over.")

At that moment, I had understood that I had to gather all my strength in order to endure the interrogation, in order not to answer the questions: "Who are your contacts (who is in command)? How do you decipher the code? From where did you obtain your I.D.'s which are forged so well? Where is your son? ..."

We had been briefed in advance that torture was always used during the interrogation of arrested resistance fighters. And all our thoughts revolved exclusively around our willpower to withstand the torture and to preserve our human dignity.

But the trap of Block 10 appeared to me to be far more frightening. Here, I told myself, it is not only death that is lying in wait, but also the danger of being used as a guinea pig by the Nazi doctors until I became similar to those women in Block 10.

I have to admit that on that evening in Block 10, behind the thick wooden boards barricading the windows, I had very little hope of returning one day a free person.

But there were also other moments. Once, my eye caught a ray of sun through the barricades which penetrated my heart and filled me with sadness. I took a vow: On the spot where my infamous Block 10 was situated, a monument would be erected for all the martyrs. One day, free people from all over the world would come and prostrate themselves on this sacred soil. Free people—because they would be free (I did not doubt this for an instant)—would visit this camp by the thousands together with their children and their loved ones and would pay homage to the martyrs and swear never to forget.

My ardent and fervent vow was fired by an immense hatred for the henchmen, and an immense love for those who suffered. In my mind, I saw the accomplishment of this dream. But, would I see it realized? Impossible, impossible to believe.[8]

Then there were the "girls," my comrades of the resistance group with whom I had been connected in Paris.

Not all, but the majority, were communists.

Thanks to them, the spark of hope was not extinguished. Thanks to them, the small flame of energy was rekindled in me.

How did Fanny, so full of vitality, perhaps with Irene's help (she had arrived with an earlier transport) find a needle and some thread? Fanny was sewing a gown out of some rags for me and also a shawl. With her sweet smile, she told me,

"I know you cannot sew, so please sing something."

Good hearted Guittele almost forced me to take a morsel of bread from her meager ration.

Soon, we learned that doctor Slavka[9] had discovered, in the men's camp, an old comrade in arms from the days when she had fought in Spain. Clandestine activities were organized, comprising Jews as well as non-Jews.

All of this, of course, was strictly secret.

We breathed more easily and gentle Gina whispered to me, "You will see, Eva, I have the feeling that we shall be liberated."

The first song which Gina, Regina and I sang stupefied the hundreds of Jewish women, deported from many different European countries. They admired us for the solidarity which we manifested toward each other and, later, for the way in which we organized help for the sick women whom the Nazi Clauberg had already "treated."[10]

They called our group, "The French Colony," and many times they asked us, "French Colony, please sing some songs."

Thus, during the months we spent together in this Block, we occupied ourselves intellectually each free moment.

We did our best to keep up the morale of those women doomed to despair. Together with some comrades, we tried to evade the experiments with the assistance of a woman prisoner physician and a young woman from Greece.

When we could not elude the experiments any longer, and in retaliation for doing so, we were transferred to Birkenau in June 1944, to Block 27 in the "Aussenkommando" (heavy outside work).[11]

This was not a rare occurrence; as if carried by a raging sea, prisoners were often transferred from one camp to another. I stayed a few days at a block for the sick and, afterward, was sent, together with a friend of mine, to Rajsko where I met Marie-Elisa Cohen.

On January 18, 1945, the evacuation of Auschwitz started. During the so-called "death march," I dragged myself, with my last strength in the icy wind which whipped us, across the snow-covered fields with my group of friends. I tried not to distance myself so that the SS would not kill me and leave me at the road-side, the way they did many others.

They took us as protection, and hoped to return to the center of Germany, thus avoiding the punishment which was hanging over their heads.

A rumor spread that warmed our frozen joints; the SS had escaped in panic from Auschwitz.

This would mean that the camps had not been destroyed.

This would mean that our comrades who had remained; Cyporka, Regine, Rose, Gina, Mira, Macha, Annette and the others whose fate had so worried us were still alive.

It was really the case.

The Red Army liberated the camp on January 27, 1945.

I, myself, had to drag myself along for a long time, death at my side, until May 1, 1945, when I also was liberated.

I still remember our mixed feelings; a feeling of relief and joy at the idea that Hitlerism, the murderers of our people and of many other people, had been forced to their knees and vanquished!

But, also a feeling of sadness because who among us had not lost their dearest during the years of death and destruction?

I was lucky to be reunited with my son and my husband after the war. In 1952, we had another son. Jean, the first born, is married and has three children.

My husband and I take care of our health and continue to be active in organizations such as Former Fighters, and former Concentration Camp Prisoners, Jewish and non-Jewish.

After liberation, we were sure that a new era of peace had started and that all traces of Fascism had been extinguished.

Who could imagine then that forty years later people would try to erase the Nazi crimes and would organize campaigns, not against the Nazi henchmen, but against their victims, the resistance fighters.

Who could imagine that we were hearing once again, just as before the Second World War, the hateful slogans of anti-communism which the bloodthirsty dictators have used since time immemorial.

Who could expect that even in France we would re-encounter the same demagogues, politicians like Le Pen, and that there would be people who would accord him the democratic seal.

It is our duty as survivors to incessantly keep alive the memory of those who forget. And our testimony should be heard as long as there are witnesses in the hope that future generations will learn a lesson from it.

We have to tell about Auschwitz in order to block the road to nostalgic memories about Nazism.

❖

Part Two

RAJSKO

RAJSKO

After the Polish inhabitants of Rajsko had been deported, the camp authorities established an agricultural satellite camp in the village. Particular attention was paid to the possibility of cultivating the kok-saghyz plant brought there from the conquered Ukraine, which in its roots contained a caoutchouc-like substance, an essential ingredient for the artificial rubber produced at the I. G. Farben factory in Monowitz.

In the second half of 1942, women prisoners were employed there. Under the guidance of Russian and German scientists they were busy growing one variety of this plant, among many, which would contain the highest percentage of the latex substance.

The women prisoners were employed in the work details of Pflanzenzucht (plant cultivation) and Gaertnerei (horticulture). The skilled work of the prisoners was to further widely designed economic plans incorporated within the Four Year Plan (Vierjahresplan).

The director of the agriculture enterprise at Rajsko was SS-Obersturmbannfuehrer Dr. Joachim Caesar.

Kommando Gaertnerei (Horticulture)

This work detail consisted of women prisoners mainly comprised of Polish, Russian and Yugoslavian political inmates. They sowed and cultivated different types of vegetables, such as cucumbers, tomatoes, onions, peas, garlic, etc., for the SS-kitchen as well as for the Wehrmacht (armed forces). The women also raised flowers, which were shipped to Germany.

Kommando Pflanzenzucht (Plant Cultivation)

The major purpose of this work detail was to grow, study and improve taraxacum kok-saghyz, a plant that contained a rubber substance in its root.

The first women prisoners, a group of Polish political prisoners, all of them biologists, arrived in May 1942. Gradually, the work squad expanded and then it was moved to its permanent quarters in June 1943...some newly-erected barracks close to the experimental station in Rajsko...it numbered about 150 women.

The prisoners were divided into six working groups: the greenhouse, experimental fields, chemical, botanical and microbiological laboratories, photography, drawing and sewing.

In the greenhouse, seeds were planted and plants tended until transplantation to the field, which took place in May. The task of the experimental fields group was to transplant the plants and nurse them until the formation of roots. Jozefa Kiwalowa, Zofie Abramowiczowa and Riwa Krieglowa worked here. The director of the chemical laboratory was Ruth Weimann (later the wife of SS-Obersturmbannfuehrer Caesar), but the French prisoner Dr. Marie-Elisa Cohen-Nordmann, from the Sorbonne, was responsible for the work...soil analysis, pH measurements, adjusting of fertilizer, chloroform extraction of latex by different methods, estimation of latex percentages, as well as the study of the microbiological makeup of cellulose in the latex-containing root. The botanical laboratory was directed by SS-man Dr. Boehme and Dr. Claudette Kennedy-Bloch, a French prisoner also from the Sorbonne, was in charge of this group to which belonged Simone Floersheim, Jacqueline Odru and Hélène Parreaux. They did straining and cross-sectioning of different parts for detailed study. Inge Schlesinger-Kochmann and Wanda Jakubowska worked in the photo laboratory, documenting the kok-saghyz story, and Wanda Ladniewska-Blankenheim and Eva Gabanyi did the drawings. The sewing detail made covers for the plants.

All the experiments were carried out by women prisoners. Sabotage was rampant. Seeds were burned, careful numbering was disregarded and sometimes plants were watered with harmful chemicals.

❖

CHAPTER FOUR
Laboratory Research

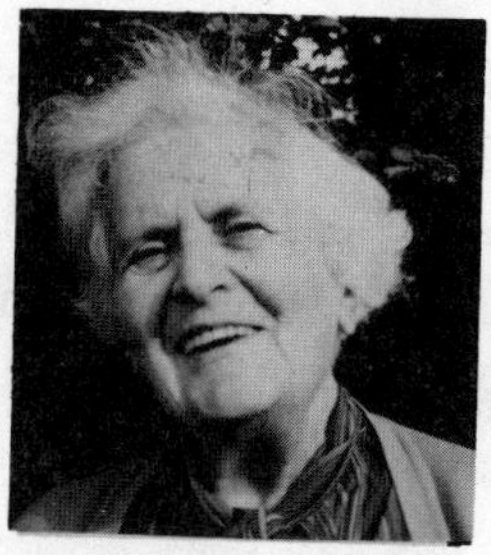

Dr. Claudette Kennedy (widowed Bloch, née Raphael)
Oxford (England)

My name is Claudette Kennedy (née Raphael).[1] I was born in 1910, at Bourg-la-Reine near Paris, where I grew up and lived until 1937. I was educated in a little school where many pupils like myself were daughters of school teachers. After my Baccalaureate I went to the Sorbonne, where I studied biology; in 1934 I was Licenciee and in 1938 got my Doctorat-es-Sciences.

In 1938 I married Pierre Bloch, ex-Polytechnician and engineer in charge of the bridges and traffic on the Seine between Rouen and Paris. When the war broke out he was called up by the army and I went to stay with friends in Caen, where our son, Maurice, was born in October 1939. In November I went to Bordeaux, where I did some scientific war work with Laure Gatet (later deported to Auschwitz for activity in the Resistance). In June 1940, when the French army was routed, Pierre and his men arrived in Auch, where I joined him with my baby after a grueling journey. Pierre still had a job in the army, but in September he was summoned imperatively to Paris in order to restore the barge traffic on the Seine, which was necessary for the provisioning of Paris, since so many roads and bridges had been destroyed. Pierre thought it his duty to obey for the sake of the Parisians. In November, like all Jews occupying public positions, he was dismissed.

In the early hours of the morning of the 12th of December 1940, two German soldiers came to the flat to arrest him. He was among the first batch of French-born Jews to be taken. Three hundred men were arrested that morning. Pierre was selected for having refused to indicate the location of the explosives concealed in the bridges. He was taken to Compiegne and deported to Auschwitz on the 27th of March 1942.

I tried to carry on without any news of him, supported by my parents, my mother-in-law and my baby, now two years old. But in May, I got so impatient that I decided, naively, to go and try to find out where my husband was. (Later I learned that in fact he had died on the 8th of April 1942, having been left outdoors in the snow because he was too weak to work.) I went to the German Kommandantur in Paris whence they sent me to Gestapo headquarters on Avenue Foch. There I was taken before Captain Danecker, who was then in charge of dealing with the Jews of Paris.[2] He received us by shouting insults, which I could not understand, and the kind man who had accompanied me as an interpreter had great difficulty in getting out free. I was taken to a small adjacent room where I sat for hours. Toward evening two civilians came to fetch me and take me to the nearest civil police station where I spent the night, and the next morning in the custodial cells beneath the Palais de Justice. There I met some friends: in particular, Marie-Elisa Nordmann, whom I was to meet again in Auschwitz, and France Bloch, who was decapitated in Germany. My next destination was the Detention Center established in the barracks known as "Les Tourelles."

Life was relatively comfortable there, but after six weeks we were ordered out, without any warning, to stand in the yard. To my horror, I saw Danecker arriving. He proceeded to conduct a roll call and, without looking at us, selected seventy under-forties and sent us to a big hall in another building. We spent two nights there without any toilet facilities or beds. We received the food in the first parcels that had been sent to us, but we were not allowed to see our parents when they came on the visiting day, and they had to go home again with full hands and heavy hearts.

At dawn on the morning of the 22nd of June, we were ordered out into the yard where buses were waiting for us. We started to sing, and the prisoners who were left behind joined in from behind the closed windows which they were forbidden to open. We were driven to Le Bourget Station, where some men prisoners were standing. Seventy women did not merit a train and the men were to make up the required number. German soldiers now took us over from the French police. They pushed us into the cattle cars in which we were to spend three days and three nights. We were packed in with hardly room to lie down, and a single bucket. While we were still within France we managed to throw out bits of paper with a few words and our addresses. Some of these messages reached their destination, thanks to the French railwaymen who gathered them up and posted them. We stopped at a station in Germany, where the doors were slid open and we could see, on another platform, some German Red Cross women in grey uniforms waiting with provisions for a train of German soldiers. We were desperately thirsty and shouted in various languages, "Water, please!" They turned their heads away.

When we finally arrived at Auschwitz, they slid the door open and soldiers with dogs drove us out of the cars, forcing us to leave all our luggage including our handbags. There was a small truck for those who absolutely could not walk, but some women who were working above the railway line shouted "Walk! At any cost, walk!" We did not understand why, but the small truck transported our unfortunate friends to the small gas chamber already existing at that time.

We were made to form up in ranks of five, surrounded by soldiers with guns and dogs. After a short walk, we passed through the gate of the camp, past stone buildings which we learned later were the offices, and finally stopped in front of some long trestle tables manned by prisoners. They told us we had to undress completely and give them all personal possessions, such as watches, necklaces and even our wedding rings. As clothes, we were given the uniforms of Russian soldiers who had perished from disease and hard labor in Birkenau before our arrival, but we were not yet allowed to put them on. There we were, standing naked in the open air with the thin uniforms over our arms, completely stupefied.

We now had to wait like that a while; the Camp Commandant, Hoess, had ordered the proceedings to stop. He wanted to enjoy the sight of the first French women to enter his camp. He and his retinue especially enjoyed the spectacle of red-painted toenails. We were then entirely shaved, given a succession of hot and cold showers and then, hardly dry, we put our "new" clothes on. When we looked at our companions we could not recognize each other! We were then each given a scrap of material with a number…my number was 7963, subsequently tattooed on my arm. This was to be our only identity from then on. How to fix the label on our tunics, which was compulsory, seemed an insoluble problem. Somehow it was solved…otherwise I would not be here to tell the tale…but I don't remember how.

We were shown the barracks and the bunks on which we were to sleep, but we were not allowed to stay there. The rest of the day was spent carrying bundles of laundry. Every step required an incredible effort and some of us collapsed. Later (how much later? it seemed an eternity) all the outside "Kommandos" (labor squads) came in and we began to hear about the sort of place we were in. There were no French speakers among our new comrades but several of us could understand Slovak and they translated for us; we could not believe them. Suddenly, everybody and everything came to a standstill, after the repeated words, "C'est l'appel"…at least that is what we understood. In fact, what they shouted was "Zaehlappell." The whole mass of prisoners had to stand, in ranks and motionless, in order to be counted. This took another eternity during which many fainted but had to be left where they lay in order not to disturb the counting.

When at last we were dismissed there was a rush toward the barracks. The bunks which had been so tantalizing at our arrival were now to be fought for. There was no hope of getting one for oneself; they had to be shared. After having received, in another struggle, some bread and some hot liquid they called tea, we dropped onto our half-bunks and fell asleep. Not for long...it was still dark when there resounded the shout "Aufstehen!" It was easy enough to understand what they meant, and if you didn't obey fast enough, a lash from a leather belt supplemented the order. After some of the same hot liquid as the night before had been swallowed, we were pushed out of the barrack and found ourselves carried along by the crowd hurrying to line up for another Appell. This one didn't last very long; soon we were dismissed and turmoil set in again. The women were running in all directions and we didn't know what to do. Groups were forming, each around one or two guards and their dogs. Each group was assigned to a particular job. This scramble was in fact a race for a light job known to be the responsibility of such or such "Aufseherin" (SS woman guard); so the main thing was to reach her before she had made up the number of workers allotted to her. Of course we newcomers did not know about this and the result was we ended up in a group whose job was especially onerous.

The Aufseherin organized her group into ranks of five, and we started to walk toward the gate. There stood a bunch of SS, watching us moving painfully, dragging our wooden clogs and bending our shaven heads, which did not feel as if they belonged to us. Shortly after the gate was passed, a new order pierced our ears..."Shoes off!" And now we advanced barefoot on the dusty, stony road. Further on we passed close to a house and in the garden a woman was hanging out diapers. Such a homely action seemed extraordinary in this nightmarish world; surely a real woman could not bear the sight of these zombie-like women treated so cruelly. I expected her to phone the police and alert them! She was the wife of one of the guards; she paid no attention to us.

When we arrived at our destination we found ourselves on derelict ground. Our job was to level it. We were given picks and shovels, and like most of the newcomers I received a pick-axe. I did not know how to use it and could hardly lift it; a blow with the butt of a gun taught me how. We had only one break, to eat some soup brought from the main camp. By that time the sun was high and our shaven heads felt as if they were burning. At the end of the day (what time? One never knows the time in a concentration camp; anyway, it was still hot), we went back to the camp and had to stand for the Appell with more and more women collapsing. In the distance I saw a prisoner called out of the ranks by the

Oberaufseherin, Mandel, for what reason I don't know. Mandel then set her dog on the woman, commanding it to bite her and then to let go. The woman fainted and fell to the ground. Mandel proceeded to slap her face hard to bring her round and ordered her back to her place. I was aghast.

Once dismissed we managed to summon up enough energy to seek out our friends with whom we had arrived, and together we resolved to meet every day thereafter. The ensuing days followed the same pattern, but every day we were fewer. Every day we heard that one of us had been picked out and taken away when passing the gate where the SS checked out the condition of their work force. We knew now what it meant to be taken away…the gas chamber. We had no time or strength for mourning, feeling that soon it would be our turn.

Those selections of prisoners for the gas chamber were often quite arbitrary, adding bewilderment to our pains, like much else in the camp, including the personal sadistic whims of the guards. Two such incidents stand out in my memory. Once during a break at work when we ate our soup, a male guard, wanting to show off in front of his female colleague, called one of us over, a pretty young girl who was with her mother. He took off his cap, threw it some distance away, and ordered her to fetch it. As she went after it he shot at her and missed (whether intentionally or not) and then explained he could have killed her for attempting to escape; I heard of other cases when this was actually done. It might have been better for the girl if she had died then and there. She caught typhus later and was taken from her mother's arms to the gas chamber. The mother then lost her reason, wandering around reciting poetry. She tried to touch the electrified fence on several occasions but was pulled back each time, surviving for several weeks before she was taken to the gas chamber.

The other instance of a guard's personal initiative that I remember vividly took place when he was escorting us along the top of a low ridge on our way back from work. Below us there was another kommando going the same way and at the rear of it were the older and weaker women, supporting each other as they dragged their feet painfully and slowly along. Suddenly ordering us to stop, our guard scrambled down and laid about him with the butt of his gun among these poor women, hitting them and ordering them to go faster, faster. Obviously pleased with himself, he rejoined us and ordered us to proceed.

Then, for three of us, a miracle happened; at the end of the Appell our numbers were called out and we stepped forward, to be taken directly to an "Aryan" block. Later we learned that this was the doing of Anny Binder, secretary to Obersturmbannfuehrer Caesar, head of the "Landwirtschaft" (Agriculture) section. Anny had noticed our qualifications in the office files and thought she could save at least three of these French women who were in a tiny minority and seemed especially vulnerable. In this way we became members of another tiny minority, those with a chance of survival. Realizing this, Andrée Weiler (who, like me, had left a small child behind) implored me, "Tell them [at home] what they did to us."

Conditions in this block were not at all splendid, but we had bunks to ourselves and the food was distributed in a more orderly way. Together with eight Polish women who had come from Ravensbrueck, we were charged with the cultivation of a species of dandelion, *Taraxacum kok-saghyz*, from which the Germans were hoping to extract some natural rubber to improve the synthetic rubber being manufactured in a factory nearby in Buna. So every day we walked to Rajsko where they were already growing vegetables for the guards and their families. An area had been set aside where we were to proceed with our cultivation. It was rough ground and our first job was to dig and transport soil to make beds. Our work was supervised by two Ukrainians, civilian detainees. They favored the Poles and we three Jews got the toughest jobs. But what mattered above all was that at Rajsko we had water every day!

Each evening we were marched back to stand throughout the Appell like everyone else. Being now in an "Aryan" block meant that we were allowed to wear the camp uniform, a striped shift which was more comfortable than the miscellany of ragged garments we had been given in place of the Russian uniforms. Nevertheless, these new clothes were anything but waterproof and when it rained we were soaked. Our guards put on their big capes as soon as they felt the first drops. With nothing to change into back at the camp, we had to stand wet as we were through the Appell. That is how Anya Litvak (previously Professor Faure-Fremiet's assistant at the College de France), with whom I had come and whom I knew before the war, developed bronchitis and was taken to the "Revier" (Sick Bay) where she became weaker and weaker and was accordingly sent to the gas chamber, in full knowledge of what would happen to her.

After work one day in August 1942, we were surprised to be led along a new route. The road we were following took us near to the new railway line. On the platform a group of people were standing...men, women and children all wearing a big yellow label with "Jude" written on it in thick black letters. It was one of the first mass convoys, arriving from Poland. It was the beginning of the mass deportations from occupied Europe, the start of the Final Solution. We continued on our way and arrived in Birkenau (the place where they had built the gas chambers and crematoria). The long sheds ("barracks") we were to live in from now on were so low that we could only see what they were when we were almost upon them. They were spread over a huge area. We were dumbfounded at the sight of crowds walking in all directions, including our guards, who did not know the place. As we were special we were allocated a barrack with bunks, but all the others were distributed at random in barracks furnished only with boards set at three levels and divided by partitions. In each section three or four persons were to sleep under a thin blanket. Lucky were those who got this accommodation, since many barracks were not finished and the boards not yet in position. The following Sunday we had to work on completing them.

Life in Birkenau was beyond description. There was no water; when it rained women were crawling about lapping up the muddy water in the puddles. The only two latrines, which consisted of long trenches surmounted by planks with holes on which we were supposed to sit when we could find room, were at the end of the camp...quite a distance to go when one suffers as we all did from diarrhea. So the ground was covered with excrement. And we were covered with lice. Typhus spread all over the camp. In the evening, when we came back from Rajsko, I went to the block where the few survivors of my transport gathered, fewer every day. Even Tamara Isserlis, the doctor, who worked in the Revier where for the doctors life was more possible, caught typhus and therefore suffered the same fate as all other prisoners contracting the disease. She was my best friend.

One evening as I was on my way to visit my friends, I noticed a group of women standing around a huge wooden tub. They pushed me away but I had time to see what they were doing...tiny fingers were grasping the edge of the tub. In order to save the mothers who had secretly given birth, these women were drowning the infants. They had told each mother they knew a place where her child could be put away, where it would be safe. Only in this way could the mothers continue going to work, essential if they were not to be sent straight to the gas chamber. Much later I met a woman who had been saved in this way and in spite of everything, was confident her baby was somewhere safe. She died afterwards, never knowing the truth.

Typhus was now spreading among the SS; our great chief Caesar caught it, and so did his wife, who died of it. He recovered, and finding us so dirty and weak (one of us, a Polish woman, had already died), he decided for his own sake that we should be moved out of Birkenau. He managed to persuade the Administration that, for the sake of the rubber we were to provide for the Third Reich, we should be protected from the filth and live in the same conditions as the secretaries, who had been taken out of louse-ridden Birkenau so as not to be a source of infection for the SS with whom they had to be in contact for their work. They had been installed in the basement of the building ("Stabsgebaeude") where the Aufseherinnen lived, and we shared their accommodation from late September 1942.[3]

When we got there we could not believe our eyes. These women were "Haeftlinge" (prisoners) like ourselves, but clean, in decent clothes and looking almost fit. The food was distributed properly, the Appell was short and there was even a washroom! At first we were looked upon as intruders but this did not last and I had the pleasure of finding Raja Kagan again. She had come in my transport and I didn't know what had happened to her. Besides, that was when I met Anny Binder (now Urbanova), Caesar's secretary, the one who had picked out our names when we arrived and persuaded Caesar to take us into the "Pflanzenzucht" (Plant Breeding) kommando, thus saving our lives. Anny and I immediately cemented a friendship which lasts to this day. Other members of our group also found old friends and Eva Gabany was re-united with her cousin, Lily Tofler, later shot for refusing to give the name of a man to whom she had sent a note hidden in a bouquet of flowers.

Life being easier and our evenings "free," our minds were waking up. We chatted, recalling our past lives, and we endeavored to exercise our brains by undertaking intellectual activities. Anny taught me some German, which was so necessary to understand the orders we were given (as we couldn't understand what we were supposed to do or not do, the guards took us for imbeciles). I gave some talks on biology, but the most striking recollection I have of those evenings is the reading and translating of Goethe's *Faust* by Ella Schliesser, who had found a copy of it in the mud.

During the day we still worked at Rajsko, digging, carrying wooden trays of soil...until one day Caesar arrived with a microscope! He didn't know what to do with it but had thought it would look good to have a scientific instrument. Such a familiar object filled me with contradictory feelings, but I had been in camp long enough not to be sentimental, and to think instead of what advantage could be gained from this new acquisition. To impress Caesar, I showed him a drop of dirty water under the microscope; placing his eye clumsily on the ocular he marveled at the sight of the corpuscles floating in the water. I explained then that we could find which kok-saghyz plants were the richest in latex by making sections of the stems, and then we could cultivate the seeds of these high-yielding plants and only those. Up till then we had simply been planting the specimens received from the Ukraine, and each successive generation was thinner and thinner, and poorer and poorer in latex. (No wonder...Ukrainian soil is basic and Silesian acid.) I said I would need a razor, glass microscope slides, and some elder pith. To my surprise, some of these requests were granted. The next day I was taken to "Canada," the name given to the place where all the possessions of the new arrivals were brought and sorted...clothes in one heap, shoes in another, toothbrushes in a third, luggage, everything. From each heap anything that could be useful to the Third Reich was set aside. It was an extraordinary sight. Hardened as I was, I stood there stupefied, forgetting why I was there. After recovering my wits, I mentioned my request and was quickly provided with a razor. In front of all these riches of which we were utterly deprived, I should have liked to take something of everything, but I was warned that I would be searched at the gate and I had to be content with a piece of soap, which even by itself was a treasure!

On my return to Rajsko I proceeded to make a section of a tomato leaf. As stain, I used red ink, and to clarify the section I used the crystals of potassium chloride which served as disinfectant in the latrines. Some glass slides had been provided with the microscope, so I was able to show Caesar under the microscope a bit of tissue colored red in various parts. He was full of admiration and called the NCO in charge of the gardeners to admire this wonder. This won me a bit of respect from this gentleman who until then looked on me with suspicion because I was not sufficiently submissive.

From that day Caesar decided to have a real laboratory and enlarge the Pflanzenzucht kommando. One day on returning to our lodgings, we found a French woman who had been sent to work with us. She was a communist who had arrived in January with the first and only batch of non-Jewish Frenchwomen. They had created a profound impression on everyone by singing the "Marseillaise" as they were marched into the camp. Among them was Marie-Claude Vaillant-Couturier, who had established contacts with the internal Resistance and had managed to have the youngest of them, Madeleine Dissoubray, sent to us at the Stabsgebaeude. She told me the names of some of her comrades; what joy when I heard that my friend Marie-Elisa Nordmann was there! She was a chemist who, like me, had worked in the Sorbonne. The next day I told Caesar what a piece of luck it would be to have a renowned chemist with us; she could follow the changes in the nature of the latex in the course of the year. He agreed to get hold of her, together with another chemist (Mimi Dechavassine) and the daughter of the physicist Paul Langevin. After this easy success my secret preoccupation became the finding of as many requirements as possible for gardeners or scientific specialists, for whom I invented special qualifications. It was not always easy and sometimes dangerous.

Living in the Stabsgebaeude and working in Rajsko where the soup and bread were provided regularly, was quite a bearable life in comparison with what we had experienced and thousands were still living through, with a life expectancy of no more than weeks. Even so, it was not safe, as I was to find out. Jewish women were not allowed to wear underpants. I had obeyed this rule since Birkenau. One of my friends, having discovered my lack of underwear, managed to "organize" a pair of striped pants such as those which were distributed to the favored Haeftlinge. I was very pleased but a bit scared, having always been too clumsy to keep anything concealed. Worse luck, the very day I was at last enjoying the comfort of not suffering a draft down below, a clothes inspection took the fancy of our Blockaelteste (jailed for prostitution). In the evening she ordered us all to undress, and her eyes fixed on me. There I was, standing in my beautiful underwear! Seeing this she was furious and decided that such a crime should be reported to higher authority. A few days passed, during which I tried to imagine what sort of punishment I would have to endure. Then during the Appell the Aufseherin announced that I was to spend a week in the "Bunker" (the jail within the camp where they locked up and tortured resistants and other camp offenders).[4] So I was not to go to work the next day, and later in the morning a soldier from the main camp came to collect me.

As I was leaving, the Blockaelteste probably felt some remorse, for she gave me a loaf of bread to take with me, which turned out to be very useful indeed. At the door of Barrack No. 11, just next to the wall where executions by shooting took place, we were received by the Blockaelteste of the Bunker. His name was Jacob and with me he behaved quite decently (his reputation has been the subject of contradictory statements), allowing me to keep my bread. He led me to the cell which I was to share with five other women. There were no beds, only a few blankets on the concrete floor with just enough room for us all to lie down at once. The other women had backgrounds completely different from mine and I found it very instructive to live so closely with them. They were "Aryan" German prisoners and, like the majority of German women prisoners in Auschwitz, were there for prostitution or crimes under the civil code. Belonging to the "Master Race" entitled them to prominent positions and special rights. But there were limits to what they could get away with. One was there for trading with a soldier some jewelry which she had collected at "Canada;" another one had been caught sleeping with a soldier; another had been involved in disseminating forged banknotes among the soldiers.

On the whole we all got on very well. Their complaint against me was that I couldn't sing, which they could, and it helped to pass the time. We received food every other day, and in spite of being completely inactive, we were very hungry. My loaf divided into six had not lasted long. Most of the time I kept very quiet, remembering pleasant or funny events in my past life. My main vision was of grapes...they were so clear that I could taste them in my mouth! Ever since, I have had a passion for grapes. Every other day we were led to the washroom. Once there was blood along the passage. I was told that men had been shot in the back while washing, to make room for new prisoners. But I saw the various torture chambers only when I visited Auschwitz four years later as a free woman.

I really had very little hope of ever getting out of this hole of desolation but, it turned out, exactly a week after my incarceration I was summoned and taken back to Rajsko, leaving behind my unfortunate companions whose sentences were much longer. Back at the Stabsgebaeude I received a warm welcome from my friends; to the joy of being reunited there was added great relief for them because there had been a rumor that any Jew in the Bunker would be sent to the gas chamber. As soon as they came back from work they climbed up to the edge of the upper bunk where I lay recovering, to see with their own eyes that I was really back. I remember them as birds on a branch.

So I resumed my life in the lab. The kommando grew, and we were moved to a new little camp built near the work-place for the Pflanzenzucht along with the Gaertnerei Kommando, who grew flowers and vegetables for the SS and their families.[5] The Pflanzenzucht now comprised about ten of us on the Botany side, ten in Chemistry and ten working in the greenhouse or outdoors, where our precious plants were trying to acquire straight and thick roots. The proximity of the onions and carrots in the field and tomatoes in the greenhouse made it possible for us to help ourselves to these riches. Not without risk, though; two of us were sent back to Birkenau having been caught red-handed. I escaped the same fate thanks to Caesar, who had my punishment commuted to spending a Sunday emptying and cleaning the latrines of the SS. We were so deprived of vitamins that we would risk anything to get some raw vegetable. And to send some to our friends in Birkenau; this was achieved by giving it to the kommandos who worked in the same fields but still lived in Birkenau and did some petty pilfering on their own account. Carrying such contraband was very dangerous for them since there was always the risk of being searched at the entrance to the camp. The problem was to learn that a search was going on in time to get rid of your precious load in haste.

For us, the problem after having stolen some goodies was to store them. There were many hiding places in the lab, but from time to time the Aufseherin would undertake an inspection and she was accompanied everywhere by her dog, who could sniff out anything odd, even carrots. As soon as her arrival was signaled we had to throw away our precious booty. I developed a means of defense against this invasion of our privacy…the technique used to stain the latex included treating the slides with bromium vapor, the smell of which, if released in time, kept our visitors at the door until we had gotten rid of our merchandise. From time to time we had official visitors from Berlin who were sent to see what was going on in this bizarre research laboratory inside a concentration camp. We were warned in advance by Caesar, who was nearly as keen as ourselves to dazzle our visitors. They were all completely ignorant scientifically, and a slight smell of bromium contributed to creating a mysterious atmosphere for our demonstration that followed...some brilliantly colored slides which the visitor was invited to look at through the microscope...some of our best roots dried up and used again and again, etc.

Once we even had a visit from a Frenchman called M. Lecomte, who had been sent by his firm to inquire about this marvelous dandelion which could improve synthetic rubber. A White Russian officer who spoke French was present during my whole conversation with the Frenchman, so I could not inform him about what went on in the camp. All I could tell him was that I had worked at the Sorbonne, and with this information he succeeded in finding my parents...after the liberation of Paris. He made no effort to do anything while the Germans were still there. Anyway, he had not seen anything, nor asked any questions about the smoking chimney, nor asked who lived in the rows of barracks which he had certainly seen on his way to Rajsko. All he seemed to know was that I worked in a lab and was wearing a white lab coat. As there had been so long a time between his visit to Auschwitz (in the early spring) and his going to see them (autumn), my parents didn't get much comfort from his visit. Just as well, because things were going to be worse and worse and they could have been very disappointed indeed if I had not come back, which seemed more and more likely.

The SS eventually found a real German scientist to take charge of the lab, a Dr. Boehm, who had studied not only in Germany but also in England. How such a highly educated man could have sunk to joining the SS in order to supervise the work done in Auschwitz is beyond my understanding; but he had, and did the job wholeheartedly. Inevitably he found out that, if our work in the Pflanzenzucht lab was accurate, it was, to say the least, slow and not very original (in fact, when we received books we discovered that what we had done was already known in the Russian literature). Naturally, he held me responsible for the mediocrity of the work and developed a keen dislike for me. I suppose psychologists could find an explanation of his special hate for me, whose background was similar to his own. Anyway, he decided that now we were to endeavor to produce polyploids which would be very rich in rubber. Genetics was not my strong subject and I became more of a technician than a research worker. Not a very good technician either, in his eyes, which was not very surprising. At every opportunity he reminded me of my prisoner status, while he was one of the masters. To illustrate his point, he sent me spreading manure in the fields on a cold winter day. The freezing cold did nothing to improve my skill as a chromosome counter.

Early in 1944 I came down with malaria, which was spreading through the camp, among the SS as well as among the prisoners. In order to restrict the spread of the disease the authorities decided to send all infected Jewish prisoners to the gas chamber. I was still in Rajsko when the result of my blood test came back from the Hygiene Institute, where smears were examined; an SS doctor came to check the results and look at the slides himself. When it came to my slide, which our doctor knew to be positive, she, Stephanie Schrameck, with the assistance of Mela, another doctor, managed to get rid of my specimen and substitute a healthy one. I don't know how messages were passed so quickly through the resistance network of the main camp, but the word went round that I needed quinine if I was to survive and the next day or so I got enough quinine to cure me and more, while the Germans themselves were short of it. I was very weak indeed and only regained some strength thanks to the ingenuity of my friends who provided me with extra food, which they stole from everywhere right up to the SS kitchen. I especially remember a spoonful of stewed cherries!

But in August 1944 we suffered a terrible blow to our morale. Following a speech on the B.B.C. naming some of the (non-Jewish) French women in Auschwitz, all the non-Jewish French women were to be transported to another camp. Where to? Nobody knew. And what was going to happen to us? Of course we feared the worst and tried to think of some way of defending ourselves if they attempted to exterminate us all. When our comrades left us, they were loaded with messages for such of our dear ones as they could find...if they themselves ever reached home.

The departure of these friends, who formed a "family" with whom I had lived and struggled, left me limp and disheartened. However, they were replaced, and among the newcomers was Simone Franck (now Floersheim). She had been a youthful member of the Resistance in Savoy, and was to be my constant companion during my last months of slavery until we finally gained our freedom. Life was getting tougher and tougher, but the good news of the advance of the Soviet troops in our direction and of the successes on the western front filtered through to us, and the prospect of an end to the nightmare we were living through seemed faintly more possible. What would this end be? We could not imagine, and the hope of getting home seemed less and less realistic. We did not much care; the end was what mattered.

However, on the 17th of January 1945, more and more rumors spread through the camp and anxiety mounted while orders and counter-orders were issued. Finally, toward evening, we learned we were to be evacuated. I had no shoes at that time and the ground was covered with thick snow. Suddenly, the door of the barrack opened and I heard a voice saying, "These are for Claudette Bloch." I rushed to the door but my benefactor had disappeared, leaving a pair of real boots! I couldn't believe my eyes! It was just in time, for not many hours passed before we saw columns of prisoners from Birkenau and elsewhere arriving slowly in ranks of five. We were made to join them and this was the beginning of the march which was to be the very last stage for so many of us. How many died during that march I do not know, but something I do remember is having to step over their fallen bodies as we marched.

We arrived in Ravensbrueck in such a state of exhaustion that I cannot describe it. I lost my senses entirely in the cattle car in which we finished the journey, and I remember it as being in a boat. On our arrival in Ravensbrueck we learned that there was no room for us and we had to wait in the snow for a decision as to what they would do with us. I laid down in the snow and if Simone had not forced me to get up it would have been the end for me. Finally, we were packed into tents, and the next day we were found by our friends from Auschwitz. Marie-Elisa, having heard that people from Rajsko were among the new arrivals, searched everywhere until she found us. She and all those who had left us in August had been there ever since. What emotions, to meet again! And they had brought us some food from their own meager rations.

We stayed in Ravensbrueck only a couple of weeks or so, then were transported by train to Malchow. There was not much work for us there, and still less food. We had come close to the point of death by starvation there when we were moved on yet again, to various camps. Our group was sent to a small working camp in Leipzig…a women's annex of Buchenwald. There, in what we thought to be the height of comfort, we received food, somewhere to sleep and to wash. And we found French women who took care of us and explained how to survive in that camp.

But a couple of weeks later, as the Allies were approaching, again we were on the road. Our destination was unknown even to our guards! Their morale was breaking; and if some of them were becoming harder and harder, many of them were thinking of their own skins. As luck would have it, the guards who were walking alongside us themselves deserted. Simone immediately realized that we also could escape and together with our new friends we leaped off the road and hid behind bushes. We waited until the column had disappeared, came out of hiding and gathered together. There were thirteen of us, too many to undertake any plan for what we were going to do next. So we divided ourselves into two groups, making sure that in each group at least one of us could speak German or English.

Our little group walked until we found a village made up of farms. We asked for shelter, pretending that we had been working in a German factory and had been bombed out. We had some civilian clothes that had been thrown to us by Ukrainian women working in a village we had passed through the day before. The first houses shut their doors in our faces, but in one of them we found a Belgian war prisoner, Victor, who had worked that farm while the master of the house was in the army. When he opened the door and realized we were French women on the run, he dropped his arms in awe. He had never dreamt that the first French women he would meet after five years would look so awful. He didn't seem to know very much about what had been happening during the years he had spent looking after the farm. Anyway, he let us in, led us to the pig shed and decided the most urgent thing for us was to wash. How surprised he was when he came back with a pail of water to find us bending over the pig trough devouring the potatoes cooked for the pigs! He didn't trust the farmer's wife enough to tell her of our presence. So he led us to a further outbuilding, where later he brought us some soup. The floor was hard, concrete I think, but we slept nonetheless, though not yet confident we were free.

Early the next morning Victor woke us up, and we could see at once he was upset. He explained why. In that village there was a post of Germans who had not yet given up; they had heard that some women had escaped from the column of prisoners and gave orders for the village to be searched and the women brought to them. We got up in haste and Victor showed us the direction we should take to find bushes where we could hide. We ran as fast as our poor legs could carry us and found the bushes; from our hiding place we could see the front of the farm and soon we distinguished the silhouettes of soldiers talking to Victor. He was gesticulating, pointing in the direction opposite to the one we had taken. By a stroke of luck an air raid alert sounded at that moment and everyone, including the soldiers, took shelter. Not us, however; we crept into a ditch and when the alert finished we were already at a good distance from the village. We were saved for the time being, but what to do next? We decided to keep walking, trying to head in the direction of the front in the hope of finding the Allies. How we were to cross the front lines we had no idea, but we would see. In fact the sound of the guns became more and more sporadic and crossing the front lines proved no problem.

The problem was how to survive. We were in open country without money or identity, and anybody we met could be an enemy. But it was freedom and we felt very happy. When we reached a farm we told them the same story of being bombed out, and that we were trying to get back to France. In fact, the morale of many of the farmers we asked for hospitality was not very high and some of them thought it might be a good idea to shelter these French people, whoever they were, as this would be a reason for indulgence on the part of the victorious Americans, who were expected at any time now. Many of the Germans were hoping the Americans would go on to fight the Russians.

In fact, it was a long time after the fighting had ceased before any ally penetrated this part of the country (between Leipzig and Dresden), because of the lengthy negotiations between the Americans and the Russians to settle who would occupy what. For us this meant that for a fortnight we walked on westwards, stopping at farms who allowed us (which many did not) to sleep in barns where the hay made comfortable beds. We had seed potatoes collected from the fields where the farmers were planting them, and many of the good people who harbored us gave us something to eat with the potatoes they cooked for us.

Finally, after various adventures, we reached Torgau, where by chance we found the other group with whom we had escaped. They were installed in a hotel converted into a hospital for French prisoners-of-war. The major in charge allowed us to share the dormitory which our friends occupied and the meals which were cooked for the men. What a life! It was heaven. Not for long, unfortunately. The men were to be repatriated by air. The French major asked the Americans, who were responsible for the air lift, whether it could include us, but the answer was negative. So the thirteen of us were left in the big hotel, inhabited only by the proprietor, who had never left the premises. There was some food remaining in the kitchen and the soldiers gave us some money. So we could survive for the time being, but the question was what to do next?

This question became more acute two mornings later when we woke to found the Americans who had been occupying the town had left and been replaced by Russians. We had heard scary stories about Russian soldiers pillaging everything on their way and raping women. So in the evening as we were eating our supper, we were frightened when a group of Russian soldiers came into the kitchen uninvited and sat down around the table. They started talking with those of us who understood Russian, proudly displaying their loot, in particular the watches...but doing no harm. However, they were becoming more and more familiar and we were getting more and more tense, when an officer arrived and ordered them out. Later we had another fright when, as we were ready for bed, there was a knock at the door and two Russian officers appeared; they asked for an interpreter and two of us got dressed after the light had been switched off because the officers stood there waiting for them. We watched them going away with tightened throats...and a short time later saw them come back, with immense relief. In fact they had simply been asked to tell the hotel proprietor what the new occupiers were expecting from him and in particular to show them where he had hidden his wine. After that the only disturbance was the noise of the bottles being carried away.

In the evening of the 8th of May we knew that the armistice had been signed and we demanded a radio from the proprietor. He was so frightened by that stage that he would obey any order. He lent us a radio set and we heard, pressed together in a little room, the bells of Notre Dame and the rejoicing in the streets of Paris.

For us the problem of getting home was as pressing and unsolved as ever. Our interpreter (Lise London) went to the Soviet Army Headquarters established in the town and asked what help they could give us. The answer was that if we wanted to be taken to Kiev, from which we would be sent back to France one day or another, they could do it, but they had no means of sending us back directly. This solution didn't appeal to us, so it was decided that we would be escorted up to a small river which we could ford, and beyond it we would find ourselves again in the American zone. That is what we did, but it took a lot of walking before we found anybody who could help us. There were people walking in all directions: ex-prisoners-of-war, non-Germans who had been doing forced labor, and also SS tearing off their insignia and silently running for cover. In short, it was a shambles; and it was difficult to find anywhere to sleep or anything to eat. Among the milling crowds, at some stage we met our friend Victor, who gave us some tins of spaghetti that he had taken with him on leaving the village where he had worked; that was all he could do. Later we passed through a village that was not only pretty but whose inhabitants were kind; the mayor even gave us some bread coupons which we proudly exchanged for real bread at a bakery. There was not much bread to be had but the kind woman shopkeeper supplemented it with some soup! It tasted so good that I still remember it.

After a lot of walking, a short way by horse-drawn cart and a longer way by train thanks to a friend of my family met by chance among the American soldiers (he was their interpreter), we arrived in Leipzig. We expected to be promptly put on a train to France and that would be the end of our ordeals. But we were not the only ones with this hope; there were thousands of us and there was no organization. There was just a big camp where we were given food after lining up, vessel in hand. However, after three days we found ourselves…exactly how, I don't know…in a cattle car attached to a train repatriating ex-prisoners-of-war. We had a lot of room and were given enough blankets to make our car comfortable for sleeping; but we were given hardly any food, only cigarettes. The journey took a week. The train progressed so haltingly that the men had time to jump off, run to a farmyard, kill a few chickens and at the next stop make a fire and cook them. We received a fair share of the products in these exercises and it was very welcome indeed. When we arrived on French soil women came from the villages with baskets of eggs which we sucked out with relish.

At the frontier we had to get out of the train and go to a makeshift office. There again we had to line up in spite of our exhaustion. After being interrogated about our identities and where we came from in Germany, we were given a sort of identity card and some money. This had a profound effect upon me. Until now, the struggle for sheer survival had absorbed all my energies; and now suddenly it came home to me with overwhelming force that I was going home at last, but…whom should I find there? The question became unbearable and I put it out of my mind by planning what I would do if my little boy and my parents were not there. I decided I could continue to fight, probably in China.

When at last we arrived in Paris, at the Gare de l'Est on the 17th of May, there was a band playing and a crowd on the platform welcoming us with open arms. My heart was heavy, though: all these embraces…and not a soul I knew. A bus took us to the Hotel Lutetia, a journey as in a dream. I remember only the women's tall hats and barrow-loads of cherries. At the hotel there were volunteers to help us find out what happened to those whom we had left behind. When my turn came to be asked who I was, I had hardly given my name when the girl who was asking leaped to her feet shouting, "Claudette Bloch! I am going to phone them!" "Who are you going to phone?" I asked with anguish. "Your parents, your mother-in-law. They are with your son!" I nearly collapsed, my eyes full of tears.

A short time later my parents arrived. After embracing me, they explained that they had not stood at the door like many other people had done because the day before they had stood there expecting to meet my sister's husband among the survivors of Mauthausen, in vain. When they heard more survivors were arriving (they didn't know where I would be coming from), they couldn't face it. then my mother asked me if I had met her brother or his wife in Auschwitz. Coolly I answered, "How could I? If they were deported they surely went directly to the gas chamber." My mother collapsed and I understood how cruel I had been. I realized how wide was the abyss that separated the world in which I had lived for three years and the civilized world. But it took a long time to adapt to my new situation. On the one hand, I felt it my duty to tell people what had been the fate of the dear ones whose return they were awaiting in vain; on the other hand, I had to re-learn the values of a civilized world.

Together with my parents, I went to my flat, where I found my little boy and my mother-in-law. There also the emotions were mixed. She put on a brave face but my mother-in-law was only then realizing that her son would never come back. And for Maurice, my son, now aged five, what a disappointment it was for him to find a Mummy, whose picture he had been shown many times, arriving now dirty, in rags, and careful not to embrace him too closely for fear of giving him her lice.

Gradually, an ordered sort of life returned. I went back to my old research job in the Sorbonne while my mother-in-law or my parents looked after Maurice, now starting school. In 1949, at a scientific conference in Cambridge, England, I met John Kennedy, a member of the scientific staff of the Agricultural Research Council (now Professor Emeritus). A year later we were married, and settled with Maurice in Cambridge, where two more children were born. The three of them are now married and parents themselves, one an anthropologist, one an applied mathematician, and one a biologist. So now, after teaching French for many years, I enjoy the normal life of a wife, mother and grandmother. Without my husband's help I should never have been able to write down these recollections, which still give me nightmares.

❖

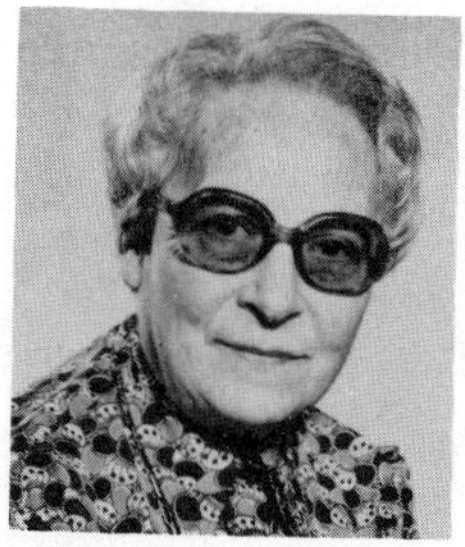

Dr. Marie-Elisa Cohen (née Nordmann)
Paris (France)

I was born on November 4, 1910, in the Eighth Arondissement (district) of Paris. My father had a good position in a Russian bank, which failed due to the 1917 revolution. Having failed to find a better alternative, he accepted an inferior job in another bank. Thus, our lifestyle changed drastically. Nevertheless, I was able to study at the university and obtained a Ph.D. in chemistry. In 1942 I was employed by the National Center for Scientific Research, working in the field of physical chemistry. I was divorced and lived together with my six year-old son as well as with my mother, who had been widowed in 1937.

Already in September 1940, I had started to fight the occupation. I belonged to the resistance organized by the Communist Party for intellectuals. In 1942 I transported, mailed and distributed "l'Universite Libre," sheltered those members of the resistance who had been warned, "Don't go home, the cops are waiting for you!"; and collected funds for the National University Front.

I was arrested at my home on May 16, 1942 by special gendarmes who had just apprehended France Bloch-Serazin (the daughter of Jean-Richard Bloch, who was decapitated on February 12, 1943, in Hamburg) by having followed her for several days. I was not in the same organization as France (who belonged to the F.T.P.) but I was caught in the same trap in which Politzer, Solomon and their group had been taken during the months of February and March. France was a friend as well as a colleague and...disregarding advice...I had helped her in certain missions of the F.T.P.

From the Prefecture of Police I was transferred to the depot. A note written on cigarette paper in a package informed me that my mother had been arrested by the Gestapo as a civilian hostage on August 7, 1942. My mother had remained in her apartment, although being Jewish she should have saved herself. But how could she abandon her grandson, her daughter and her daughter's friend, France, to whom she delivered packages in the Sante? Under torture she revealed that she was Jewish.

On August 24, 1942, I was transferred to the Sante and on September 29, 1942, I was sent to Romainville. There I learned that my mother had preceded me and had been deported on September 3. As a civilian hostage, my mother should have been released after four weeks (a rule which was rarely followed, but it was still the rule). The Germans discovered that she was Jewish and she was therefore transported to Drancy.

After a few days in Auschwitz I realized what happened to old Jewish women upon arrival...straight to the gas chambers from the ramp.

I arrived at Birkenau in January 1943 with the only transport of French "Aryan" women. Fortunately, I was using my maiden name since my divorce. The SS never suspected that "Nordmann" could be a Jewish name and in France, neither my mother, my brother or myself were registered as Jews.

The majority of us, who were going to be known as the "31,000" (because all of us were tattooed with prison numbers in the thirty-one thousands), had worked in the resistance movement against the Nazi occupation. More than half were involved in communist activities, while one-fourth were Gaullists who came from various regional networks.

No selection took place at our arrival. The "Marseillaise," which we sang when entering the camp, made a big impression. However, selection started immediately the next morning at roll call and continued in the work kommandos.

We passed quarantine in Block 14, a difficult block, whose occupants were Slovakian. Two of our comrades were no longer with us...Danielle Casanova worked as a dentist and Heidi Hautval as a physician in the Revier. Once, in February 1943, after the evening roll call, Magda, our Blockaelteste, asked for biologists, botanists and chemists to register. Danielle had to convince me to report. If I remember correctly, three of us applied as chemists.

After the quarantine, during which many comrades had been selected for the gas chambers, the 31,000 were transferred to Block 26, which was adjacent to the notorious Block 25, the death block. The new Blockaelteste was Stenia, a Volksdeutsche whose cruelty was well-known.[6] We had to work in Aussenkommandos (doing hard work outside of camp). However, those who had registered with Magda, including the three chemists, were assigned to the Canada kommando, which sorted clothing while they awaited their departure. We had to sleep with the privileged prisoners, who were so disagreeable that once we stayed up all night. Although Stenia[7] had warned us that she would send us to Block 25 if she ever saw us in her block, we spent each evening with our comrades. Jacqueline Odru was the first of us to leave as a botanist.

From February 28 until March 21, 1943, I was ill in the Revier of Birkenau with bronchitis, perforated otitis and dysentery. I was present when a great number of the 31,000 whom I loved, died. I saw how a new-born baby was drowned in a bucket of water.

One evening, Danielle Casanova came to see me and brought me a message from Claudette, an old friend of mine who had been arrested about the same time I had been. She informed me that she too, was in Auschwitz and Claudette strangely assured me that she would take care of me. Indeed, on March 21, 1943, Gerda Schneider, the Blockaelteste of the Revier, a German communist who had been imprisoned since 1934, called me and told me to get ready to depart. I left Birkenau that afternoon to go to the Stabsgebaeude along with Hélène Solomon, another friend of mine, Madeleine Dechavassin, the other chemist, who had registered after the roll call, and Alida, a seamstress. Fortunately, they helped me walk, though the distance was not great.

Stabsgebaeude, March 21 through July 1943

What a joy to meet Jacqueline and Claudette again. Immediately next morning, I was admitted to the Revier of the Stabsgebaeude with a high fever. It was typhus, which many of the 31,000 contracted. I was very lucky that it broke out in the

Stabsgebaeude and that none of us had exhibited suspicious spots when we were examined by the SS doctor; otherwise they would have sent us back to Birkenau. This was the case with a green-triangled German inmate who never returned. For me, the Stabsgebaeude was a place where one forsook the madness of extermination. Nevertheless, from the windows of the Revier one heard, day and night, the noise of maneuvers and the whistle of trains.

The Polish physician was no Francophile and I seem to recall that she spoke no French at all. She was saccharine as well as hypocritical with the Polish inmates, who received vials of calcium from their Polish kochanis (boyfriends). The physician gave the injections and got a share of the provisions received in the packages in return.

I was a future chemist of the kommando Pflanzenzucht. Claudette introduced me to Anni Binder, the secretary of SS-Obersturmbannfuehrer Dr. Caesar, the head of the department. At the end of April 1943, I started to work in Rajsko. I was extremely thin, suffered from hepatitis and was pulled along on the march by Hélène and Jacqueline. Since there was nothing for me to do in the beginning, I spent my first days warming my right side next to the ceramic stove which was still lit.

The Camp of Rajsko

The camp of Rajsko was officially opened on July 1, 1943. There was a wooden building with dormitories for both the Pflanzenzucht and the Gaertnerei as well as a room for the Blockaelteste. The first one was Gerda Schneider. Another barrack contained two dining rooms and a large work hall where the women of the Pflanzenzucht sorted the Kok-Saghiz grain during the winter. The block next to the dormitories contained our showers. The camp kitchen, which was operated by Polish inmate personnel, and the room where packages were distributed were located in the only pre-war building.

The Pflanzenzucht

The task of this kommando was the study of the culture of Taraxacum Kok-Saghiz, a kind of dandelion whose root and juice contain latex. The Soviets grew it in the Ukraine. In order for synthetic caoutchouc (India rubber), which the buna factory manufactured in Auschwitz-Morowitz, to be elastic, it had to be mixed with natural caoutchouc. One could use the latex of the Kok-Saghiz instead.

The effective personnel of the Pflanzenzucht consisted of a great number of Poles. The ones in responsible positions had previously been in Ravensbrueck. Their Auschwitz numbers were very low, only four digits, indicative of how early they had arrived. They were Wanda Dulczynska, the Kapo, Marichna and Zofia Grochowalska.[8] I am certain that the last one was still alive in the summer of 1987, although perhaps Wanda Dulczynska, our Kapo, who supposedly emigrated to South America, was too. They encompassed the entire kommando, which was supervised by Herrn Doktor Schattenfeld, an agronomist. He was a middle-aged man who promenaded around, usually inspecting everything without malice, except in the chemical laboratories, which did not concern him.

The purpose of the chemical laboratory was the chemical analysis of latex. Ruth Weinberg (or Weimann), a young woman, was in charge. She had studied chemistry at the University of Strasbourg (naturally after 1940). She was pretty much a zero and supervised the large chemistry laboratory, where about eight prisoners worked, among them Madeleine Dechavassin. These French women had arrived before us or with a transport in February 1943. Since I was the most qualified, she assigned me to her personal laboratory, where I, together with two Polish inmates did research on her dissertation. All three of us always seemed to be busy in front, continuously running the machines. She never realized that we did not renew the contents of our experiments. And our results? They were great, since we knew what we were supposed to find, thanks to Russian journals which were translated by two of our colleagues.

Naturally, we had to do numerous calculations and I requested a calculator, which was delivered from "Canada" and placed into Ruth's (or "Juliette's" as we nicknamed her) office. Incidentally, she had become Frau Caesar in December

1943, so we prepared little rails of goose feathers which had come from Harmense for the wedding.

Juliette never realized that we were play-acting. She was very proud of her future dissertation.

The layout in the laboratory building, which was situated on the left-hand side when entering Rajsko from the main road, was approximately the following:

There was the photo-lab with Wanda Jakubowska and one aide; the botanical laboratory; the SS-kitchen, which prepared the meals for the Doktor and for "Troutrou" (about whom I am going to speak later), with one Bibelforscherin (Jehovah's Witness) as cook and one "31,000" as assistant; the large chemistry laboratory; and the small lab of Juliette. In addition, there were two Polish prisoners who worked as cleaning women. In all, there were about 22-25 persons in the building.

The other female inmates of the Pflanzenzucht worked for three seasons in the Kok-Saghiz fields, whereas they toiled in a hothouse situated in the aforementioned dining room barrack during the winter. Those Polish women whom Kapo Wanda liked were assigned to the hothouses that were located behind the laboratory. Every day, a kommando of male prisoners also came to work in the hothouses and among them were a few survivors of the transport that had received prison numbers starting with 45,000, i.e., the only transport of French resistance fighters. (Of course this does not mean that there were no members of the resistance in the racial (Jewish) transports.) These men brought us the "Voelkischer Beobachter" and the "Oberschlesische Zeitung" which they hid in a predetermined place, from where we fetched them at propitious moments. One of us translated the news into French and we followed the Nazi defeat at the Eastern front and later the progress of the Allies after the invasion of Normandy on a small atlas, which these same comrades had given to us. The atlas was hidden in the laboratory's attic above the kitchen, where only those of us who were allowed to look for new glasses were permitted to enter. The atlas was underneath these glasses, hidden under some straw.

Immediately after the arrival of the men's kommando, on June 6, 1944, we knew about the debarkation. When Caesar arrived at 9 A.M., we heard him say to the Doktor, "Der Teufel ist los" (all hell has broken out).

The Gaertnerei

This was the second kommando which was lodged at Rajsko. Its purpose was the cultivation of vegetables for the SS. It consisted of young female Russian and Ukranian inmates commanded by a German Kapo with a green triangle (a "criminal"). One of the 31,000, Germaine Renaudin, belonged to it. She passed away in 1968. The corridor which separated the dining room of the Gaertnerei from ours was the ideal meeting place for exchanging bread and package contents, which we were allowed to receive at a later date, for onions, garlic, cabbage, tomatoes, etc. One of the Russian prisoners, a teacher, gave us Russian language lessons in the winter of 1943/44.

SS-man Grell, a non-commissioned officer, was in charge of the kommando. His office was at the right-hand side of the entrance. Lilly Toffler,[9] a cousin of Eva Gabany, one of Claudette's designers, was his secretary. We have never forgotten Lilly's departure to Auschwitz and her tragic death.

Joachim Caesar

Dr. Caesar was an agronomist, held the rank of Obersturmbannfuehrer when I knew him, and was in charge of all agricultural kommandos which belonged to Birkenau, whereas the Hygiene Institut (Institute of Hygiene), about which I will speak later, belonged to Auschwitz. The other agricultural kommandos were at Harmense, where poultry were bred; at Budy, where cultivation of potatoes had replaced the Strafkolonne (punishment kommando); and at Plawy, which was involved in fish breeding. However, the only kommando that interested Caesar was the Pflanzenzucht. He had been able to prove the importance of Kok-Saghiz for defense purposes. Oswald Pohl[10] had visited Rajsko and, if I remember correctly, it was after this inspection...of which I cannot give the date...that Caesar became Obersturmbannfuehrer.[11] He managed to avoid being sent to the Eastern front and enjoyed a family life.

Even if our life had the appearance of normalcy, we nevertheless, always saw the red sky over Birkenau. We could smell the odor of the crematoria. Caesar had no scruples about returning us to Birkenau for punishment. This happened to

Germaine Pican, one of the 31,000, who was caught "organizing" onions to send them to our starving comrades in Birkenau. The same fate befell Berthe Falk, a French woman who had arrived in camp long before us. Troutrou surprised Berthe, who was writing after D-Day about the liberation of Paris, which she had put on the Quatorze Juillet (14th of July). Consequently, Berthe was sent to the Strafkolonne.[12] Caesar did not intervene in either case. He also did not do anything for Lilly Toffler and had great difficulty in replacing her for SS-man Grell.

I never understood how Caesar could profit from these strange prisoners who were termed "dienstverpflichtet" (obliged to serve). They could circulate freely and even had permission to go shopping in Kattowice. There were two Ukrainians, experts on Kok-Saghiz, and one German, an old communist who was a specialist in fish research.

Thus, Caesar was adroit and knew how to play the game very well. We were extraordinarily lucky that we had the opportunity to profit from our jobs.

Das Hygiene Institut

About three hundred meters away from the laboratory were the headquarters of the kommando of the Institute of Hygiene. It consisted of physicians and scientists who were specialized in producing serums to make vaccines. We knew some of the French prisoners among them: Landau, Lewin, Lettich, and later, Marc Klein, who had been arrested together with his colleagues at Strasbourg University and subsequently had been transferred to Clermont-Ferrand. The only woman in this kommando was Mrs. Seemann, who…by another miraculous contradiction…had been able to save her young son from the gas chamber. This laboratory was under the supervision of SS Dr. Bruno Weber. Their equipment was quite sophisticated and this gave us the pretext to go there every once in a while, escorted by our SS-Aufseherin, to feign centrifuging the latex samples which we were studying, just so that we could see our friends. We brought them…hidden in our vast pants…tomatoes of the season and they reciprocated by giving us jam and sometimes blood, with which we made blood sausage, while the Aufseherin flirted with the SS-guard. But a superb new centrifuge in our laboratory, furnished by the best Parisian specialist who collaborated, caused the discontinuation of these excursions.

Thies Christophersen

Thies Christophersen had been seriously wounded during the 1940 offensive in France. Not being able to return to the front, he took some agriculture courses in 1942/43. Thanks to this newly-acquired knowledge, he was sent to the Ukraine in order to raise India rubber plants. When the Nazis lost the Ukraine, Christophersen was transferred to Rajsko to work under Caesar, where the 31,000 met him for the first time in January 1944. He received the nickname "Troutrou" because of the deep scar on his face. It was Troutrou who sent our friend Berthe Falk to the Strafkompagnie in July 1944.

In 1973 Christophersen published a little brochure entitled "Die Auschwitz Luege" (The Auschwitz Lie) in which he denied the existence of gas chambers and crematoria at Birkenau. "...During all the time I was in Auschwitz I never in the least observed anything that ever indicated mass killings in gas chambers. Also, the story of a smell of burned flesh that allegedly hovered over the camp at times was an infamous lie. In the vicinity of the main camp there was a smithy whose horse's hooves were shod. The burning of the horses' hooves when fitting them with shoes naturally caused an unpleasant smell...(p. 19).

Thies Christophersen, alias Troutrou, an old Nazi, succeeded in escaping all difficulties after the war. His brochure was not innocently written. The idyllic life of the Rajsko inmates and of Troutrou himself takes up three-quarters of the book. The other quarter is a manipulation of scientific sounding history by a false witness who abuses the fact that he really belonged to the camp personnel of Auschwitz. This is an abuse of confidence which culminates in intellectual swindling.

The millions of those who were gassed at Auschwitz have left profound traces in people's memories. And we, the survivors, as long as we have enough strength, represent our dead comrades. We must speak for them.

Ravensbrueck and Mauthausen

Our group of eighteen 31,000 Rajsko inmates left Auschwitz for Ravensbrueck on two different occasions. The first eight women departed in January 1944; the second group, to which I belonged, on August 14, 1944, i.e., after the August 2, 1944, transfer of our comrades who had remained quarantined in Birkenau. In Ravensbrueck I worked as a lab technician doing urine analysis. Mass killings occurred, but there was a laboratory to analyze the urine of patients.

In March 1945, the NN inmates (most of the women of the transport had been classified as NN [Nacht und Nebel], signifying extermination as our fate) were sent from Ravensbrueck to Mauthausen. I joined them, although I could have avoided it. In Mauthausen I worked as a nurse. I was liberated by the International Red Cross and repatriated to France via Switzerland.

I arrived in Paris on the evening of April 30, 1945, and was reunited with my son, whom my sister-in-law in Rennes (Bretagne) had brought up. My only brother, a professor and founder of the F.F.I. in Morbihan and Cotes-du-Nord, had been arrested in Rennes in April 1944 and deported to Neuengamme with the penultimate transport which left Compiegne. He died of typhus in Bergen-Belsen on May 1, 1945, two weeks after the British liberated the camp.

I returned to work relatively early, i.e., in October 1945, and readjusted quite quickly. This was especially due to the fact that I remarried in 1948. Francis Cohen was a journalist who had three children (two sons and one daughter) which, in spite of the fatigue, helped to rejuvenate me. Nevertheless I had great difficulties in taking up research again. After six years at the Commisariate of Atomic Energy, where I directed the documentation service, I re-entered teaching. I only re-started publishing scientific papers in 1960. Asthenia (debility), which does not interfere with work, does, however, disturb the creative process. Other medical problems are: stones in the bladder (supposedly a side-effect of typhus), rheumatism and intestinal problems.

Since June 1945, I also have been active in a concentration camp survivor organization.[13]

❖

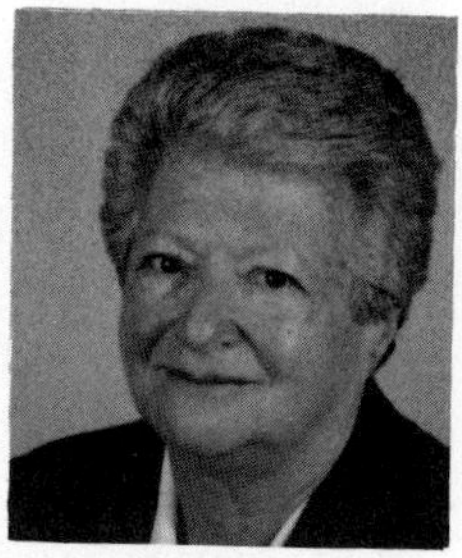

Simone Floersheim (née Franck)
Chambery (France)

I was born on October 10, 1920 in Albertville (Savoie) in the Alps, a very small town of six thousand inhabitants at that time. (That number has diminished significantly since then, although it will be the place of the 1992 Winter Olympic Games.)

My Family

My family is of Jewish-Alsatian origin. My great-grandparents left the Alsace in 1871 when it was annexed by Germany. After having lived in Switzerland a few years, they moved to Albertville which was close to both the Swiss and the Italian borders.

This was how my mother's family arrived in Albertville. My father's family left Eastern France and settled in Dijon.

When my father married, he joined my mother in Albertville. My maternal grandparents had lost a son in 1917 during the First World War and wanted their daughter and son-in-law close by.

One of my great-grandmothers was still living when I was young. She had been born in 1837-38 in the Alsace and died in Albertville in 1926. Thus, my family memories cover a large epoch of one and a half centuries.

My maternal great-grandparents were modest people who had been horse dealers in Alsace. My grandfather, whom I knew well and with whom I conversed much, passed away in 1947 after my return from the concentration camp.

Throughout his life, he regretted never having studied at the university. He was the second of five children. His father died young, and therefore, my grandfather had to help his mother at an early age. He was a good man, quite intelligent, who always remembered his difficult beginnings in life. He founded a dry goods store in Albertville which is still in existence today.

My mother was sixteen years old when World War I broke out. She interrupted her studies to help her father, whom she closely resembled in physique and character. When she married in 1919, my father took over the family business in Albertville. He was more educated, having completed his secondary studies. Toward the end of World War I, he served as an interpreter for the American troops in France.

My Studies

Since there were no secondary schools in Albertville, I attended school in Chambery where I graduated from high school (obtained the Baccalaureate) in 1938. I would have preferred to study science, but my father would not allow me. I, therefore, studied law at Grenoble against my will. We were on the eve of World War II.

Religion

The family members who influenced me most, my grandfather and mother, were for the most part atheists.

If they had been religious, they would not have settled in Albertville where there was no possibility of practicing the Jewish religion in the traditional way. We were the only Jews in the village. My father was a believer, but was unfamiliar with the practice of religious law.

My uncle, who was killed during battle in 1917, was not even bar mitzvah. When he died, a Catholic priest wanted to conduct the funeral service. His

Christian childhood friends, who were in the same regiment, informed the priest that my uncle was Jewish, thereby preventing the occurrence of a Christian funeral service.

We did not adhere to any of the Jewish ritual or dietary laws, nor did we keep the Shabbat. In fact, we celebrated Christmas at our home, although in a pagan way, but Christmas, nevertheless.

Religion was not taught to us children, nor was it of interest to us. I had two brothers and one sister. We were never asked any questions concerning religion. In Albertville, the world was not divided into Jews and Gentiles.

Friends

Under these conditions, we children had practically no Jewish friends. We were assimilated and invited to first communion and other various Christian rituals by our Christian friends. We did not suffer from anti-Semitism. During my entire childhood, I can remember only one incident. There was an old spinster who taught catechism at a local school. She forbade her pupils to speak to us. The parents of the school children were indignant over this and made amends to us by welcoming us even more into their homes.

Another example: My grandfather's best friend was a chanoine (a Catholic dignitary) whom I knew quite well when I was young. He had insisted that my grandparents live in his house and he sold them his house saying that, because they had children and grandchildren, he knew to whom the house would go after his death.

The Jews that we knew at that time, i.e., until the last pre-war years, were family members or friends of our parents and grandparents.

Hobbies

My parents worked hard and I don't remember their hobbies. We walked a lot, hiked in the mountains or went on vacation annually for two weeks at the seaside. We children did a lot of skiing. We were on the trails all the time and became really good skiers. Moreover, we had a rule: at six we learned to swim and at 18 to drive a car. But we were not great sportsmen.

Curiously, the men in our family were musicians. We, of course, studied the piano, my mother, my sister and I, but we were never more than poor performers. My father and my brother loved music and they were better flutists and violinists than we were pianists.

Pre-War Years

Since 1930-32, a few Jewish families had come to the region. They had escaped…not from Nazism, since it was before Hitler's coming to power…but, from the climate in their countries of origin: Poland, Hungary, Czechoslovakia. In general, they were poor people; artisans and factory workers who had come to our area because there were factories. They were more pious than we, but not excessively so.

I suppose the real pious people had not stayed in our area because one could practice one's religion only in a restricted, non-Orthodox, way.

Starting in 1933, a few German Jewish families arrived who had run away from the Nazis. They had lost almost everything. They were merchants, industrialists and professionals.

We helped them a lot, but today it seems to me, in retrospect, that we felt little empathy with their troubles. We were persuaded that they were safe from the minute they set foot in France. Here nothing like that could happen.

And, nevertheless, in 1938 we met a German Jewish family of industrialists. They had lost everything and had started assiduously to build a new life in Grenoble. They were weavers, and taught the French stocking manufacturers the art of elastic threads.

The monsieur, or father of the house, always had had a chauffeur in Germany. In 1938, shortly after Munich, we learned that he had made a wrong turn while driving and that he and his entire family had drowned in the lake. Later, we realized that it had not been an accident but suicide. How could we have prevented this? I often think of them.

My brother had met a nephew of Einstein in school in Grenoble. He trained to become a chef in order to emigrate to America. This also surprised us; were we not secure here in France? That happened in 1937.

The First War Years

And war came, inexorably. We had felt it even at Albertville since Munich. Despair gripped us. I was not yet nineteen, and I was the oldest child of the family. Our friends were mobilized, risking their lives. Since World War I, we had been brought up with the fear of another war. Perhaps, that is why we did not want to see or believe the new one. But, after the despair of the first few months of "quiet" war (if one can call it this), there occurred the catastrophe of defeat. The Germans had invaded France, almost reaching us. But in order to finish France off, the Italians had Allied themselves with the Germans. and thus we were "occupied" by the Italians.

Leaving aside our disgust at their cowardice, the Italian occupation was a smaller evil for us. You could not compare it to the German occupation. Immediately, people arrived in this Italian occupation zone for different reasons; they were refugees, Jews, Germans, anti-Nazis, etc., who wanted to escape the German occupation. They were well received and found lodgings easily. In spite of everything, our region had some cultural distractions and was not overcrowded. Restrictions were felt here less acutely than in the cities.

But the laws that were imposed by the Nazis also contained the statute of the Jews: withdrawing French citizenship from those naturalized less than three years; prohibition to practice certain professions, *numerus clausus* in the universities, etc., etc., and the obligation to declare oneself as a "Jew" at the Police Commissariats. All of this was dangerous, but what could one do?

The Resistance

The Resistance was organized very quickly. First of all, the region lent itself; one could hide in the mountains, sabotaging electrical pylons, railroads or perform other clandestine activities which were less difficult here than somewhere else.

My father was contacted by an envoy of a group called "Liberation Sud" (Liberation of the South). between the end of 1940 and the beginning of 1941. They were looking for a correspondent in Albertville. He had volunteered for this job. But by preference, they chose a Non-Jew who was less exposed in the public eye. Father died in August 1942, but the Resistance functioned perfectly already by that time. My brother and I were "liaison agents" of the Resistance. It was our task to operate as couriers to deliver papers and messages, etc.

The region rapidly became a region of refractoriness for Forced Labor in Germany. The young men joined the maquis. My brother was suddenly forced to stay in one of these maquis.

But we also carried the brunt of these acts of sabotage: the arrest of hostages. At first, foreign Jews were arrested in August 1942. In our region, warned in advance, on the lookout and helped by the population, there were not too many arrests.

Then came individual arrests, either of persons who had been denounced and who were suspected of being resistance fighters or terrorists, or again as hostages.

Without a trial, they were deported or executed.

At the end of 1943, beginning of 1944, the arrests intensified, and so did the acts of sabotage. One could sense the imminent debacle.

One evening, toward the end of February 1944, the secretary of the sub-Prefecture visited us. He had been sent by the sub-Prefect to tell us that the Gestapo had asked for the list of Jews which the sub-Prefect had not relinquished. The Gestapo, however, had managed to obtain the list through other channels. He asked us to warn the refugee Jews in the region whom he did not know, and to advise them to go into hiding.

That's what we did. The population of the region was understanding and compassionate. It was very easy to go into hiding. I was, together with my mother and sister, at friends' not very far from us. My grand-parents stayed with other friends, etc.

Unfortunately, my mother, who was usually quite healthy, fell ill at the friends' house. She did not want to let the doctor come to them. That's why we returned home. She had an ear infection. The doctor, who knew that we should not be at our home, advised us to return to our friends. My mother wanted to wait for her complete recovery. The others, when they heard that we were in our own home, also left their hiding-places. One evening, we had another visit of the envoy of the sub-Prefect who once more reminded us of the risk we were running. We promised to warn everybody and to return into hiding, but we could not do it before the following morning. There was a curfew. One could not go out and we Jews did not have a telephone any longer. The next morning at seven o'clock, we were arrested. It was March 7, 1944.

The arrests were not carried out according to an official list. Some people, for example my grandparents, were overlooked, and others, although they had not been registered, were arrested. We had been given away by a spy. After the war, there was a trial and I appeared as a witness. He was sentenced to life-long imprisonment. I do not know what became of him.

Twenty-five were arrested that day in Albertville. I was the only one who returned.

Prison and Camp

We were first taken to the "Kommandantur" in Albertville and then transferred to the prison in Chambery. There we were kept in cells and condemned to deportation.

I was together with my mother and sister in one cell. My 33 year old aunt was together with her two young sons (five and eleven years old).

Conditions of life were very difficult. We did not leave the cells and it was very cold and damp. Compared to what I later encountered in camp, it was Paradise.

One day, we, the Jews, left our cells. We were transferred to Drancy, the concentration camp for Jews in France. I have a horrible memory of Drancy. It was the antechamber of the camps in Poland. Just as one began to realize this, people fought in order to remain in Drancy. Some of them behaved abominably. Perhaps they were justified, but they probably suffered pangs of conscience later. Nevertheless, it was an unbearable atmosphere.

We stayed at Drancy approximately three weeks. On March 27, 1944, we departed with a transport to Auschwitz. The conditions of the journey were dreadful: freight cars, men and women of all ages mixed, suffocating in the cars, the buckets that spilled their contents of urine and feces on the tiny amount of straw that covered the floor, the saving of the little food we had because we did not know how long the trip would last, etc., etc.

My mother was 46 years old. I saw how her face was deteriorating during the three days and three nights in the car.

We knew that we were going to Poland, but we did not yet know what was in store for us. One morning, we stopped at a sort of station with a sign "Auschwitz." We had heard the name before from the BBC broadcasts which had warned us about this camp in Poland. It was too late.

I encountered the shrieking at the arrival of the train, the beatings because we did not descend fast enough, and I found myself, stunned, with my sister in a small group which the Germans counted and recounted and which had to walk into the camp. We saw our mother climb on a truck. They wanted to spare these people the effort of marching, we understood and believed at the time. Considering the shortness of the distance that separated the "Rampe" (railroad station) from the camp entrance, I was surprised by this exaggerated complaisance, but we were in a secondary state.

When we entered the camp, we were assailed by creatures in rags or in striped prison uniforms who asked us in all European languages, incomprehensible to us, how many we had been when we left Paris and how many at arrival. And, they explained that all those who had not entered the camp had already been reduced to smoke which we saw coming out of the high chimneys a short distance away. They informed us about the gas chamber and the crematoria but we did not want to believe them. Even on location, seeing and feeling everything, one balked at believing the truth. I, myself, refused to accept this truth for several days. It was difficult if one had left a mother of 46.

And then one had to admit it.

And, I'll say something terrible; when I learned about life in Auschwitz-Birkenau and when I finally had to admit my mother's death under the conditions I have described, I did not regret any more that she had been gassed at our arrival. She would not have survived. She had suffered enough already, and finally, it was almost a privilege not to have entered the camp. Auschwitz was monstrous.

Auschwitz-Birkenau

We were in Birkenau, the extermination camp of Auschwitz. I do not want to dwell on living conditions in camp, others have done it already: the lack of hygiene, the lack of food, the incomprehension (we French Jews had never learned Yiddish in our families, where it had not been spoken for several generations) and the Poles, Hungarians and Czechs did not forgive us for this, the waking at dawn, the interminable roll-calls, the inhuman work.

My sister, Janine (not even 19 yet), and I did not have any scientific or medical qualifications that would have permitted us to leave the masses. I had studied law and she had worked as a secretary but did not know German. We were, therefore, put into an Aussenkommando to do very hard outside work.

And, there I passed one of the most difficult times of my deportation. My sister was immediately convinced that none of us would survive, and she would not do anything to prolong life under these conditions. The sooner she would die, the better. The disappearance of our mother and of the rest of our family only reinforced her determination.

Friends helped me and tried to keep up her morale...without success. Moreover, she did not have a chance; she immediately developed enormous abscesses on her hands, her breast, all over. She did not eat any more, and had no strength. (She was very tall, and when she did not work, she was easily visible.) She insisted on going to the hospital, which she should not have done, but one could not prevent her.

At the Revier (hospital), she risked a selection process similar to the one that took place on our arrival, but from here one left for the gas chamber fully aware. She died a natural death before there was any selection. The last day I saw her at the Revier, she was standing naked without a cover and resembled those images of concentration camp prisoners which one saw later. I could not hold back my tears. She was the one who consoled me, telling me, "You know quite well that's what I wanted." She died the morning after our last encounter.

It was July 13, and we had been at Auschwitz a little more than three months. If ever I should get out of this hell, how would I be able to explain to my brother and my grandparents what happened.

Rajsko

Curiously, it was the day following these events that my life changed. I was in such bad physical and moral shape that I didn't believe I would last long. When we were marching out to work, the Kapo of our Kommando had too many women. The same number of people always had to march out. Doubtlessly, our Kapo had recruited too many girls on the "Lagerstrasse" and had a surplus, something which had never happened before. She had pity on me and took me out of the Kommando. I stayed in camp and met a woman from my transport to whom I explained why I was left behind. She told me, "Come with me, they are asking for chemists, and we are going to apply." She was really a chemist, but I was not. She dragged me along, saying that this did not mean anything. There would not be any verification with the declaration we had given upon our arrival in camp; I should just answer the way she did.

Anyway, I was so desperate that I was not afraid of anything; neither punishment, nor selection, nothing at all. And without a fight, luck and chance came to my aid.

Erica had dragged me into this adventure. Of course, there were far more applicants than places. Later, we learned that it concerned replacing the communists at Rajsko whom the Germans were transporting closer to the center of Germany as a result of Soviet advances.

When Hélène Parreaux and Claudette Bloch-Kennedy heard that Birkenau had sent them young French girls, they came to see the candidates. Hélène still tells me today how pitiful I looked with conjunctivitis, wounds on my legs, and that I was nothing but skin and bones. And my morale!! Claudette came to see me at the Pflanzenzucht, where we stayed temporarily.

Claudette Bloch-Kennedy

She was only ten years older than I. But the trials she had endured, and which I had escaped except for the last six months, gave her maturity, whereas I, in spite of my 23 years, still remained a little girl. She had an instantaneous affection for me which I returned, attempting to replace the mother whom I had recently lost.

She interrogated me as to my itinerary, posing profound questions and pondering a lot. I told her everything I have described so far, and Claudette asked herself what she could do to save me: I was not a chemist, had practically no more family, and I did understand her doubts that I might take the place of another one who, perhaps, deserved more of a chance to return home. I did not fight any more, I had become fatalistic: going back, or not going back after what I had seen was of no more importance. Anyway, we had more chances to return to France by staying in Rajsko. There was, of course, no guarantee. This was until I told her that my family and I, myself, had worked for the Resistance, and that my brother was fighting in the Maquis in the Alps.

I had always considered that what I had done for the Resistance was really very minor, missions without risk, or at least I had not been aware of the risk, lighthearted how I had been. On the eve of my arrest, I had gone 10 km on my bicycle to warn a resistance fighter leader of his imminent arrest. I saw him when I returned, tormented by remorse because he had not impressed upon me enough to take care of myself. These missions, this transport as courier of letters and of clandestine newspapers, seemed to me very little. And, nevertheless, that is what weighed in my favor, and thanks to this activity, Claudette could plead my cause. Even today, I often think of this; of causes that have such big effects.

Thus, thanks to Claudette, I remained in Rajsko. Interpreting for me, she succeeded in persuading Dr. Boehm (her worst enemy) of my efficiency and I was installed in Rajsko.

I am not going to talk much about Rajsko, about the work we were supposed to do, but did not. The real scientists will do this better. They had explained the work in Rajsko very superficially to me, about the research of dandelion roots which should furnish latex for the caoutchouc the Germans needed very badly toward the end of the war. I was not impassioned by the scientific aspect of the problem and did not want through assiduous and diligent work to prolong, even for a few minutes, this infamous war. How much trouble we caused Claudette, who was responsible for our work, or rather of our non-work, and had to listen to often well-deserved reproaches.

Life in Rajsko was Paradise after hell. We could wash ourselves and keep ourselves clean. The roll-calls were short and we had time to think, though this may not have always benefited us, and we were able to have friends. I cannot name them all, but I would like to repeat the quasi-filial affection which united me, and always will, with Claudette.

And then, we received news. A male comrade from time to time brought us a newspaper. We followed the retreat of the German Army which had been considered invincible for a long time. I even had the joy at Rajsko of meeting a family friend among the Frenchmen who had been arrested after me and who gave me news about my family. And through him, I met another, the commander of a network, older than us and a Polytechnician, who had been arrested in Lyon and who had been in charge of the Maquis unit in which my brother served. Like my brother, he had heard of our arrest and he knew that at the time of his own arrest, my brother was still in the Maquis.

These two men, unfortunately, did not come back. They died during the evacuation of Auschwitz.

Evacuation of Auschwitz

Rajsko was a small satellite camp which belonged to Auschwitz but was located a few kilometers from the main camp.

Already, since January 16, 1945, rumors had been circulating that Soviet troops were approaching and that the Germans evacuated the camp. That was a good omen. There were many of us who had thought that the camp would be exterminated, but where would we go? At first we believed they had forgotten us at Rajsko, but on January 18, at 6 p.m. we were on the road like all the others. It was -20° celsius in Poland. We were, of course, in better shape than the others, and a little privileged because we were the chemists. Before our departure, bread had been distributed and we risked death by drinking 90 proof alcohol meant for our experiments.

But we were very scantily dressed, and had less adequate footwear than the others. Everything is relative.

We marched 80 km on foot in three days, stopping from time to time for two or three hours in barns. We had to walk without looking right or left. There were corpses all over, men and women. Some probably died a “natural” death.

Others, who could not keep up, were slaughtered by the SS who accompanied us. We were extremely tired. I am certain I slept while walking. We were convinced that we had already encountered the worst, but physically this was even worse. As to our morale, we wondered whither we were marching, how much longer did we have to march, how long would we be able to keep it up before we would finish in the ditches which lined the roadside? And all this at the very moment when the war was coming to an end.

We were again mistaken. After three days of this infernal march, we passed a border and were in Czechoslovakia. We arrived at a railroad station where trains were waiting. We, the "chemists" had the right to a freight car with a roof. The others climbed on flat-bed cars without a roof. With -20° or -30° you really had to be of iron to survive.

Madness spread in the cars. There was no place, and we had not eaten anything for a long time, and where were we going? We traveled for three days, passing Berlin, and finally arrived in Ravensbrueck. We remained outside the camp an entire day, we were too numerous. The Commandant did not want us. In the evening, we finally entered the camp. They had erected giant canvas tents; we were about two thousand in each tent.

But at Ravensbrueck, we also found friends, former Auschwitz inmates who had been evacuated before us, and who had been here for several months. Then there were fortuitous encounters: for example, the nurse from the hospital in Albertville who had been arrested because she had taken care of the members of the Maquis. She recognized me, and called me Mademoiselle Franck. It had been a long time since I had been called this.

Ravensbrueck also signified lice. We had forgotten about them because, at Rajsko, we had disinfectants. But here we were devoured by them, their origin was controversial. The Ravensbrueck administration claimed that we had brought them from Auschwitz, and the Auschwitz prisoners held that we got them in Ravensbrueck. As if this would have been of major importance; but we were pitilessly bitter. And, we did not have the right to wash ourselves.

We remained, I believe, three weeks in Ravensbrueck, and one day in the beginning of February, the "old-timers" of Auschwitz departed. Where to? Who knew? American troops were advancing in the West, Soviet ones in the East. The relatively short journey was made totally in cattle cars. We arrived at a railroad station in Malchow.

Malchow

Malchow is a small town between Schwerin and Neubrandenburg. There was a small camp which was not an extermination camp any longer, no more gas chambers or crematoria. We were in a forest. We saw French prisoners of war passing by. But, soon we realized that they no longer needed the artificial means of extermination. We were going to die of natural causes: hunger. From time to time, they distributed moldy bread which we ate. Even more seldom did we receive soup…made of what? We stole the bones thrown to the dogs for food. Then one of our friends oxidized them and reduced them to powder which we used as medication against our diarrhea.

And there, during our free time spent delousing ourselves, we started to think of possible escape. We were now in Germany, in a small camp, without the organization of Auschwitz and Ravensbrueck. We needed civilian clothes since we were still wearing striped prison uniforms. I was the least clumsy of the group and I was able, more or less, to make some skirts out of blankets. I'll pass over the difficulties of the undertaking, but in order to sew we had to pull threads out of the fabric with only a single needle, among other difficulties. When the skirts were ready, we put them on underneath our dresses. We were so thin that one did not notice the underlying clothing.

One day, I believe it was April 1, 1945, there was a new order; we were leaving Malchow. We put our prepared skirts underneath our dresses, and I don't know why, probably because my skirt was showing, the Camp "Commandant," a superb German woman, gave me the last, and undoubtedly, the most terrible slap in my face I ever got in camp, but she did not take my skirt away.

We were again transported in cattle cars. At the railroad station of Magdeburg, we encountered a terrible air-raid; the bombs fell all around us, but miraculously, our train was not touched and we arrived in Leipzig.

Leipzig

We arrived in a labor camp with many French women who had worked in a factory. But the factories did not exist any more, there was no more raw material. By coincidence, I met a young woman with whom I had celebrated New Year's Eve 1942-43 together with ten other friends at Antibes. We were both surprised to see each other under these circumstances.

We hoped to see the end of the war in Leipzig, but it should not be. On April 13, one could hear American cannons from the West and Soviet cannons from the East. A new order; evacuation of the camp.

We departed, with empty stomachs, for Dresden, on foot of course. Trains were no longer available. Dresden! For us French nationals, we turned East, while liberation was here at our doorsteps. And, again we marched 70 km in two days. But the season was more favorable, it was nice weather and our guards were less eager to kill us than during the evacuation of Auschwitz. Because we were dying of hunger, we ate herbs, and rape flowers. The guards shot into the air to make us return to the ranks. And suddenly, dispersed in a rape field, we perceived that nobody was shooting, our section of the column was not guarded anymore. We had to avail ourselves of the opportunity. We crossed the field and found thirteen of us on the other side on a small road.

We were too numerous and divided ourselves into two groups; each group had to try its luck on its own.

Liberation

It was April 15, 1945. From that day on, luck smiled upon us. We had no major difficulties and were not caught again. French prisoners of war whom we met hid us in barns. The German peasants felt it more advisable to give us shelter and feed us and help us. It was just at the right time. Thus, we lived for about two weeks until the American front arrived. War was still going on. They could not do much for us except provide us with cigarettes and food items when they were available.

We joined the meeting of the American and Russian troops at Torgau. It was joyful for them and for us. We celebrated the event.

Then we were transported to Leipzig, and from there we were repatriated faster than we should have been, thanks to a comrade who had met an acquaintance in the repatriation office.

We again traveled in a cattle car. But this time we were less numerous and in supreme luxury. The floor was covered with straw. The journey from Leipzig to Longuyon, where we were sorted out at our arrival in France, lasted one week. We were together with prisoners of war and were surprised that they were completely ignorant of what had happened to us.

We were happy but restless. Whom would we find at home? And the closer we came to France, the more our restlessness grew.

At Longuyon, I left my friend Claudette. She absolutely wanted me to go to Paris. I, in turn, wanted to give her the chance of finding her young son, whom she had not seen for three years, all by herself; and, in spite of my anguish, I was in a hurry to find out what had happened to my family after my departure.

So, I left in the direction of Dijon, where I met two of my uncles and where I learned that my brother was alive. But he was stationed in Germany since he had joined the regular army after having participated in the battles to liberate the Alps. I found my grandfather, but my grandmother had died of a heart attack at Albertville, practically on the same day her daughter had died in Auschwitz.

Immediate post-war period

Readaptation has been difficult. We arrived in France, which had already been free for several months and, of course, we were happy. We arrived with our terrible memories, with horror stories. There was total incomprehension between those who returned from camp and those who had been fighting in France or in the FFL free from the tribulations of arrest.

They did not believe us, how could they believe us? We who had experienced these events had great difficulties ourselves believing them. I have said it already. How could one believe that young people aged 19, 23, 26, 30 would never come back? How could one believe what really had happened?

I, for my part, found my grandfather an older gentleman of 83, who had already suffered a terrible loss during the war of 1914-18. I was forbidden to tell him what had occurred. They said it might kill him. I obeyed, but nobody thought how it would affect me to play the permanent comedy to let him believe that my mother, my sister, uncles, aunts and cousins would one day return. It was total miscommunication, thus we did not speak to each other and became more reticent.

In this respect, the Nazis carried away the victory. We were not the same any more, and now, even after almost 45 years, we still are not the same.

And, I have to admit that we were difficult to live with. When I had left, I had still been a little girl and I had lived under exceptional conditions. All values such as openness, modesty, and honesty with which I had been brought up, were put into question. We had to try to make the best fit possible between the upbringing we had received and that which we had been forced to learn.

I returned to a family who materially wanted to spoil me, but who morally did not understand me at all. How could one forget? Impossible!

I was in good health. I was an exception, and this was also difficult to admit. How can one be in such extraordinarily good health after so much suffering? I was sent to several specialists to have it confirmed.

I also was lucky being French, thus without any emigration problems, I returned to my home in France. When I came back to Albertville, I was celebrated as a heroine, which I was not; I had just been lucky. But this also seemed suspicious. I had been lucky because I was only 23. Probably, I had used survival techniques in little accordance with the morals I proclaimed. But how could one make these good people understand how we had been humiliated; how our torturers rejoiced when they saw us argue over a sip of soup; with how much disdain we had been treated; that our guards walked around while we were naked like a herd of cows. And that our physical aspect (our looks) had played no role whatsoever in our survival, so much less so since we had rapidly lost this physical aspect after our arrest, only to regain it quickly after our liberation.

Post-Auschwitz

Finally, my brother was demobilized and we decided to live together in Albertville. My parents' apartment existed, but was completely empty. Friends lent us furniture and linen.

And, we had practically never worked before, not my brother and not I. We recovered a store equally completely empty, as well as employees who were faithful and attached to us. They depended on us for their livelihood. We felt indebted to them. So we both went to work without enthusiasm and without much fervor. I could have finished my law studies; in my case it would have been only a formality. France offered us examinations. But this would have meant that my brother would have had to take care of my upkeep; I could not stand that idea. And what would that have changed?

My brother understood me well, but he was a shy young man, rather reserved, and had been deeply touched by losing what he held dearest in life. He listened to my tales without asking any questions or making any comments. Today, I still believe he is certain that, if he would have been together with us, he would have succeeded in avoiding the arrest of our family.

Then I got married. My husband was a childhood friend whom I found again very shortly after my return. He always understood me very well. He spoke, asked questions, listened and was silent when it was necessary. He accepted my friends like his own. I believe, without modesty, that he was a very good husband.

Different trials were waiting for us. We lost three of the four children whom we had great difficulties in having. The shared grief drew us closer together. But, we had immense satisfaction with the daughter who remained, we accepted her with great joy. She was a brilliant student, and both of us had every reason to be proud of her.

Now, she herself has two children who are my joy and my raison d'etre because I suffered another terrible blow; my husband died of a heart attack which came without warning when he was only 56 years old.

At that time, I almost cracked up myself. It was too much. When I was younger, I had the strength to fight to survive. My life seemed definitely finished, useless. Now, I was not so young any more. But, in the last analysis, one is always indispensable to somebody. My old aunt, whom I had found when I returned from Auschwitz, was still alive and needed me. My daughter and my grandchildren needed me also. I survived.

And thus, in conclusion, I have to blame the deportation for everything which I have said so far. But, in spite of everything, there are some positive points such as a new value scale, primordial qualities: truth, generosity and just causes. I continue to fight for truth, individual human rights, brotherhood and, naturally, anti-racism. Politics interest me also, though less than before.

On the other hand, I am tolerant of religion, no matter which one, for others, but I, for myself, don't want to hear about it. Life in Auschwitz has been for some among us a test of strength, a test which, no doubt, we had to endure. For me that has been a complete and irreversible detachment, there is no God who can permit Auschwitz.

Well, that's the gist of what I had to say and write. After 43 years, it was the first time that I dared to make such a profound analysis. It has not been easy.

❖

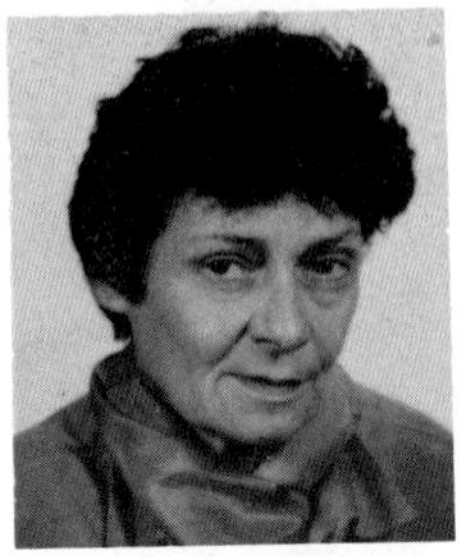

Madeleine (Jacqueline) Odru (née Dissoubray)

Montreuil (France)

I was born on November 25, 1917, in Morienne (Seine Maritime) and grew up in Aumale and Rouen. My father was an agronomist.

I completed my studies to be a high school teacher but taught only a short time since, in 1941, I decided to put myself entirely at the disposal of the resistance movement. I participated in the first organized sabotage activities of the secretariat of the communist section of Rouen.

On February 20, 1942, I was arrested. A policeman equipped with a special pass-sign (for example a torn postcard of which two persons each have one half...probably confiscated from a comrade who was arrested earlier) presented himself at my apartment where I lived under a false name. I did not suspect anything, and just told him, "Make yourself at home and wait for me. I'll be back in a short while. I have to see somebody." The so-called comrade had posted his colleagues outside. As soon as I met my contact person, we were both arrested.

I was transferred to Paris and imprisoned in the disciplinary section of the jail, doubtlessly because I had attempted to escape several times during the arrest and while being transferred from Rouen to Paris. On August 24, 1942, I was sent to the fortress of Romainville from where I was deported on January 24, 1943 along with 229 French women of the resistance, as hostages, to Birkenau.

Conditions in Birkenau were indescribably horrible. After all our belonging had been taken away, our heads shaved and our arms tattooed (my number was 31660), we were given some thin, dirty, lice-infested clothes, and finally led to our block where we slept on the bare floor. There was very little food and no water at all, either for drinking or washing, so that after a few days a dreadful stench emanated from us. Typhus and dysentery were rampant in camp and the latrines, which were surrounded by seas of excrement, could be used only at certain times. Thus, feces were everywhere, running down our legs, in containers meant for receiving our watery soup once a day, and in the bunks where we lay down to sleep. In addition we endured the constant beatings and long roll-calls that lasted for many hours in the bitter cold, during which women fainted and were later carted off to Block 25, the antechamber of the crematorium.

In the beginning, I did "Aussenarbeit," hard work outside the camp. At the end of February, or beginning of March 1943, I was recruited as laboratory technician for work in Rajsko and was transferred to the Stabsgebaeude. Hygienical conditions were much better here. I received clean clothes and even a pair of passable shoes, and although I still had fleas and lice I, at least, could take a shower every evening. Shortly after my arrival, I fell ill with typhus, from which I recovered very slowly. Life in the Stabsgebaeude was much less rigorous than at Birkenau. One risked less beatings here and the roll-calls were held indoors and were much shorter.

Here I met Claudette Bloch, a French Jewess who was responsible for the laboratory at Rajsko, as well as the other Jewish prisoners who spoke French and belonged to the same kommando with whom we formed a solidarity group.

Every day we went to work in Rajsko. We had a clean and heated laboratory. Working conditions here were infinitely better than at Birkenau where we had been working outside in the cold, snow and rain on a daily basis. Finally, when the installations for our lodging...which had been under construction...were completed, we moved to Rajsko. There were eight French women from our transport of January 24, 1943 among us.

Our work consisted of the following: It was our task to find the means to manufacture caoutchouc from latex found in a sort of dandelion plant. There was a chemistry laboratory and a botanical laboratory. I worked in the latter. There were hothouses and outside plantations of dandelion. In my laboratory, we prepared cross-sections of the roots which we examined under the microscope in order to select those plants that were richest in caoutchouc according to different modes of cultivation, different seasons and different selection of grains. We organized sabotage by giving incorrect information or by sabotaging the selection. A German specialist, who supervised our work for some time, never discovered what we were doing.

We also had to supervise, irrigate and maintain the plantations. Thus, we had access to the greenhouses and the gardens where vegetables and fruit trees were growing. In spite of the fact that the camp was surrounded by watch towers and the risks of being discovered by the Germans who guarded the kommandos, we succeeded in stealing practically every day in order to improve our diet.

On the other hand, this allowed us to encounter male prisoners who came daily from Auschwitz to work in the garden. I was responsible for the liaison with a responsible French communist. We received news of the war developments. We pondered the question of finding means to liberate the camp in a propitious moment.

Like the other French women of my transport who survived (49 out of 230), I owe my return to France to the marvelous solidarity that we had organized. We formed special groups for this purpose. In Rajsko, we were (without counting myself) 3 French communists from my transport, four French Jewesses, two Polish Jewesses, two Czechoslovakian Jewesses and one Polish communist. The only criterion to belong to the group was to rigorously practice the solidarity of sharing everything honestly and helping each other. We equally practiced this mutual solidarity with the French male prisoners who came to work in Rajsko, and with a kommando of French women prisoners who also commuted to work there.

On August 14, 1944, the eight French women of my transport who worked in Rajsko (including myself) were transferred to Ravensbrueck. In February 1945, I was in a women's transport that was sent from Ravensbrueck to Mauthausen. We were the only women in this men's camp. All the French women were liberated on April 22, 1945, by the Red Cross and we were returned to France after some transit in Switzerland.

After the war, I continued my activities in the departmental secretariat of the Union of French Women; in the federal office of the communist party of the province of Seine-Maritime; and later in Paris as instructor for the Union of French Women and as vocational counsellor for scholastic and professional education.

At present, I am retired from secondary education, married and have two children. My son is an engineer and my daughter is a veterinarian.[14]

❖

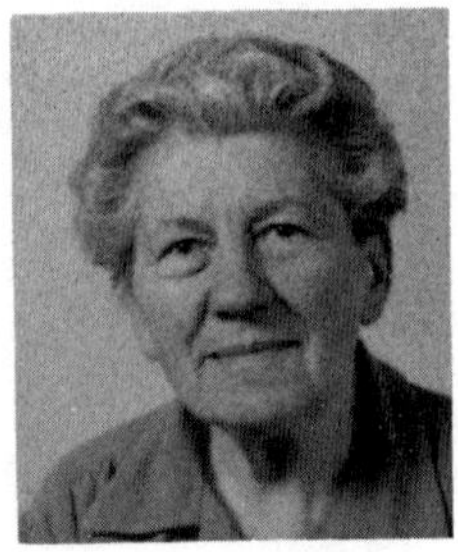

Hélène Parreaux (Widowed Solomon, née Langevin)
Paris (France)

I was born on May 25, 1909, in Fontenay-aux-Roses and was brought up in Paris together with my sister and two brothers. My father, Paul Langevin, professor at the College de France, was a well-known physicist and member of the Academie des Sciences.[15]

I attended elementary school in the rue Monge, then I went to the Lycee Fenelon, where I received my high school diploma. In 1929, I married Jacques Solomon, who was in charge of research at the Centre National de la Recherche Scientifique.

My father, Paul Langevin, aged 68 at that time, was arrested at his home on October 30, 1940, by Boemelburg, Speidel's[16] adjutant, and imprisoned in the Sante. Protests and student demonstrations on November 8, 1940, in front of the College de France, demanding "Liberez Langevin" must have provided food for thought to the Germans, who released him on December 15, 1940, and placed him under house arrest in his residence at Troyes.

In 1942, my husband and I belonged to the Front National Universitaire...the editors of l'Universite Libre...which had appeared since November 1940 and which had already published 50 pamphlets. "On Freedom of Thought" was in preparation when we were both arrested.

Jacques Solomon was arrested on March 1, 1942, in Paris. He had been tailed by policemen of the special guard since Georges Politzer's arrest on February 14, 1942. I was arrested the following morning when I was about to pick up a suitcase which I had checked the previous evening in order to make an emergency switch of apartment because of the multiple arrests in our group which had taken place during the last two weeks.

After a few days in the general investigation office, I was taken to the Depot and stayed from March 10 until March 23, 1942. Subsequently, I was at the Sante until August 24, 1942, and later at Romainville.

My husband was shot on May 23, 1942. I had the opportunity of saying goodbye to him at the Sante. I was deported with the convoy of January 24, 1943, and arrived in Auschwitz on January 27, where I received the prison number of 31,684.[17]

At the beginning of February 1943, an SS-guard mustering our ranks during roll call asked if there were biologists and chemists among us. Along with four others, I reported and on March 21, 1943, I was sent to the Stabsgebaeude in order to join the kommando Pflanzenzucht. In July 1943 we were transferred to the newly built barracks in Rajsko. Here I worked in the company of Claudette Bloch-Kennedy and Marie-Elisa Nordmann-Cohen in the laboratory, investigating the Kok-Saghyz plant. Our Rajsko group of French political prisoners was transferred to Ravensbrueck on August 14, 1944.

I left Ravensbrueck in the autumn of 1944, along with a convoy of Polish women arrested by the Germans after the insurrection of Warsaw. I was separated from my comrades and it was very hard for me. We were the survivors of a group, united before our arrest by identical Resistance activities; we then suffered the same tribulations (French "Depot" in the caves of the "Conciergerie", quai de l'Horloge, Paris) from where the French police which had previously arrested us delivered us to the German police. Then, Prison de la Sante (Paris), Fort de Romainville, Camp de Royallieu (Compiegne). Thus, in the autumn of 1944 I went on a transport as a nurse. Other nurses and a doctor were expected to be at the small station of Dreillinden when we arrived. We got out there and walked to a big factory nearby; it was guarded like a fortress and divided into big shops hidden, as best as possible, under the trees of a huge park. In the park there was an enclosure of electrified barbed wire which isolated one of the big shops, where we were expected.

I was horrified when I discovered that I was, temporarily, the one and only medical attendant available on the spot. I was supposed to organize an infirmary; it was totally devoid of any surgical implements or medicines. One of the SS who accompanied the convoy, when he saw my horror, took me to the central infirmary of the factory. There, a kind and portly nurse helped me find my way through the German technical vocabulary, of which I was totally ignorant.

I went back to the small camp where I was staying, equipped with the minimal necessities, to try and disinfect the aftereffects of our railway transport. Fortunately, a Yugoslavian woman doctor and two nurses arrived a few days later. Later on, a Polish woman dentist was added, equipped with a dentist's mill. It made me think of an old sewing machine when I was a child.

That winter was very severe, but we heard the Russian cannons come nearer and nearer. So did the Allied bombings, which became more precise and frequent...we were extremely close to Berlin. The only place where we could hide was a cellar underneath the workshop. The walls and the floor vibrated every time there was an explosion until the day when all the windows and the power plant itself collapsed so that no one could work any more.

A few days later (in the beginning of April) we were evacuated toward the camp of Sachsenhausen, situated at Oranienburg, from which we were administratively dependent. There, the different "nationalities" were segregated from each other and I arrived in a hut where I knew no one but where I found some French and Belgian women. There was some heavy bombing, and the next day I heard that some huts had been destroyed and prisoners killed.

Berlin was very close by and the Red Army was victoriously finishing the siege. The camp of Sachsenhausen was evacuated...men first, then women. Everyone was walking in a file along the roads, guarded by SS. They gave us some "camp bread" and a slice of "paté"...the ration for three days...and a gray blanket. It is impossible to describe the horror of this march to nowhere where the password was: no stragglers!

That's the reason why, almost immediately after our departure, we started to see corpses in the ditches. They had a bullet in the head and a blanket had been thrown over them.

Of course, very soon we were left with nothing to eat (it snowed on the First of May, 1945) and we suffered from the cold and exhaustion. Sometimes we stopped in one of those huge barns of Northern Germany, and sometimes some straw was left.

When we had to walk at night, we saw on our right the light of Russian cannons, on our left the Allied ones; they kept us company because they heralded our liberation.

We heard the cannons come nearer and nearer. We had stayed in a swampy wood under an icy rain for a day and a night without anything to eat. At dawn, we discovered that the SS who were guarding us had disappeared.

With some difficulty, we managed to get to the nearest farm, where we found a barn with some straw. There, the women who couldn't walk any more were able to lie down. Immediately after that, we met French prisoners of war who took care of us, and we went to the Red Army "Kommandantur"...the Red Army had just freed us.

An officer offered us the choice: we could stay with the Red Army and go back home through the U.S.S.R., but in that case, it might take us about a month to get back to France. Moreover, we would then have to go across some countries which had been totally devastated by recent battles. There was another solution; we could wait until the Allied Forces and the Red Army had met and then cross the bridge made of boats which enabled people to cross the Elbe. So, we couldn't cross that bridge until May 8, 1945, and even then we were taken by trucks along the few roads that had been cleared by mine-sweepers. It was, of course, better not to stray from the indicated path. One of the trucks in our convoy was delayed. It took a shortcut and exploded on a mine.

We arrived at the Dutch border, where we boarded a train. It crossed the Netherlands...they had been devastated, especially the harbor of Rotterdam. It was nearly annihilated. Then we took another train. It went to Lille, where we arrived on May 15, 1945.

In Lille I went through extremely tedious repatriation formalities...receipt of wardrobe, identity card and reparation premium (200 marks). I succeeded in phoning my parents, who were in Paris at the Gare du Nord when I arrived the next morning, provoking a small incident...I had taken a gray Luftwaffen coat and German military boots because it had been so cold.

We had survived and were now free at last, and so exalted by our joy that...at that moment...we did not yet feel the consequences of our ordeal.

How did I readjust to post-war (normal) life? With great difficulty! In the beginning, I thought I could do everything at the same time...study, militant activity (work for our cause), work, etc. I was elected member of the Assemblee Nationale (the French Congress or Parliament) in October 1945 and was re-elected in June 1946, but I was exhausted by the night sessions and the campaigns in the provinces, and had to give up running for re-election in November 1946. After several months of medical care and some recuperation in Switzerland, I entered as a part-time tenured technician at the C.N.R.S. (Centre Nationale de la Recherche Scientifique). Only in 1952 was I capable of working full-time. In 1958 I remarried.

For all these years I have been suffering from severe asthenia (great fatigueability), cervical and lumbar arthrosis and decalcification. These conditions are getting more and more acute as time goes on.

❖

CHAPTER FIVE
Kok-Saghyz Cultivation

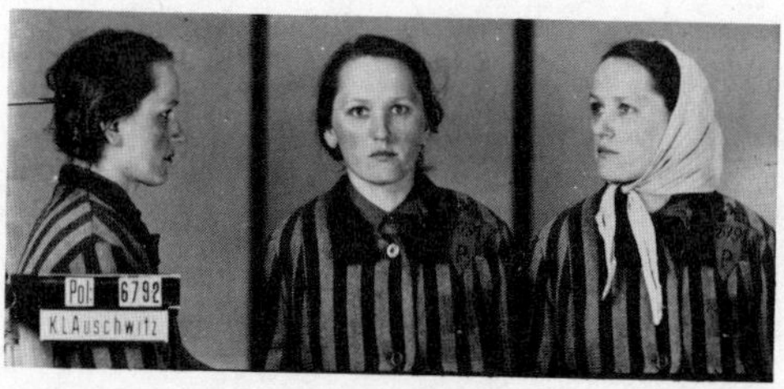

Jozefa Kiwalowa (née Kaleta)
Cracow (Poland)

My Auschwitz number was 6792. After the relocation of the women's camp from Auschwitz to Birkenau on August 6, 1942, I was sent to Block 12, a wooden barrack.

In the women's camp in Auschwitz, I already used to go with the "kommando" SS-Waescherei (laundry detail) to the Stabsgebaeude, located outside the camp in one of the buildings of the tobacco monopoly. The kommando had 40 prisoners and the kapo was a German inmate called Frieda.

For three weeks, we walked every day from Birkenau, accompanied by an SS-guard. At the end of August 1942, we were transferred to the Stabsgebaeude. We lived in the cellar where the SS-Waescherei was. In the first room on the right were the big tubs with cold water for soaking the dirty clothes. The next hall was the ironing place which was later divided to provide a room for drying. Across the stairs, there were a sewing room to mend clothes, underwear and socks as well as another wash room with tubs. On the left-hand side were the place to rinse and also the actual laundry. There were huge pots, similar to the ones you cook food in. There the clothes were boiled. Under the side staircase, in a narrow space divided by a wall, were two washrooms and toilets for prisoners. On the other side of the staircase was a room for the SS-Aufseherinnen on duty and a narrow place with showers for the SS. Sometimes we used to sneak in and take a shower when nobody was watching. On the opposite side of the cellar were our sleeping quarters. There was even a little Revier (hospital) for the inmates. The physician was Dr. Janina Aydukiewicz Kosciuszkowa, a Polish prisoner.

Forty women worked in the kommando SS-Waescherei and SS-Naehstube, eight of them were Polish:

Wanda Blachowska-Tarasiewicz #6883
Zofia Augustyn-Pajerska #6884
Irena Glowacka-Zakrzewska
Eleanore Piekosz
Zofia Dyl
Zofia Kranz
Janina Klich
and myself.

All these women were from the Tarnow transport, i.e., all having prison numbers in the six-thousand range except myself who had come from Cracow on the same day. The German women had black triangles (characterizing them as "Asoziale"), only Frieda was a political prisoner.

The clothes we washed were the personal clothes and bed linen of the SS and of the Aufseherinnen. I remember the names written under the shirt collars:

Palitzch, Stiewitz, etc. Before the division was constructed in the ironing room to create a dry-dock, other prisoners used to come to dry the clothes outside while the blouses of the Aufseherinnen were dried in the attic.

In the beginning, I worked exclusively in the washrooms, but in January 1943, I was moved to the ironing room.

The roll-calls took place in the hallway at 6 a.m. and 6 p.m; but we worked until late at night. Our food was brought from the men's camp in Auschwitz. We did not leave the premises of the Stabsgebaeude.

Milan and Franz were our Blockfuehrerinnen. Sometimes we took their laundered clothes to their rooms. Their rooms upstairs were at the entrance of a big auditorium. I heard that there was a "rusznikarnia" on the first floor.

Jewish prisoners from Slovakia also lived with us. They worked in offices, such as the camp administration and the political section of the camp. I remember Vera, now Plaskura, and Lilli Toffler, a Slovakian Jewess who was shot in Block 11 because she was caught with "gryps."

There were also five Polish women prisoners who had come with a transport from Ravensbrueck about May 1942, and whose Auschwitz numbers were around seven thousand. They were the first members of the future Pflanzenzucht in Rajsko. Wanda Dulczynska,[1] Maria Raczynska, Emilia Gastkowska and two who died of typhus and whose names I do not remember. They were engineers and agronomists.

Zdzislaw Palasiuski, a chimney cleaner, who also was working in Birkenau used to come at times to the Stabsgebaeude and through him we kept in contact with our girlfriends in Birkenau.

On May 8, 1943, we received an order stating that all Polish women had to leave the Stabsgebaeude. From work...we could hardly take our personal belongings...we were taken to the women's camp in Birkenau. At the gate, we were met by SS-man Taube and taken to Block 7 whose block elder was Stenia Starosta.

We attempted to be admitted to the kommando Pflanzenzucht since we had been together with some of the veteran members of this work detail in the Stabsgebaeude and we had connections to get into the kommando Gaertnerei in Rajsko. On the first day we came to work, Wanda Dulczynska, the kapo of the Pflanzenzucht, took us into her group. Thus, when we returned to Birkenau in the evening, we were already bona fide members of the kommando Pflanzenzucht. Every morning we marched out to work in Rajsko and returned in the evening to the women's camp in Birkenau until we were permanently transferred to the newly constructed barracks in Rajsko on June 13, 1943. The Gaertnerei (gardening) grew vegetables for the SS and the Pflanzenzucht (plant cultivation) cultivated the Kok-Saghyz plant.

There was a Geraetehaus (tool shed) where the tools were kept, handed out and fixed. It also contained wooden signs for the plants and other items. When we arrived, work was in process to enlarge the existing hothouse near the school building for the Pflanzenzucht and to construct a new hothouse, part of which was designed exclusively for the cultivation of Kok Saghyz; the prisoners were also tending the beehives.

The main camp consisted of five barracks: two with windows to live in; one for the kommando Gaertnerei and for the Pflanzenzucht; one barrack was the kitchen, one was for washing ourselves and one was the toilet.

In addition, there was an Arbeitsbaracke (work barrack). It contained a kitchen to boil the Kok-Saghyz seeds; the Schuettelmaschine (shaking machine) to extract the gum (rubber), analytical scales and a special room to count the seeds.

The camp area was fenced in with single wire without electrical current. There were reflectors on the fence posts but no guards were on duty. However, during the day while we worked in the fields, the large Postenkette (sentry chain) was in place on the hills on the way to Birkenau and around our work area. After the evening roll-call and until morning, SS-men patrolled outside the fence and the camp area.

The order of the day was as follows:

Up at 5 a.m.; washing, making beds and eating breakfast. The morning roll-call was at 6 a.m. and afterward we worked until noon. We returned to camp for lunch and from 1 p.m. till 6 p.m. we went back to work. Then there was the evening roll-call in camp and afterward we received dinner. At 9 p.m. the lights went out. During the winter, we worked till dark.

The high season of the Pflanzenzucht was from October to December, and we worked in three shifts of 8 hours each to separate the Kok-Saghyz seeds. The work in the Pflanzenzucht was experimental and intended to cultivate plants whose extract could be used for the production of caoutchouc.

The plants were sowed in the winter from seeds selected the previous year. Each seed had a separate planter and was under constant observation with strict record keeping. In the spring, each plant was taken out and planted in the field. Each woman prisoner had to take care of one thousand plants. Each plant had a sign and was properly numbered; for example, one inmate had from 1000-1999, the next from 2000-2999, etc. In our records we noted, for each of the 1000 seedlings, the exact date when the leaves appeared, the size of the leaves, the appearance of the flowers, the size and quantity of the flowers and when they started to seed. The seeds from each plant were placed into separate little sacks and numbered.

While the plants were growing and before they started to bloom, our supervisor, SS-officer Dr. Schattenberg, would select some plants. These were then separated in a wooden frame, covered with cheese-cloth or glass, so that they had a chance for better growth and would not be pollinated with pollen from inferior plants. The selected plants were pollinated by hand with a brush dipped in alcohol after each plant. For this purpose, each woman had a little bottle of alcohol. If nobody was looking, we did not dip the brush every time. We used to keep the alcohol for making "kogel-mogel" for a birthday party.

After we collected the seeds from each plant, we put them into separate sacks, each properly numbered and recorded. In October, we dug up the roots, cleaned sand from them and marked them with signs and numbers.

After approximately two to three weeks, when they had dried, they were put into boxes ready for the separation process in the fall. In order to determine the amount of rubber in the roots, we had to cut up the roots lengthwise, weigh and number them and place them in glass tubes filled with a liquid. They were then put into water-filled pots in a certain way so that they would not touch each other, and boiled in the working barrack in camp. After about 20 minutes, they were taken to the Schuettelmaschine in the next room where the back and forth shaking motion separated the rubber from the roots. Next, the glass tubes were taken to another room where the percentage of rubber for each tube was established and recorded according to number. The purpose of this procedure was to select specimen with the highest amount of rubber. These seeds were used for the following year's crop.

The rest of the roots from which the samples with the largest quantity of rubber had been taken were sent to I.G. Farben in Dwora for the production of synthetic rubber. In the laboratory, there was a big tire made of this rubber.

In the main laboratory, there was also a photography room. Here, pictures were taken of the different stages of the cultivation of Kok-Saghyz. Wanda Jakubowska and a French Jewess worked in the photographic laboratory.

A copy of Jakubowska's original photo is shown in the appendix. It was smuggled out by Anton Mencher of Wilczkowic, a civilian employee. It shows Kok-Saghyz plants in a box in a stage of pollinating.

Quite frequently, there were inspections by the SS or by civilians to observe the experimental cultivation of Kok-Saghyz. The guides were usually SS Obersturmbannfuehrer Dr. Caesar, the head of the department, and Dr. Schattenberg.

The instructors for the cultivation of the plants were Russians: Popow, Nikitin, Zasmuzec and a certain doctor who always worked alone. They lived with their families in houses in the village of Rajsko. They supervised us at work and were friendly but afraid to have any contact with us.

Caesar was in charge of the kommando Pflanzenzucht and of the cultivation of Kok-Saghyz. He took care of the women prisoners and provided more favorable conditions compared to conditions in Birkenau. We had better food, clean clothing, change of bed linen, heavy blankets from "Canada" and white aprons. His main interest was precise and accurate work. The women workers had to have a secondary school education. He gave us more freedom and a better work environment. In time we were no longer so disciplined.

For the dirty and hard work, such as digging and clearing the roots, women from Kommando 11 in Birkenau used to come to Rajsko. Thanks to our freedom, everything worked out all right...but that brought us in conflict with SS-man Grell of the Gaertnerei.

In the beginning, there were 80 women in the kommando Pflanzenzucht, but with time the number reached 150. One-third of them, including myself, grew and took care of the plants throughout the cycles...from the time of planting to the selection process. After that we were busy counting the seeds and packing them into bags. Part of the women prisoners worked in the main laboratory. They all had diplomas in chemistry, biology, pharmacology or agriculture. A large group of them was from the Sorbonne in France.

Some women worked with us in the hothouses. In the old as well as in the new hothouse, there was another SS-man whose name I do not remember. He worked under Dr. Schattenberg and we called him "dziurawiec" (hole-man) because he had a hole in the bone of his forehead.

In addition, there was SS-man Lettmann, who used to take our group to Auschwitz when we took the clothes and aprons to be washed at the SS-Unterkunft or when we had to see a dentist.

The supervisor of the laboratory was a German civilian woman called Weimann. She married Caesar after his wife had died from typhus.

The Aufseherinnen in Rajsko were Bormann and Cichon. In 1944, SS-women Hasse, Franz and Orlowska were alternately on duty.

In the beginning, our block elder was a German prisoner called Elsa. In 1943 came Gerda Schneider, who liked to hit everybody in the face. In 1944 she was sent to Birkenau for punishment. In her place came Dana, a Yugoslavian woman. One of our "sztubowas" (room servant) was Ludwika Makuch from Bialy Dunajec.

The kapo of the Pflanzenzucht was...as already mentioned...Wanda Dulczynska. On June 23, 1944, after a big search during which they discovered and transported three trucks with illegal used clothing to Birkenau, Dulczynska was taken and sent to the punishment company. From there she was transferred to Ravensbrueck after a month.[2] We did not get a new kapo.

We constantly had contact with the free world by correspondence. Sometimes a few dozen letters used to come at once. The "mail box" was in the old hothouse under a planter. The letters were taken and delivered by Anton Mencner[3] from Wilczkowic, a civilian employee with a green armband who used to work nearby. He probably was a Volksdeutscher (ethnic German) who knew some SS-men and who used to come to the hothouse under the pretext of buying flowers. Thanks to him, we were able to send letters out of camp and to receive answers. Often, he went to Cracow to deposit and receive letters for us. The contact place was Mrs. Cjankiewicz' store in Cracow. There never was a problem. We received letters until January 18, 1945, the day Auschwitz was evacuated.

In Rajsko, our group also had a cultural life. On the occasion of every holiday, we had a play. On Christmas, we had a Christmas tree and a festive supper. We had combined all the packages we had received from home. We also performed a three-act play written by Zofia Grochowalska on a religious theme. We even made costumes for the actors. On Christmas 1944, we had a puppet show and on New Year's 1944 we had a French play by Moliere, "The Holy Women." Claudette, a French woman, remembered the entire script by heart and put it together. On Christmas we used to dance our folk dances in costumes, the polonaise and the Mazurka, and we invited our friends from the Gaertnerei.

On January 18, 1945, we left the camp. In the morning, Caesar had ordered us to shut off the water in the installation of the hothouses because of the frost. We were busy doing that until the afternoon. At 5 P.M. we were evacuated in the direction of Pszczyna. At 10 P.M. we arrived in Jastrzebia Gorny and were put into a big warehouse for the night. The next morning, when we got our marching orders, Irene Glowacka-Zakrzewska, Aurelia Piekosz and I hid in the attic underneath the straw. However, many more women were hiding like us and when they started to count and discovered that so many were missing, the SS went looking in the building. At that moment, we heard screams in the attic where we were hiding. The SS discovered my friend Zakrzewska and me. We ran out, but Piekosz...probably confused...was still lying under the straw and the SS-men killed her with bayonets. We took advantage of the confusion and ran after the transport to fall in line with them. While we ran we noticed a horse and wagon on the road and a kapo standing next to it. When he saw us he asked us where we were going. We did not answer since we saw two SS-men leading one of our friends and killing her on the road. We turned around to run back, but there was no chance to return to the buildings from which we heard constant firing and screaming. When we passed the kapo again we noticed that he motioned us to go to the side. Not thinking if the SS-men who were walking toward the wagon would notice us, we jumped to the side and slipped under a sled and some machines. Then we ran to the back of the warehouse. We saw a big pile of compost and a herd of cows which was evacuated from Babice. The cows were looked after by some Ukranian women prisoners. Without thinking, we hid under the pile of compost. One of the women saw us and threw some more compost over us. We lay there for a long time. When we crawled out from underneath the compost, it was night. Everything was quiet and deserted. Slowly, we started to walk in the direction of the houses that we saw from afar. We knocked at the door of one of them and they took us in. We remained in hiding until March 25, 1945, the day the Russian army came to Jastrzebia.[4]

❖

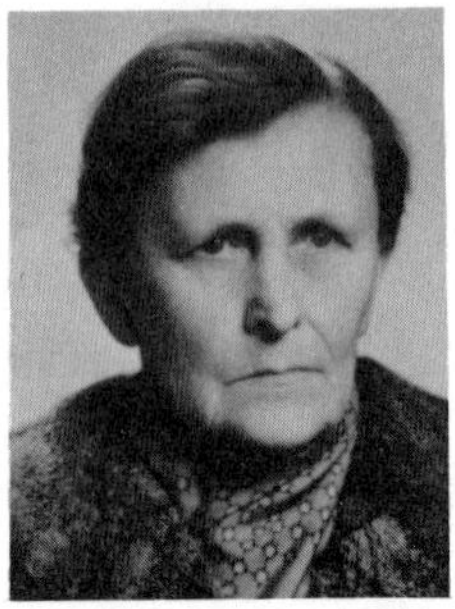

Zofia Abramowiczowa
(widowed Grochowalska, née Bolechowska)
Warsaw (Poland)

I was born on December 1, 1902 at the manor house Czerwonka powiat Sochaczew, owned by my maternal grandmother Garbolewska. My parents were Stefania Garbolewska and Boleslaw Bolechowski. My ancestors on both sides of the family belonged to titled gentry and were land owners, i.e., my grandparents and their grandparents before them owned large estates. The different manors were in the hands of the descendants until 1945 when the land was nationalized, and the previous owners were not allowed to stay in the districts in which their former properties had been located.

My parents were well educated. My mother spoke French fluently and my father had finished his studies in biology at the university of Cracow. My uncle had studied mechanics at Liege in Belgium. All were active in the public sector during the first years of Poland's independence after the first World War. Two of my uncles had been in General Holler's army during the war of 1914-1918, and my grandfather's brother had been killed in 1863 during the resurrection against the Russian occupation.

I was brought up in Kownaty, my father's manor. My four sisters, my brother and I received an excellent education. In Kownaty, we children had private teachers, a French mademoiselle who taught us French, and later a German

Fraeulein for the German language. From 1916 onward, I attended the Hralianka Plater school in Warsaw, and from 1919, the national school in Lomza. The graduation certificate of such a school entitled any graduate to pursue studies at the university level.

However, I did not study...instead, I became a primary school teacher in a rural school after having obtained my teaching credentials. My teaching career did not last very long. Soon I returned home and was busy with managing the house and the garden because my mother was living in Lomza with my brother and my younger sisters. I was home with father, who had returned from a camp in Ekaterinburg, Siberia. He had been taken prisoner by the Soviet cavalry general Gaj on his march to Warsaw in 1920. After 15 months of captivity, he had come back without any teeth, all lost due to scurvy. The cause of his deportation, according to Gaj's arrest warrant, had been "bourgeois exploiter."

In October 1931, I married Wladyslaw Grochowalski, a graduate of S.G.G.W., i.e., an agricultural university. He was an engineer in ichthyology. We had acquired some land in the district of Suwalki; our farm was called Pojezierze. On August 30, 1939, my husband, a reserve officer, was mobilized and went to war. At the end of September, he was taken prisoner by the Soviet Army in Lvov and held at Starobielsko. On April 1, 1940, he was taken to Katyn and murdered by the Soviets.

Together with Bronislaw Czarnocki, I traveled to Lithuania. At night we attempted to cross the border between Poland and Lithuania. It was November 1, 1939. We had been sent by Stanislaw Bielicki, the leader of the underground movement in the district of Suwalki, to the French consul in Kowno. Unfortunately, the Lithuanian border police arrested us. After a week, they handed Bronislaw over to the German border station. I was set free at the border at night after ten days.

On April 7, 1940, I was arrested by gendarmes in my home on orders of the Gestapo and charged with having offended the German Army. At first, I was taken to Gestapo headquarters in Suwalki, then to prison and later, for two weeks, to the transit camp Dzialdowo. Many people were arrested on the same day. The Germans had a list of members of the Polish intelligentsia: teachers, doctors, judges, land owners, priests, officers, et al, whom they merely suspected of resistance activities. If somebody claims he or she was arrested because of membership in an underground organization, they seldom tell the truth. Organization members were usually arrested on other grounds and sent to concentration camps. If, after some months or even years, the Gestapo discovered that they had been members of an underground movement, they were investigated or even returned to prison. People arrested for participating in A.K. (Armja Krajowa, a Polish partisan organization) went to prison, were tortured and executed, or were sent to concentration camps with specific death sentence instructions.

On May 8, 1940, I was sent to Ravensbrueck concentration camp, together with fourteen other women. There, I received the prison number 3499. At the beginning of 1942, a Gestapo official from Suwalki came to interrogate me in Ravensbrueck. He questioned me about members of the underground. Somebody in Suwalki had been recently arrested and must have revealed something. The other woman, Lucja Brenneisen, who was also interrogated on the same subject died after three days.

I was brought to Auschwitz from Ravensbrueck in June of 1942, in a group of twenty-five women prisoners. We were to work in the vegetable gardens or in the kok-saghyz (taraxacum kok-saghyz) experimental fields. The Germans had selected women with several years of experience in agriculture or graduates of well-known agricultural schools to work there.

SS-woman Langefeld, who admitted us to Auschwitz, asked whether we had any experience in agriculture. One woman, who was German, said that we had no experience. Therefore, we were sent to a regular block. I do not know why that German woman was in our group, or why I, trained in that Ravensbrueck rigor, did not object at that time.

We were in one of several blocks that were set aside for women in the men's camp in March of 1942. Our group was one of the first Polish women prisoners who were brought there. The month of March 1942 had been the beginning of the women's camp in Auschwitz. Later they started bringing women from other Polish prisons and from all over occupied Europe. Everything was moving fast. The first transport in March of 1942 began with prison number 1; on June 24 of the same year, I was given the number 7943. Several months thereafter, the numbers already had five digits.

In Auschwitz, they would send us to various work assignments, such as removing bricks from torn-down buildings or cutting reed in the swamps. Several women from our group were sent to work in Harmense, a chicken farm.

On August 1, 1942, we were moved to Birkenau (or, in other words, Brzezinka). There, I worked in the kitchen. It was a very difficult time from me.

My hand was injured because I had to carry steaming cauldrons of soup, weighing about 100 kilograms, without handles. An abscess developed between two of my fingers. My hand was swollen and I was sent to the camp hospital.

We did not have running water nor restrooms in Birkenau. (In the kitchen, at least, I had been able to wash myself). All the women there had lice. After two weeks, I already had spotted fever. During the sixteen days that I was in the Revier, my temperature was between 40° and 41° celsius. I had terrible headaches and felt pain in my thighs. I was tortured by thirst. Later, my temperature dropped to 35°. I could barely speak. After I got my strength back, I became a block servant (Stubenaelteste).

In March of 1943, I went to work in the fields. Later, I was assigned to a group that worked in the vegetable gardens in Rajsko. I had to weed and harvest everything that grew there. We came in the morning, had our lunch delivered from Birkenau and returned in the evening to camp. In September 1943, I was transferred to the Pflanzenzucht (plant cultivation station) in Rajsko.

The sub-camp in Rajsko was formed at the site of a former village. Some of the buildings were transformed into living-quarters for the guards, storage for tools and various workshops. The largest building near the road was turned into a laboratory equipped with exhausts, kilns, heaters and other laboratory equipment. Five additional wooden barracks were built. Three of them were turned into workshops and the other two into living quarters. The kitchen was located in the remains of an old building. Showers, with hot water, and restrooms were in a large brick house. All that was surrounded by a high fence. At the entrance gate was a brick house for the guards, who would constantly walk along the fence during the night. Massive electric lamps were placed high on the fence to light the whole camp. When the construction of Rajsko was finished, women were moved into the barracks. But until it was completed, women who worked in gardening and the experimental kok-saghyz fields would come to work from Birkenau and in the evening they would go back to the camp. After they moved us to the barracks, we would go directly to our greenhouses, laboratories or to the experimental fields right after the morning roll-call.

Nevertheless, numerous groups of women from Birkenau and men from Auschwitz were constantly coming to work in the vegetable fields and kok-saghyz fields. Toward the evening, they would go back to their camps. Women would plant, weed and harvest. Men would be used to repair tools and equipment, to glaze, or to construct special four-sided boxes covered with gauze, with no bottoms or tops but covered with glass. They were used to isolate various plants in the experimental fields.

Within a radius of several kilometers, the vegetable garden was surrounded by the guards' sentry boxes, which were about 500 meters apart. The boxes were very high. Each was equipped with a machine-gun, placed in such a position that the guard on duty could shoot in all directions. The guard and his machine-gun were protected by a small roof. Each box was, of course, open. Not every box was equipped with a machine-gun; some had just regular guns. The prisoners could move only within the area surrounded by those boxes, unless they were accompanied by a guard. When going to work, we always had to walk with a guard who had a machine gun and, sometimes, a dog.

Joachim Caesar (ex-general) Obersturmbannfuehrer, and former agriculturist, was supervising the various farms where prisoners from Auschwitz and Birkenau worked. The farms included: cattle, horse, pig, and chicken breeding, vegetable gardens, greenhouses and the experimental kok-saghyz station, of which Caesar was very proud. Caesar was a fine man, as far as we were concerned. Once during his absence in Auschwitz, the Hitlerites searched our blocks and seized our irons, electric stoves, sweaters, underwear and food (we were receiving packages from home; we also were "organizing" tomatoes, cucumbers and onions from the fields and greenhouses). After Caesar returned from Germany, he ordered everything to be returned to us.

Dr. Schattenberg, who lived in a small house in Rajsko, was our immediate supervisor. He, also, was an agriculturist. Our other supervisors included: Lettmann, Tieslauch, Grell and Doerfler. There were several others, but I do not remember their names. One was a blond, young man we called Dziurawiec (the hole man, i.e., Thies Christophersen). He was extremely malicious and disliked by all. In addition to Germans, there were three Russian expert agriculturists: Popow, one of them, specialized in kok-saghyz. He was educated and well-mannered. Nikita, little, quiet, educated, experimented with vernalization of rye. I do not remember his last name. Hanna Laskowa worked with him. The third one was Zasmuzec. He was the youngest of them and without any special education, a little crude but polite and friendly.

When, in 1941-42, the Germans occupied the southern part of Russia and discovered a plantation of kok-saghyz, they brought those three Russian specialists and many kok-saghyz plants to Auschwitz.

I lived in the block of the Pflanzenzucht work squad. There were two blocks: one for the Pflanzenzucht and the other for the Gaertnerei (gardening detail). The third block was for indoor work of the Pflanzenzucht. There, I worked in the experimental mini-fields growing kok-saghyz and a special kind of rye that, when crossed with wheatgrass, could be harvested for a number of years in a row. In addition to that, I also worked on a crossing of barley and wheat.

One of my colleagues investigated the influence of temperature on the biological features of rye. I observed the hybridization of rye and agropynon (called Perennierender Roggen [or perennial rye] in German). I had to sow or plant this rye on small parcels of land. The research plants were numbered, the sheaves isolated in muslin bags and the ripe corn was counted separately for each sheaf. The weeding had to be done and a precise record was kept. I also had a little plot with wheat-hordeum crossbreeding, which was similarly investigated. I was capable of doing serious research work together with professional agronomists and botanists because as the daughter of land owners I had always been interested in growing and breeding, i.e., in gardens, fields and beasts. I knew how to handle a hot bed and had read many books on this subject.

This type of work stopped late in the fall, and from then on until early spring, I worked with the other girls of the Pflanzenzucht in conveyor belt fashion, analyzing the kok-saghyz plants: weighing, drying and measuring the seeds and extracting rubber from the roots. We worked in two shifts of twelve hours each. After the work with the selection of kok-saghyz roots was completed and the fields frozen, the hard labor for the year was almost over, except for the chemical and biological laboratories where the work still continued.

Overall, conditions in Rajsko were much better than in Birkenau. They wanted us to do very precise work, so they could not let us be hungry or dirty. We could not have lice because, constantly working under German supervision, we would pose a threat to their health. Also, our kitchen was supplied with vegetables so the soup did not taste like that awful mash from the main camp. The Germans would shut their eyes to our "organizing" of cucumbers, tomatoes and onions. The male prisoners who would come to work there would bring us irons, scissors, sewing supplies, electric stoves, and also clothing, mainly sweaters, nightgowns, pajamas and underwear. Although we had to wear uniforms, we could adjust them so they would fit better and we also could wear little white collars.

We would teach other women, and they would teach us. We would celebrate the anniversaries of major national events, do Nativity plays, contemporary plays, write poems and lyrics. We would also make little puppets which, to this day, are in the Auschwitz museum. I still have the poems I wrote in Rajsko. My girlfriends hid the poems in a bottle, which they locked and then buried somewhere near Rajsko. After the war, the bottle with my poems was dug up.

The French women from our group would often do Moliere plays; I do not remember which ones. They would teach me French history with more specific details than it was taught in Polish schools, I, in turn, would teach them Polish history.

In the meantime, terrible things were going on in the main camp. Someone was always missing from the group of men that would come to work. What happened to them? Were they transferred? Killed?

In the evenings, we would see smoke coming from the gas-chambers. They would burn all those that died in the gas-chambers, and all those whom they murdered in some other manner. The wind would carry that terrible smell of burning bodies and bones. I remember when they once brought a wagon of ashes from the crematorium to fertilize the soil near Rajsko. I remember seeing pieces of human bones that did not completely burn up. We often could hear the shouting and yelling of the Hitlerites who would drive people to the gas-chambers. On January 18, 1945, I was evacuated with the Rajsko women. We went on the deathmarch to Ravensbrueck (where, this time, I received the prison number 102146). After a short time, we were transferred to Malchow. Here, we received nothing but a tiny piece of bread and a cup of soup with a few potato peelings or some leaves of beetroot. The last two weeks of imprisonment we spent in a small camp near Leipzig. After wandering around in Saxony for about ten days, the Hitlerites left us in a barn adjacent to a large farm house.

I was liberated together with Aniella Gutt. We decided not to wait for a transport and to return home to Poland by ourselves. Sometimes by auto, and sometimes by truck, we crossed into Czechoslovakia. The last stretch, from Bratislava to Katowice, we went by train, which we also did from Katowice to Warsaw. After leaving the railroad station, we saw nothing but a stone desert. All around us were mines. From far away, we saw a house without roof and windows. We wept...

At the beginning of July 1945, I was already in Lomza, where my mother lived after she had been expelled from Kownaty manor, which had already been expropriated and nationalized. I was so happy that I was free, that I could go wherever I wanted to and that there was no SS-man with a rifle or Aufseherin with a dog behind me, that I did not feel the loss of Pojezierze, which was also nationalized. I began to walk from town to town to see my school friends and my sisters, who worked as teachers in different places. They were happy days. I covered 30-40 km. per day.

In September 1945, I traveled by various trucks to Suwalki, and became a teacher in Zlobin. There, I met Lucjan Abramowicz, my future husband. He was the son of peasants and many years my junior. There was an uproar among my family and friends, and everybody said that I was stupid and that our relationship would not last. Now, we have been married for over forty years and are happy.

In 1947, we left Zlobin. I worked as a teacher in Otwock, and my husband completed a course in auto mechanics. Later, we moved to Warsaw. I became a clerk at Ciech, an export and import company of chemicals. I was responsible for the purchase of a variety of chemicals for laboratories. Lucjan worked in auto repair shops. He had an accident (one of his legs is shorter than the other) and retired. I remained childless and am now on disability.

I am in contact with many friends from camp all over Poland. We correspond and visit each other, and have interesting discussions. I also welcomed, in

Poland, some of my French friends from Auschwitz such as: Marie-Elisa Cohen, Claudette Kennedy, Mimi Dechavassine and Hélène Parreaux. I exchange letters with Marie-Elisa and Claudette, and I was at Claudette's house in Cambridge and Ascot during my stay at Mrs. Ryder's Foundation in the United Kingdom.

I participated in some gatherings of ex-prisoners. When I was younger, and when the schools requested it, I gave more than twenty lectures about concentration camps to the senior graduating classes. I wrote about the camps I was in. The book was written in Zlobin in 1946, and published in 1960. Its title is *Tak Bylo* meaning *That's the Way it Was*.

❖

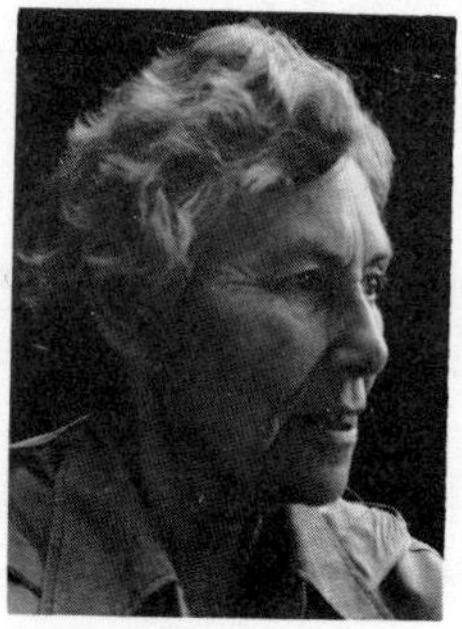

Riva Krieglova (widowed Friedova)
Prague (Czechoslovakia)

I reminisce upon a long life and recall more and more frequently the good and the evil which I have experienced. My imprisonment under the Fascists during WWII belongs to the evil. I do not want to remember those years, but, unfortunately, it is impossible to forget them. The memories are too profoundly imbedded in my soul and always resurface.

Many books have been written and movies made about the inhuman conditions under which political prisoners lived in prisons and concentration camps. All of them are truthful, yet they do not grasp the atmosphere of the environment which an "also-human-being" had created for his fellow human-beings. I remember the film director Wanda Jakubowska,[5] herself a former prisoner, who recounted the efforts involved in re-creating the camp environment as true to life as possible in her film "Auschwitz." For approximately three months, they mixed dirt with water to simulate, at least in part, the muck in which the exhausted prisoners got stuck with their Dutch wooden clogs. How often one could hear desperate screams for help. It was equally difficult to portray the walking skeleton inmates in the film.

Jakubowska told me that she visited almost all Polish hospitals in order to attempt to portray reality, even if only partially. In spite of all this, although the result was a powerful, deeply moving film…I myself did not want to see it…the film could not come close to capturing reality.

I am entirely incapable of describing the horrors of the concentration camps…I do not even want to do so. I solely intend to relate some of my subjective experiences as well as events that occurred in the prisons Pankrac, Karlac, Little Fortress of Terezin and in the concentration camps Auschwitz and Ravensbrueck. Even under the worst conditions, the spark of humanity was not extinguished. There were people willing to risk their lives under extremely hazardous conditions in order to help prisoners. There were prisoners, though constantly oppressed themselves, who, nevertheless, attempted to assist their fellow prisoners with small humane acts of advice, kind words, and empathy to overcome spiritual crises and to rekindle the will to live.

Since the late thirties, my husband and I had voluntarily joined the illegal anti-Fascistic fight. We were fully aware of the perils awaiting us in case of arrest, but knew how important it was to persist and to make sure that during the interrogations nobody would be betrayed.

And here came the first experience: What a big difference between the realization of danger and reality. At the moment of our arrest I sustained such a strong shock that I was incapable of uttering a single word.

To this day, I can recall the beautiful, mild spring night in Prague when we were arrested and taken for interrogations, and it brings back the strange feeling of paralysis that in one instant profoundly transformed my entire life henceforth.

Our interrogations and confrontations immediately after our arrest were intense and accompanied by beatings and sadistic tortures. They seemed endless, lasting from the evening of April 24, 1942 through the entire night and the whole next day In the evening of April 25, 1942 we were transferred from Peckarna[6] to Pankrac. What I remember most after all the years is the desperate effort to convince myself to withstand the tortures and, above all, to refrain from betraying anybody.

After the beatings and mental stress, I received some "strokes" in Pankrac. They came from a female guard, a "Sudetendeutsche" (ethnic German who had lived in Czechoslovakia before the war) who spoke Czech to me. Her name was Andela. While I was undressing, she noticed the wounds and asked, "Who did this to you?" Haltingly, I stammered, "Boehm." Perhaps I had won her confidence, or perhaps she pitied me, but she gave me some valuable information. I learned that in my cell a very friendly lady was waiting for me. Andela warned me not to discuss my case with her. Weren't these "strokes" in this atmosphere of hopelessness and pain? One of the methods of the Gestapo was to introduce confidantes into the cells of prisoners when beatings did not produce the desired results. And indeed, the "friendly lady" was waiting for me in my cell. She nursed me, was extremely kind and solicitous toward me, and constantly questioned me about my case. Thanks to the precise warning I had received, she was not successful.

But she succeeded with others. She was transferred to the cell of Bozenka Kostejnova, whose fiance was Jewish and had been deported. The Gestapo was interested in his valuables: money and jewelry.

During the interrogations, the Gestapo requested the surrender of these items, or the address where they were hidden. Bozenka refused to provide this information and demanded to see her sister. The request was granted. In the meantime, the confidante "worked" in her cell. She acted so likable and friendly that Bozenka confided in her that during her sister's visit she would hand over the location of the hiding place of the money written on toilet paper. Of course, the Gestapo received the information immediately, and the day of her sister's visit Bozenka was asked to surrender the paper. She refused and succeeded in swallowing the "kassiber" (secret note). As punishment, her sister was arrested and Bozenka had to stand for two weeks in the hallway of Pankrac prison facing the wall. After a few days, she had swollen legs and could stand no longer. She asked to be interrogated in order to divulge the hiding place of her fiance's valuables.

By coincidence, Bozenka was placed into my cell the night before her interrogation. When she had recovered somewhat, she started to cry and berate herself for requesting the interrogation. After the experience with the "confidante," she was cautious. She did not explain anything, only cried. However, in the end, she trusted me and told me everything. The problem was that her fiance's valuables were hidden with her parents in the country. The parents were 70 years old, and Bozenka knew that they would not survive a razzia by the Gestapo. Incessantly, she repeated the question, "What now?" I devised a "plan of action" for Bozenka; she would go to the interrogation and would refuse to give the address.

In case the pressure should be too great, she would give a fictitious address and state that the money and valuables were hidden at Mr. V. Zizkov's, Taborska 5. Of course, she would have to take into consideration that the items would not be found at Mr. V's. Then she should claim she did not know any details, never having been there herself. She had merely received the address from her fiance before he was deported. Bozenka carried out the plan successfully. The parents were saved and she and her sister were transported to Auschwitz. They were extraordinarily lucky and both returned home after the war.

▼

In the Little Fortress in Terezin, a rumor spread among the prisoners that we should announce that we suffered from toothache. In Borusovice, approximately three km. from Terezin, there was a dentist. We walked there with a guard. After 8-9 months of desperate conditions and isolation, this was a unique event. Today I still can feel the beauty of this free-nature walk alongside the river. There was a further surprise in store for us in the hamlet; the guard led us to a cafe where we received hot cocoa and other sweets. Then the guard took us to Dr. Nerad, the dentist. He not only took care of our teeth, but enabled us to send letters and "kassibers" (secret notes), and even to meet family members and friends. Until today, I do not know who financed and organized this operation. Even after the war, I was incapable of finding out more about it. It was a heart-warming feeling and replenished our strength during those horrible years to know that there were human beings ready to help in spite of the enormous risks.

In May 1942, the Reichsprotektor Heydrich was assassinated in Prague. There were mass arrests and the prisons in Prague and in the Little Fortress of Terezin were overcrowded. The Germans made preparations for a large transport. Some of the major characteristics of a totalitarian regime are lies, half-truths and secrecy. All of these were used against us in the Little Fortress. They told us one day that an amnesty had been declared; we would go with our husbands to Germany where we would work together in freedom. It was nothing but a deception; our husbands did indeed accompany us on the transport, but the majority of us never saw our spouses again.

Auschwitz

Today it stands for horror, distress and hopelessness...We arrived on January 28, 1943, during a gloomy dusk while a mixture of rain and snow was falling. We first observed two gigantic heaps of personal belongings, clothing, blankets, suitcases, etc., covered with mud and snow. Most likely, these were items left behind by transports of Jews who had been gassed. Like ghosts, exhausted inmates milled around us. They carried bricks and stones here and there. Their faces were as gray as the uniforms they wore.

It forced the question, "Where are we? Have we reached the end of civilization?" Only then did we realize that we were in Birkenau, Auschwitz II, an extermination camp with four crematoria. We were led into the camp to a wooden barrack without floors or ceilings. There were some dirty bowls for food and also several buckets for our physiological needs. And, steadily, more and more transports arrived. We were squeezed one over another, and so we stayed for three days and three nights.

Then, in the middle of the night, they took us to the Sauna for "processing" where we were shaved completely bald and tattooed. They sprayed ice-cold showers on our shorn heads. It was still dark when we had to stand for the roll-call. It was a frightful sight; exhausted women who could not stand up any more and were lying in mud and snow. The SS-women and kapos forced them to get up with beatings. After the roll-call, they led us to work in the swamps. It was bitter cold and we were poorly clothed to do the exhausting work.

While marching to work, an orchestra played in the men's camp that was separated from us by barbed wire. I saw exhausted male prisoners marching to work and upon returning, many carried their half-dead or dead comrades on their shoulders. I thought, I will never be able to listen to music again.

A few days later, we were again told a great deception. Before we went to work, an SS-woman asked those prisoners who did not feel well to step forward; they would not have to go to work. We greeted this as a humane gesture. After returning, however, we discovered that these women had been taken to the "preparatory block for the gas chamber." There had been young, healthy women among them who had only suffered from a slight indisposition; for example, Mrs.

Weidmann (45) and her daughter (17) from Pilsen; Irene Lorencova-Strnadova (about 20) and many others. All of them were gassed except Irene Lorencova-Strnadova who immediately understood where she was when she entered the Block. During the subsequent medical examination, she had sufficient presence of mind to declare that she was healthy and had erroneously been placed among the sick. So she saved her life.

How little was needed to lose one's life. Under the pretense of performing a count of prisoners of the whole camp, a brutal selection was undertaken. In the beginning of February, they took us out to a meadow for nearly a whole day's general roll-call, neglecting to feed us. Plagued by hunger and frost, we had to perform "physical fitness" exercises in Dutch wooden clogs. After each individual prison number had been checked, we had to run a considerable distance on the Lagerstrasse (main road in camp). SS-women stood on both sides of the road, holding heavy canes in hand and observing us. Exhausted women, incapable to continue running were pulled to the roadside with the canes. They were later gassed. The same fate was in store for those women who gave up, not realizing that they were running for their lives and that they had to run regardless of the sea of mud and their unbearably sore feet.

One day, a few numbers were called out during roll-call; mine was among them. We had to step out and march...where to? and why?...Again a "secret." The explanation was better than I had expected. The SS was about to start a research institute in Rajsko to cultivate and analyze Kok-Saghiz, a kind of dandelion, whose roots contain caoutchouc. Rajsko was a satellite camp, approximately 4 km. from Auschwitz. They needed laboratory technicians and chemists, so they selected male and female prisoners according to their occupations. We were housed in the Stabsgebaeude. It was a very lucky coincidence for me. Living conditions there were far superior to Birkenau. Each one of us had her own bunk as well as bed linen. There also were showers at our disposal. Whereas, in Birkenau we had only dirty "kojen" (berths) which had been woefully overcrowded. If there were any blankets, they were filthy, no water, but on the other hand, epidemics of typhus and dysentery.

In Rajsko we could move around more freely as the allotted work allowed. I worked in the greenhouse. Once, I noticed an exhausted, sick male prisoner lying under the table of seedlings. He coughed pitifully and was in a state of deep depression. I wanted to know why he was lying there. He replied, he did not want to live anymore and had decided, after work, to go voluntarily to the gas chamber in Birkenau.

I, myself, did not believe that I would survive the concentration camp, but this I could not permit. The man told me that he came from Pisek, where his wife and son lived. I do not remember what I told him. I only know that I kept talking to him. "Is it not enough that the Fascists exterminate us, why should we give in to them and commit suicide?"

I begged the head of the greenhouse to take care of this man and not to leave him alone in such a condition. I could not do any more for him. I did not know the man's name and did not think that he knew mine. I had only noticed that he had one eye glued shut with mud. I did not understand why.

After the war, a friend of mine who had been in Buchenwald concentration camp related that he had met Honza Soukup, a Czech prisoner there and that supposedly I had helped him when he had been in a deplorable state. I insisted there must be a mistake since I did not know any Honza Soukup. My friend gave details and I did not believe it could have been the man from Rajsko until he reported about the eye that was glued shut. Soukup had one glass-eye, and since there was no water in Birkenau, it was cemented with mud. In the end, I met with Honza Soukup and his family in person when they came to see me at my house. We all rejoiced.

Everybody experienced the Fascist prisons in a different manner: it was different for the young and different for the old; different for those physically and emotionally better prepared than those who encountered the type of hardship and suffering for the first time. There were prisoners among us who comforted and helped however they could. One of these many was, for example, the Czech physician Dr. Zdena Nedvedova.[7] Because of her special relationship with the patients, she was called "Sunshine."

It is not by accident that we survivors keep in touch even after so many years. We are united by our common experience and we love each other.

❖

CHAPTER SIX
Design and Photography

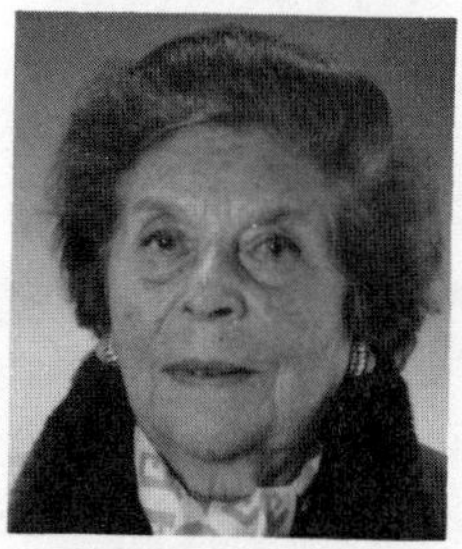

Wanda Ladniewska
Paris (France)

I was born on June 13, 1905, in Lwow (Lemberg) Galicia, then Poland and today the Western Ukraine. Dr. Simon Ladniewski, my father, was a physician in Lwow and died very young. I, therefore, spent my childhood at my maternal grandparents' house. My mother's maiden name was Erdheim. My grandfather was director of a bank and a respected man. We lived in a small but important town at the Russian border.

I attended secondary school in Vienna almost until graduation since World War I had forced us to escape. I had neither brothers nor sisters. My mother's siblings were very talented; one of the brothers was a gifted architect and an extraordinary designer, assistant at the Institute of Technology in Vienna. He was shot by the Nazis, together with his wife, in Poland. The entire family was very musical, played the piano and gave concerts at home to which many guests were invited. I played tennis, went skiing and swam a lot, the latter I am keeping up even today.

I studied German philology and art history at the University of Lwow as well as draftsmanship and anatomy at the Art Institute and passed all prescribed examinations required for the position of an instructor of art and design. I had studied according to the Austrian system and, after passing all state board tests, I carried the title "professor." I taught German at a Gymnasium, mostly in the higher grades and also taught design. In addition, I studied at the Universities of Vienna and Graz as well as architecture at the Institute of Technology in Lwow.

In 1928, I married Stefan Blankenheim. My husband was an electronic engineer. He died in the concentration camp of Mauthausen-Gusen II on April 6, 1945, just one week before liberation. We did not have any children.

The German-Soviet Pact of 1939 granted Russia the eastern half of Galicia, which was incorporated into the Ukrainian Soviet Socialist Republic. In June 1941, when it was occupied by the Germans, my husband and I immediately lost our jobs. For a short while we were hidden by my husband's secretary, Janina Popkiewicz, who now lives in Canada. After New Year 1942, when it became too dangerous, we went to Rzeszow with false papers. Two persons from Lwow recognized us and we had to run away again, this time to Zakopane in the High Tatra. Here my husband worked as electrical technician for the construction of a new power plant until he was denounced by a 17 year old co-worker. This young lad told a Gestapo officer he had an inkling that the technician was Jewish. Of course, that sufficed. Both of us were arrested and taken to the Gestapo jail, located at the Palace Hotel. Here we stayed for four weeks. The cells were the former servant quarters.

After approximately four weeks, we were transferred to Montelupi prison in Cracow. There we remained another month, still without any interrogations, and were then transported in open trucks to Auschwitz on March 17, 1943.

I saw how my husband, with a group of other men, marched through the notorious gate with the inscription "Arbeit Macht Frei." The women remained in front of the gate for quite a while. Then we were marched to Birkenau, guarded by a SS-woman.

I received number 38091.

The very first evening, when we were waiting for our camp clothes and the tattooing, I saw huge chimneys emitting black smoke and flames from time to time. Other inmates informed me immediately that human beings were burned there.

When I was still in the quarantine block, SS-physician Dr. Rohde was looking for prisoners to work in a laboratory. I could do microscopic drawings and knew how to handle a microscope...just by coincidence I had helped a friend of ours, a very talented scientist, to do the illustrations for his doctoral dissertation shortly before the war. Like a miracle, I remembered this during that decisive split second. As a matter of fact, the block elder and a co-prisoner, a former student of mine from the Gymnasium in Lwow, attempted to hold me back at the block entrance. Energetically, I pushed them aside. It was just fate.

I thus joined the Pflanzenzucht Kommando in Rajsko which worked under the direction of Obersturmbannfuehrer Dr. Joachim Caesar. The head of the botanical section was Dr. Boehme who was my boss. Besides, there were Dr. Schattenberg and Thies Christophersen, called "Troutrou."

It was the task of the Pflanzenzucht to cultivate the Kok-Sagyz plant which comes from Central Asia and whose roots contain caoutchouc. This latex, i.e., the liquid contained in the root, was examined in the chemical laboratory. Here Marie-Elisa Nordman, now Cohen, was in charge while the botanical laboratory was directed by Claudette Bloch, now Kennedy. Ruth Weinmann, a German civilian...later Mrs. Caesar...was responsible for the chemical laboratory. She also came to the botanical laboratory. Her doctoral dissertation was prepared by Marie-Elisa and I did the illustrations. She received her doctorate at a famous university, I believe it was Weimar.

The female co-prisoners were educated French women and Poles: among them were many Jewesses. All were occupied with the examination of Kok-Sagyz. The Germans needed rubber for tires to conduct the war and could not obtain it abroad. Already, Stalin had planted Kok-Sagyz over vast areas of land. This rubber was supposed to replace, at least in part, the imported one. The experiments lasted for years.

The Pflanzenzucht-Kommando had much better living conditions than Birkenau. The lodgings were clean, the washroom always had warm water and we could take showers. The food was better because the cooks were allowed to cook vegetables in the soup which were grown in Rajsko.

The day started with the roll-call, which usually did not last very long (and ended with a roll-call in the evening after work). Then we received a coffee-ersatz type of drink and our portion of bread. There was an additional bread ration for everybody which was very important. Afterward, we went to work in the laboratory, tool-shed or in the fields, according to one's job.

I had no possibility to commit sabotage; that was easier for those who did the plant cultivation. For example, especially good seeds were burned in the oven, or the numbers of the plants were mixed up on purpose. By the way, I, myself, never witnessed any acts of sabotage.

Because of my work, everybody referred to me as "Micro-Wanda." I had numerous friends in camp. I was friendly with the French women, such as Claudette to whom I really owed my job as draftswoman because I had to pass a sort of examination, with Hélène Langevin-Parreaux, et al. I was also on good terms with many Poles and am still corresponding with some of them even today and send them packages, especially medication.

For a few days, I was sick with sciatica in the Revier. I could not walk, and our inmate doctor, Dr. Stephane Schramek, treated me with vitamin-B shots which had been organized in the SS-pharmacy by some friends of my husband who worked in the Institute of Hygiene. I was acquainted with these chemists and physicians because the Institute of Hygiene was also in Rajsko not far from us and I was there a few times "on business" with my illustrations. It was one of those rare occasions when I had the opportunity to send something to my husband, particularly news. Unfortunately, Stefan came down with pneumonia twice in Auschwitz.

Flora, the first SS-woman we had in Rajsko, was not too bad; but Borman, the next one, was terrible. She was transferred to Bergen-Belsen and later hanged by the prisoners. The transfer had taken place because during her supervision a Russian inmate had escaped from Rajsko.

A dreadful occurrence was the shooting of Lili Toffler in Auschwitz. The SS had found a little note which she had written to an inmate and given to a male prisoner, who worked on this day with us, for delivery.

The last two days in Rajsko, we spent packing. The SS and our bosses thought to transport the laboratory and us somewhere else to a safe place.

Then came the death march, Ravensbrueck, Malchow in Mecklenburg and, in the end, Leipzig. When they drove us out of Leipzig, I escaped during the second night together with the Poles Lili Schneifer from Zakopane and her cousin. We hid with German peasants and at the end of April were liberated by the English and American armies.

Together with the two Polish women, I returned to Cracow, where I learned that two family members had survived the war: an aunt in Warsaw and a cousin in Cracow. I could not go home to Lwow since it now belonged to the Ukraine. In Warsaw, I immediately got a job in the Ministry of Education, the minister and his Jewish wife knew me from Lwow. I was satisfied and well-liked at work, but I was restless because I did not know anything about my husband. I had him searched for by the International Red Cross and by friends and diplomats who went abroad. Only after a year, I was informed by the Red Cross that he had died in Gusen II in April 1945.

In June 1946, I decided to emigrate to France since my aunt, with whom I was living in Warsaw, wanted to join her son in Palestine. In Paris, I worked in the beginning as professor at the Lycee Polonais. Soon, however, I resigned and worked exclusively as a sculptor and graphic designer. A terracotta bas-relief of mine is in the French pavilion of the Auschwitz Museum. It consists of three parts, approximately 1 m X 30 cm and is entitled "Rollcall."

In the sixties, I once attended the Eichmann trial in Jerusalem. It was on the day when the prosecutor, Gideon Hausner,[1] was presenting the indictment. His brother had been a colleague of mine in German philology at the University of Lwow. He was a year older than me and died quite young; his family was already in Palestine at that time. I was not impressed by Hausner's speech (listening to French or German translations because I did not understand Hebrew).

I stared at Eichmann in his glass-cage, who seemed...at least exteriorly...very calm. Neither at that time nor today could anybody comprehend the crimes he had committed. I still believe that this greatest crime in the history of mankind could have been prevented. In the meantime, more crimes are being committed and nobody knows how to put a stop to them.

❖

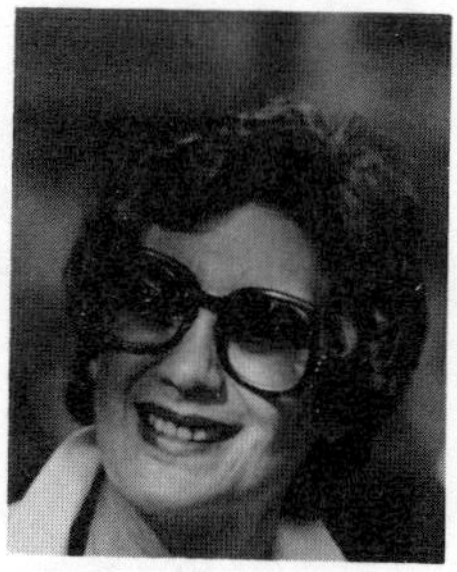

Inge Schlesinger (née Kochmann)
Bronxville, New York (USA)

I was born in December 1921 into a typical middle-class Jewish family in Berlin, Germany. We were a very closely knit, very loving family, with a lot of uncles, aunts and cousins. Being an only child I enjoyed being together with them.

I was still able to finish my high school education in the spring of 1938. The day after graduating, I started as an apprentice at the well-known Photostudio Binder-Berlin. I learned every phase of photography there, from taking the pictures to the finished product. The owner of the studio was a wonderful person whose memory I would like to preserve in this paper. Her name was Liesel von Stengel, née Aron. She was Jewish, but since she had married an "Aryan" (deceased at that time) and through her influence at the Gestapo, she passed as a non-Jew as long as her papers were hidden in her nephew's desk drawer (he was married to her niece). But one day, the nephew was on leave and Liesel was sent to Theresienstadt with a "Sonderzug" (special train). She was a fervent anti-Nazi and I met many of her friends. Luckily, she survived the camp and I heard her stories after the war when I met her in Switzerland.

I still remember the Kristallnacht...it really started during the day. I was working at the studio and, after seeing what was going on in the street, I was frightened to go home by myself, especially since I looked very Jewish. Liesel's driver took me home and that was very courageous of him.

When the war started Liesel still let me work at the Studio and, since I could not be employed officially, she paid me secretly. I stayed with her, all in all, for two and a half years, until it became impossible for her to keep me any longer, and pretty soon thereafter, she was deported.

All able-bodied Jews had to work in factories by that time and I was drafted to work at the Zeiss Ikon Filmwerk (I was sent there because I was a photographer). We were nine Jewish women there…five young girls and four older women. Some of the factory workers had never encountered any Jews and were surprised that we looked just like anybody else, that we did not have horns or tails. We had to work from 5:50 AM to 4:30 PM, five days a week and half a day on Saturday. All our work was done in a darkroom, manufacturing 35mm films. I worked there until I was deported with my parents to Birkenau (Auschwitz)in May 1943. We were deported as the last Jews from Berlin because since 1939 my father had been working for the Jewish Council (Juedische Gemeinde). This was fortunate for me. Most of the Jews that worked in factories were deported by February 1943, and most of them were sent directly from the train to the gas chambers.

I arrived in Birkenau with my parents after three or four days in a cattle car without food or water. After we stopped in Birkenau the doors of the train were opened and SS-men shouted, "Out, out," men to one side and women on the other side. They were using sticks and they had horrible vicious dogs, and this was the last time that I saw my beloved father.

My mother and I walked into the camp with the women that were chosen for their ability to work. Once inside that horrible place we had to line up to get tattooed (my number was 45226), we had to get undressed in front of the SS-men and SS-women, and all our hair was shaved off. Prisoners did the tattooing and shaving, and we were told by them what was going on in this extermination camp. We were told that the people that went by truck from the railroad station were sent directly to the gas chambers. After standing and waiting for hours, we were finally sent to a barrack with 3-tier bunks already filled to overflowing with human beings who were so emaciated that they looked like corpses.

We had no toilet facilities in the barracks or nearby, and no washrooms. The first morning after our arrival some women of our transport had already died during the night. It was unbelievable, like Dante's Inferno. Who has not been there cannot comprehend the anguish and the fright we felt. That something like that was possible is beyond understanding. That morning, after many hours of roll call, we were marched to work in the fields, always accompanied by shouting, cursing SS with their barking dogs. There was hardly any food and only heavy work. It was very hot during the day and freezing cold at night.

I was one of the few lucky ones...after being there for only a few days, a call went out for a photographer at roll call. I went forward to give my number, telling them that I was a photographer. But when I heard that I would be sent to another camp I got frightened at the idea of leaving my mother. The next day my number was called and, together with other prisoners, I was marched to meet Obersturmbannfuehrer Dr. Joachim Caesar. He questioned me and wanted to know where I had worked and what qualifications I had. He picked me as the photographer and Wanda Jacubowska[2] as my assistant, even though she was not a photographer but a movie producer. By the way, after the war she produced a movie about the camp, together with Gerda Schneider. Gerda was the "Blockova" in our barrack in Rajsko, a very fair and good person.

Something happened at that time that I will always feel guilty about for the rest of my life. Instead of following my instinct, I listened to the girls that had been with the "Pflanzenzucht," the name of our kommando. They advised me to wait to ask to have my mother with me and that they would know the right time to do it. They were all very kind and meant well but I know now that if I had asked Caesar right away, he would have let my mother come with me. I found out later that he was very impressed with my credentials...Binder was so well known. Unfortunately, I could not get my mother to join me. I saw her twice in Birkenau but she had deteriorated so much that she did not recognize me anymore. She was gassed. I will never forgive myself for what I did not do.

We left Berlin for Birkenau together with Dr. Lucie Adelsberger.[3] She had treated me for allergies and was a good friend of mine. We stayed at the same barrack and when the call came for a photographer and I hesitated to step forward because I did not want to leave my darling mother, Lucie was the one to insist that I should go, that this might be my only way to survive. Lucie was sent to the Gypsy Camp as a doctor, and after all of the Gypsies were gassed, she was sent back to Birkenau. We both survived and we met again in New York. She went into Cancer

Research at the Montefiore Hospital. When her grant was discontinued, she gave from her own earnings to go on with her work. She was a wonderful friend and person and such a dedicated physician. I will never forget her.

It is hard to believe that a photographer would be needed in a place like Auschwitz. But one has to understand that SS-men like Caesar lived like little kings in their kingdom of Auschwitz. He was the Manager of the agricultural enterprises (Landwirtschaft). That included, for instance, farming (Gaertnerei), fish and poultry. The jewel in his crown was the Pflanzenzucht.

To manufacture artificial rubber, a small percentage of natural rubber was needed (I do not know if this is still the case). The Germans did not have any access to this commodity after they lost their colonies. The Russians did not have it either. So when the German army invaded the Ukraine, they found that the Russians had cultivated a plant by the name of kok-saghyz, a relative of our dandelion. The white sap in the root contains latex. The Russians, after many years of research, had accomplished growing plants that contained a high amount of this substance. Himmler was interested in having the kok-saghyz plants researched further in Germany. He found that there was no better place to achieve this than in Auschwitz. The soil was perfect and the labor cheap and available. Himmler gave Caesar, who had a doctorate in agriculture, the opportunity to be head of this venture, which had the highest priority.

Caesar found Polish women prisoners from different camps with degrees in either chemistry or botany and agricultural engineers to carry out the research. A laboratory was built in the empty school house in Rajsko. The first prisoners to work on this project lived in overcrowded Birkenau and had to walk to and from there every day to work. Soon after, one of the prisoners died of typhoid fever, and so did Caesar's wife. Lice did not stop by biting only prisoners. A bite from an infected louse was the way to contract typhoid. Caesar decided that he had to do something to keep his kommando alive. He had the women transferred to the Headquarters (Stabsgebaeude), where the living conditions were better than in Birkenau. At the same time, Caesar started building barracks for living and working quarters, a stone's throw away from the laboratory and greenhouses. There was also a bath house and a kitchen. A completely self-contained camp. The move to Rajsko took place in June 1943, just three weeks after we got to Birkenau. In the meantime, our kommando had grown to about 150 prisoners. Now we could keep ourselves clean and get regular meal portions, which were quite small. However, we were able to supplement our diet by "organizing" (stealing) potatoes, onions, etc., because the Kommando-Gaertnerei (agriculture) with 150 prisoners lived in separate barracks in our compound.

I met many outstanding women during my two years in the KZ...interesting, intelligent and highly educated was the norm there. I met my dearest friend, who is still like a sister to me, in June 1943. Eugenia Halbreich[4] was the bookkeeper of the Gaertnerei. I do not know if I could have survived without her taking care of me. I also met Nora Mayer-Udewald there, another close friend of mine. We still meet often. Another good friend, Berthe Falk, died of cancer in France soon after the liberation.[5]

Since I was able to ask for supplies for the photo lab, I ordered items that would be useful for all of us in other ways, not only for the lab. For example, I needed an iron to flatten out the finished pictures, but it served its original purpose as well. I would smuggle these treasures into the barracks on Saturdays, together with an electric heater, which I needed to heat my developers, and we all used it for cooking on Sundays. I ordered a retouching easel which had a fairly large mirror...what a rarity to have. And I needed an "official" wrist watch to time the developing. Wanda and I would take turns wearing this "prize." All the accessories came in handy.

If we were lucky and received some newspaper, which was a crime, it was safest to read it in the darkroom. I had told the SS that they had to knock before entering, since otherwise the film or paper would get spoiled. This was really unheard of but they all complied with my rule. It was astounding how Caesar was able to obtain the cameras, one Leica and one Contax, enlarger, films, paper, etc., because it was almost impossible to get them on the outside. But apparently the work was considered so important that he got first priority.

I have to mention that we all tried to produce as little work and results as possible. I remember taking only two rolls of film, making big enlargements, framing them and hanging them on the walls of the studio. Lots of times I would wander around with the camera in my hand; I was able to do this to take pictures of the plants but also of especially large cabbage, cucumbers, etc. But most of the time I would pour the developer into the trays to make it look as though I was working and then would pour the unused liquid back into the bottle at night.

Reading this, one might get the impression that we lived a well-regulated life. This is true up to a point, but otherwise we would not have survived! But our camp was only four kilometers away from the main camp with the gas chambers and the ovens. We were always aware of what was going on in Birkenau. The ovens were burning day and night and we always smelled the smell of the crematoria.

There was only a handful of Jewish prisoners in our kommando...we always expected to be singled out at roll call and to be deported to Birkenau and the ovens. Our mental anguish is impossible to put into words. My friend Genia admonished me constantly that if the call "Jews forward!" should come, I should take the first stone and throw it at an SS-man to make sure that I would be shot and not gassed.

On Jannuary 18, 1945, we were hoarded together and marched through snow and ice toward the west to Germany. The Russians were approaching Auschwitz. I don't know how we survived the death march. Many did not. They were shot by the SS and left by the wayside. After many days of marching we arrived at a railroad siding and were herded into cattle cars.

Again I was one of the lucky ones. Most of us from the Pflanzenzucht were pushed into a car that was covered by a tarpaulin. Afterwards I found out that ours was the only car so covered; everybody else rode in open cars in the terrible cold. And I thought our trip was a nightmare! But it seems that the SS still believed that they would win the war and start another laboratory in a camp inside of Germany.

We arrived in Ravensbrueck, which was so overcrowded that unbeknownst I slept on top of frozen corpses. We were just standing outside in this cold; they had no empty barrack because prisoners arrived constantly from Poland. Days later, we were given a barrack but soon after we were on the go again...this time to Malchow (just as overcrowded)...and finally to Leipzig.

On April 13, 1945, the Americans wanted the Germans to declare Leipzig an open city. That would have meant to leave the city and surrender the prisoners, but the Germans did not want that. They poured gasoline over the barracks next to ours and torched them with the prisoners inside. We were marched out of Leipzig at night and walked around and around for ten days without any food or water.

After ten days of walking around in circles, five of us girls decided to try to run away. During the night we hid in a tiny outhouse and the next morning the SS and the prisoners were gone. We met some Belgian POWs who gave us some food and blankets. We only wore cotton dresses and had thrown our striped jackets away, so as not to be recognized as prisoners. By now everybody was fleeing...Germans, prisoners, slave workers, POWs, with one goal in common...to reach the Elbe River and get away from the Russians and join the Americans.

The Elbe was the demarcation line between the Russian and the American troops. And we found ourselves between the two armies. Since the bridges over the Elbe had been destroyed, we had to wait until nightfall to cross over pontoon bridges to the other side. Since so many people were fleeing, this seemed to take forever.

After finally crossing the river we tried to hide and sleep in a barn. But in the middle of the night we were awakened by shouts and heard the farmer tell some SS that there were Jews hiding in the barn. We were able to flee and were again lucky not to be caught and killed. We walked west, attaching ourselves to a caravan of people fleeing from the Russians, in the direction that would finally let us meet the American troops. Nobody was asking anymore who was who...we all had one goal. We would send Klarie, who was the prettiest and not Jewish looking, to get something to eat. When we finally undressed in front of each other we could not believe our eyes...we looked just like skeletons, real "Muselmaenner."

The last evening that we spent in a still German-controlled town we watched the young German girls arm in arm with wounded German soldiers. The next morning Americans came to the town with their jeeps and tanks. We could not believe our eyes, we had really made it and survived. But to come back to the German girls, they dropped their German soldiers and made out with the Americans with their chocolate and cigarettes.

We met some American soldiers who were born in Europe but had immigrated to the United States. They were very helpful to us. I remember one of them gave me a camera when he heard I was a photographer.

But since the war was not over yet, we were advised to walk to a displaced persons camp in Grimma. We stayed there for a couple of days until the war was over. I did not feel like staying in a barrack for another day. I climbed over a fence and went to the American HQ in Grimma. I told them that I wanted to work for them and did not want to stay in the camp. I did get a job as a liaison between the army and the employment agency. After six weeks I was told that the Americans were leaving the area and would give Saxony to the Russians. Since it was known that I did not want to stay with the Russians and did not want to remain in Germany, I was given an offer to join a group of Belgians. When I arrived in Liege I was told that, since I had not lived in Belgium before, I was a German enemy, even though I was Jewish, and I was sent to prison. It took days before some American liaison officer came to my help. He advised me to go back to the American zone of Germany until the time I would be able to emigrate to the USA, which was my greatest desire.

After days of waiting at railway stations to get back into Germany, I and another girl whom I met in prison traveled on coal trains, etc. It took us three to four days to reach Frankfurt am Main. There we were told that it would be best for us to travel to Bad Nauheim. A temple had been refurbished and a lot of Jewish soldiers were stationed there. Since we did not care where we would stay, providence let us go to Bad Nauheim. We went to the mayor of the town, who gave us the name of a boarding house. Next morning I went looking for work, without success. On Friday evening we went to the services in the temple, and the soldiers were all very nice and interested in us and our stories. I was one of the first to get there who had been in a KZ. I told them that I was looking for a job. One of them advised me to go to a certain office on Monday.

On Monday I went there and the man I was to see was on vacation. I met an extremely handsome and nice young man who told me to come back the next day. The next day his boss was still away and the young man interviewed me. We found out that we came from the same town, Berlin, and had lived around the corner from each other but never met. His father left Berlin in 1936 and he followed with his mother and brother in 1937. Lutz got a job for me at the American army archives. He took me to lunch at the "Kurhaus" where the Americans took their meals. A special room was set aside for a few other "displaced persons," as we were called, who also worked for the army. I met our very dear friends, Dr. and Mrs. Kelemen, there.

And the young man is my husband, Lutz.

But we still did not feel secure in our new freedom. We did not want to stay in Germany with the Germans who had killed our loved ones and had committed all the atrocities.

We were afraid we would never get out of there. It took a year for us to reach the blessed soil of America, on the first displaced persons' ship to arrive in New York in May 1946.

After finally being free and in America, another unforeseen event happened. Just before we wanted to get married in October 1946, I found out that I had contracted tuberculosis in the camp. I was sent to Denver, Colorado, to recuperate. I spent sixteen months in bed. My freedom was curtailed again!

In May 1948 we got married.

❖

CHAPTER SEVEN
Hygienic Institute

Hygiene Institut der Waffen SS und Polizei Auschwitz or Untersuchungsstation des Hygieneinstituts der Waffen SS Sued-Ost

The Institute of Hygiene was located in Rajsko, near Auschwitz. It had been planned in the fall of 1942 and was opened in April 1943. The director was Hauptsturmfuehrer Dr. Bruno Weber. His deputy was Untersturmfuehrer Dr. Hans Muench and the assistant deputy was Dr. Hans Delmotte.

The Institute was neither under the supervision of the SS physician-in-chief in Auschwitz nor under the commandant of Auschwitz. It was a branch line of the Institute of Hygiene in Berlin, whose chief was Oberfuehrer Dr. Joachim Mrugowsky.

The Institute in Rajsko consisted of different laboratories for biology, anatomy, bacteriology, chemistry, serology and others. All research was conducted by prisoners, scientists with reputations known all over the world. Many of them had been arrested especially in order to work in these laboratories.

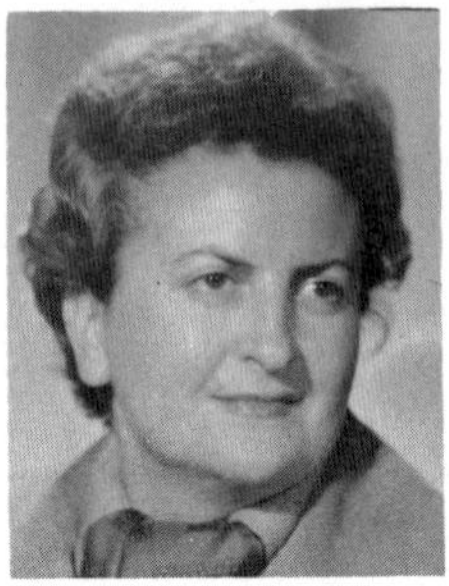

Pola Plotnicka (widowed Korn, née Beck)

Haifa (Israel)

My name is Pola Korn-Plotnicka. I was born on June 26, 1916, in Tyczyn, a little village in Galicia. My father's name was Mozes Beck, my mother's was Rywka. I had four brothers. They all had children and were married before the war. And they all (with their families) died in Treblinka or in Belzec. My youngest brother moved across the Bug (river). He returned from Russia in 1945, with his health in shambles. Then, for a short period of time, he lived in Germany. There he married and moved to Israel. He died relatively young, at the age of 48, leaving a wife and two children.

A little bit about Tyczyn

Tyczyn was only a few kilometers away from Rzeszow. The youth of Tyczyn was intelligent and talented, however without any prospects for growth and development. My father was relatively "up-to-date" despite the fact that he lived in such a backward region. He was intelligent and he read a lot. He was the one who motivated me to read all of Graetz' work.[1] My mother was the best mother in the whole world. She was good not only to her own children but to all others as well. She knew about every misfortune and disaster in the village and she was always ready to offer her help. Despite all this, I was not very happy in my youth.

My mother was very religious and not too tolerant; she was not willing to compromise as far as our religion or customs were concerned. She did not even let me belong to the Zionist organization. Here, however, I would not go along with her. I did not feel very well about the disagreement with my mother, such a good mother.

Before I managed to become independent, the war broke out in 1939. The situation of the Jews in Poland in the thirties was very difficult and was worsening as a result of the growing anti-Semitism and Hitler's coming to power. The actual repressions and persecutions began after the war broke out. The availability of places to live and supplies of food was constantly decreasing, especially when the Germans began to send us people they expelled from larger cities such as Lodz and Cracow. Those expelled were mostly poor and mostly servants. The Germans placed them wherever they could and that included our house.

Roundup and Deportation

There was no "closed ghetto" in Tyczyn. In July of 1942, we and other Jews from close-by villages were forcefully moved to Rzeszow.[2] There was only one ghetto in Rzeszow, but after our coming there they created another one for those who were forced to work for the Germans. Those who worked for the Germans had a certified work permit with an official seal. Our ghetto was the larger one, so its "members" were "sentenced" for deportation.

In Rzeszow, we lived in one very little room with many other Jews. It was crowded and very bad in all aspects. It was hell!

Everyone was extremely exhausted; no one had the strength to do anything. The packages with food and other supplies we prepared for moving were smaller and smaller. We knew we were sentenced for extermination, but our instinct of self-preservation and our will to live did not let us believe in the worst that was to happen. I believed in what was to happen to us and I was very apathetic. One morning the SS deported some people from our street. We were already standing in a row. I saw my mother standing with a bottle of juice and water in her hand; she left all her belongings in the empty apartment.

It is very difficult to describe what was happening there. Crying and lamentations. Shootings, and shouting of the Hitlerites, beating with rifles. People were looking for each other; small children were wandering not being able to find their mothers; the old and the sick were lying on the ground. Suddenly, the Hitlerites told us to go back home. Probably, they ran out of railroad-cars to put us on. We came back.

In the afternoon, I went to one of my girlfriends. I felt very close to my girlfriends since I did not have any sisters. During my absence, they deported everyone from my street and from my home. I was the only one left from my family. Suddenly, I was alone. I was close to naked and barefoot because the day was hot and I went to my girlfriend's in a summer dress and wooden shoes. So I was alone; I did not belong to anyone anymore. Actually, I did not exist anymore. I was not supposed to live anymore, but I was still alive. I could not stay in the ghetto anymore because I did not have the certificate permitting me to work for the Germans; I could not go back to our apartment because all houses on our street had been emptied. People advised me to go to the new ghetto. I went there in the evening, although I was sure that the Germans would kill me before I could reach the gates. It must have been a miracle; not only did the Germans not kill me but they showed me the way to some of our friends that lived there. Unfortunately, I could not stay with them; if I did, they would probably be deported from their home. I decided to go to one of the tents where those who were about to be sent somewhere else gathered. Those people in the tent were mostly old, sick, or children. I knew that if I stayed with them my situation would be hopeless. To die…I would always have time!

I decided to escape through the window; one of the Jewish policemen (Ordnungsdienst) noticed me but he was obviously a decent man; he did not stop me and let me go.

The Road to Life

I entered someone's house and hid in the attic. Two other girls were already there. The roof in the attic was so low that one could not stand straight or even sit. One had to lie on the floor. I cried myself to sleep. I even cried after waking up. Several days passed and I was still in the attic. Some helpful boys brought us food.

It was the time of passive noncooperation. Boys and girls with the "true Aryan look" were helping us out and giving advice. Thanks to them, I was able to get in touch with my brother who lived in the Tarnow ghetto. I received a letter from him telling me he was very happy that at least I was alive and he asked me to come and live with him in Tarnow.

Among the boys that were helping us out, there was one Polish boy who did me a great favor expecting nothing in return. I asked him to help me to get out of that attic hiding-place. He provided me with forged papers and I was finally able to leave the attic and managed to reach my brother in Tarnow. It must have been another miracle. However, the situation in Tarnow was becoming the same as everywhere else. At that time, I already had Aryan papers in the name of Janina Oles. My brother was a typographer; he did stamps and seals for different companies. Now people were running after him asking him to make stamps for their false documents. All of my brothers were very goodhearted. But the one in Tarnow was truly wonderful...he worked day and night to save people who were "dealing" and making fortunes at his expense. He did not get anything for doing what he did.

He was making stamps and seals until his last day. The Germans took him and his three little sons to the Sammelplatz. He wrote letters begging for help but there was nobody willing to help.

Before one of the round-ups, I hid in one of the bunkers and there I spent some of the most difficult moments of my life. I often thought that if I survived I would write about everything that I went through; like Anne Frank.

One experience followed another and each was worse than the preceding one. After the war, each book that I read about the occupation reminded me of my own experiences during that time. It was almost like a piece of my own life.

Among my brother's clients was one Polish woman who always used to pay me compliments whenever she was in his store to pick up the stamps she ordered. When I left my hiding place, I went to see her and ask whether I could wash myself at her home; she refused the request. In the bunker, I met a woman who gave me an address of a girl who worked as a servant in Cracow. She had Aryan papers.

With Aryan Papers in Cracow

With my Semitic looks, I could work only as a servant. I could not work among people. In one way, it was the most difficult period of my war experience. In the camps, people lived like animals; physical pain was overshadowed by emotional and spiritual pain. No one owned anything and no one had anything to lose. With the Aryans, on the other hand, I had to live in constant fear; afraid of my Jewish background being revealed. I was left at the mercy of every guard, every policeman, every man who thought that he could use a pretty Jewish girl. I never worked for long in one place. People always talked and gossiped. I was different. Once I worked for a couple who were studying at the university. The moment they opened their door, they immediately recognized that I was Jewish. They pondered long before they hired me and they did it only because they wanted to help me. I took care of their child. However, they let me go after a short period of time. They were afraid. The lady for whom I worked had a girlfriend at the university who also helped a Jewish girl and was later arrested for that. She was afraid the same would happen to her. They advised me to change places with one girl who worked for a German family. It was generally known that Germans could not recognize a Semitic look. That girl, her name was Janka, was rather happy about the exchange; she could not cook or speak German so, obviously, she was willing to trade places with me. The German family did not suspect me of being Jewish, yet everything about me seemed very different to them. Actually the same was true with every family I worked for. Even though I made up a story of my life, nobody believed me. They knew I was a professional servant. The German family asked me where I learned to cook and speak German so well; I always had a ready answer for everything.

They probably did not care too much about all that, although they were rather reluctant to register my residence at their home.

One day the Germans caught that girl Janka to be sent to work in Germany. The Aryan girls were very unhappy about this; I, on the other hand, would have been very happy to be able to go to Germany, but I couldn't.

After the incident, Janka's mother came to me and told me that if my employer would not do anything to save Janka, she would expose me and reveal my identity. And so, she did what she told me she would do. I had to quickly pack my bag and run away. And that was when my true homeless wandering began. I had nothing to eat, no place to sleep, no place to stay. There is no way to describe it. I did not exist, yet I had to live.

It was winter. One night a house manager who was hiding a Jewish child let me stay in her little room. She wanted me to give her some kind of identification, but I had left my Kennkarte with the German family. I had no choice but to telephone them and ask them to return it to me. They talked as if they did not know what was going on and they asked me to come to their office to pick up the document. Some people advised me not to go, but I went anyway. Their office was on the fifth floor. I did not have the key to the elevator anymore, so I had to climb the stairs. I would stop on each floor since I felt that I was going for a sure death; but I could not go back now. Some kind of force was pushing me forward.

A secretary was sitting in the first room. I asked her, "Wo ist der Herr Doktor?" He was a lawyer with the title of a doctor. (I think his name was Wohl.) At that time, two men came out of his office and slapped me in the face. It was the first time I was ever slapped. They said, "Marsch" and told me to go. It was the beginning of March and a pleasant spring day. All passers-by that saw us seemed to be pleased. I asked the two men where they were taking me and why they did not kill me right there. They told me that they had no plan to kill me at all. They brought me to a prison which was located in a Cracow ghetto. The ghetto was in a state of liquidation. In that prison, I saw many Jewish girls with Aryan papers that I had met earlier in the tramways or in the streets. We could recognize each other by looking into each others' eyes. I started to cry when they brought me to my cell. I was among Jews once again. What would happen to them would happen to me. I did not have to perform and play anymore. I did not have to say prayers anymore. I did not have to be a servant anymore. That's how it was with the Aryan freedom.

One Step Away from the Crematorium

Not long afterward, i.e., still in March 1943, the Germans brought us to Auschwitz. I thought about running away, jumping from the car; but I didn't. All those that tried to escape were killed. When we arrived at Auschwitz, they decided to send us directly to the gas chamber. Our group was relatively small; we all were young and healthy. All of us were in a state of shock. We could not understand and we did not comprehend what was about to happen. Wirtz was the name of the Gestapo man who led us to the gas chamber. There was one girl among us who immediately realized what was about to occur. She went to Wirtz and asked him to take us to the Lager because we were young and healthy and we could work hard. Then, he called out, "Zurueck!" Prisoners from the camp were observing us. This was a rather well-known incident. We left the crematorium alive. Usually, one left the crematorium together with the smoke.

The Institute of Hygiene

I had spotted fever and also dysentery, Lager Durchfall. I was very sick. At that time, I was in Block number 1. The block's supervisor was Edytka Blok. We had four weeks of quarantine and we felt very lucky because we did not have to work during that time. The fifth week, they started to send us to work "nach aussen" which was most difficult. Here in the Lager it was commonplace to volunteer for everything, regardless of whether you were a specialist or not.

An inmate doctor came to us one evening; her name was Ena and she was from Slovakia. She needed laboratory assistants, nurses and doctors. Thirteen women volunteered including me. She took our numbers. We were all considered to be the lucky ones. However, time passed and no one came for us. It was very, very difficult. There were moments when I thought about throwing myself at the electric wires. Every day I promised myself that after work I would have a cup of tea, I would rest a little, and then I would throw myself at the wires. I could barely stand during the roll-calls. I was exhausted and close to death. The only thing left to do was to die! But I did not have the courage to do it.

Finally, one day they came for the thirteen women that volunteered. I was so exhausted that I could barely walk. I was the last one that came. The doctor that interviewed all of us was our future boss, Dr. Weber. He only exchanged a few words with me, asked me for my number, and decided that I would be his laboratory assistant. He did not ask me to work right away; he sent me back to the block.

I was deaf and my tongue was stiff...the signs of Flecktyphus. One day in April 1943, they came for me. They washed me, cut my hair again, and dressed me in some kind of loose, long gown. Then, they took me and a group of other girls to Block 10. I had changed so much that Dr. Weber did not even recognize me. He said he did not need me anymore. At that moment I knew that if I did not do something it would all be over. I knew my life was in my hands. I pulled myself together and started begging him; I tried to convince him; I said that he could not do that to me, that he had promised to save my life and that I had counted on him. I knew he did not recognize me because they had cut my hair again. He smiled and said "Gut."

He took me to the hematologic laboratory where I was supposed to work, but in the end I did not work there. Dr. Weber assigned me to draw blood from "patients," but I told him that I could not stand the sight of blood and somehow managed to get out of the job. He then arranged for Slavka Klein, a physician, to draw the blood. She could not refuse but was successful in obtaining extra bread rations for the blood "donors." Dr. Klein was one of the rather prominent doctors there. She was very much talked and written about once. She was very active in Auschwitz. After the war, she was arrested in Prague, right before they imprisoned Slanski. Later, she was rehabilitated, but she was physically destroyed and died. Dr. Klein had two laboratory assistants, Hadas Lerner (she was called Dédé)[3] and the so-called Perelka. For the time being, I was left in the serologic laboratory that was located in Block 10.

Slavka Klein, Perelka and Dede belonged to the underground organization and had connections with the Polish resistance movement in camp. Sometimes, I delivered letters from Block 10 to the Institute of Hygiene in Rajsko and handed them to Mieczyslaw Kieta, a Polish political prisoner.[4] I never read these letters and do not know what they contained.

Dr. Alina Brewda, the resident prisoner physician in Block 10, was not a member of the underground organization. She did not take care of the sick, but if there were pregnant women among the new arrivals she performed abortions (delivery would have meant the gas chambers for mother and child).

Sylvia Friedmann, Prof. Clauberg's nurse, was an evil woman. She could have provided far less women for Clauberg's sterilization experiments...but she abused her power. Prof. Clauberg did not pay so much attention even if there would have been less patients.

When I came to Block 10, Ria Hans had already left and was in Birkenau. However, her sister, Magda, who was very sick with tuberculosis, had remained. Before the evacuation in January 1945...I had moved to Rajsko long before that time...Ria gave her sister a lethal injection and, thus, ended her life.

Later, Dr. Weber built a large Hygiene Institute in Rajsko, a village near Auschwitz. SS-men would walk us to work to Rajsko each time. Dr. Weber brought doctors and specialists from all over Europe. There were the hematologist, Dr. Jakob Lewin, a remarkable man; Dr. Landau and Dr. Lettich, as well as many doctors from France, Holland and Greece.

Dr. Fleck who worked in the serologic laboratory was the one who developed an anti-typhoid vaccine, which was supposed to be better and cheaper than the one developed by Dr. Weigel that was commonly used. Dr. Fleck worked in Lwow with a group of his assistants. When Dr. Weber found out about this, he brought the whole group with their families to Auschwitz.

Dr. Seeman worked on Wassermann's analysis, mostly for the Wehrmacht. In the group was also Dr. Umschweif, a chemist, and his wife who was a pharmacologist.

During our work in the Hygiene Institute, we did not receive any more nor any better food than before; only our hygienic situation improved. We also had the possibility of organizing more food. Prisoners who worked in the kitchens helped us. Some of our girls had friends among them. We called them "kochanis." They were usually the ones who provided us with food.

Once, when my Aufseherin was leading me to Block 10, she said, "Du, Kleine, du gehst auf eine halbe Freiheit." When compared to Birkenau, it was true. The atmosphere in Block 10 was a little better.

The Hygiene Institute originated in Block 10 with one serologic and one hematologic laboratory. Five women worked in the serologic laboratory: Dr. Anna Seeman, Natalia Umschweif, Frau Meisel, Ernestyna Fleck, and me as laboratory assistant. After some time, Dr. Weber sent Dr. Fleck to Buchenwald (I do not know why) where he probably still worked on his vaccine.

In Rajsko, there were also other prisoners who worked physically. They were gardeners, tailors, carpenters and the like who took care of animals, mostly guinea-pigs that were used for Wassermann's experiments. Dr. Seeman worked on glass sterilization that was used for bacteriological research. In those apparatuses we cooked cultures of beef for the research, but the SS-men took the beef to their kitchens and brought human flesh instead. Some prisoners did not know that it was human meat and ate it. Dr. Seeman, who was well versed in the Talmud, said that there is a paragraph which states that a difficult period will come for the Jews during which the dead will have to help those that are alive.

SS-physician Dr. Clauberg was the one who did most of the sterilization experiments of women. On the ground floor of Block 10, there were an operating room, an x-ray room, a room for the sick and a room for the personnel. There were many unqualified nurses. The "patients" slept on the first floor. The atmosphere was extremely gruesome. The windows were barricaded with wooden planks. Each woman lived in a state of constant fear; afraid of becoming a guinea-pig.

Love in hell

Often, men-prisoners were sent to Block 10 to perform various tasks. That's how I met my future husband. His name was Mikolasz Korn; he was from Slovakia and had arrived with one of the first groups sent from Slovakia to Auschwitz. He had been in such good physical condition that he had been sure he could face just about anything; he had been convinced the Germans were sending him to work; in 1942, crematoria were not yet common knowledge in Slovakia. He had come with a group of the best, healthiest and most intelligent boys.

At first, he worked as a Pfleger (nurse). Physically, the work was very demanding. He was assigned to take care of a group of sick inmates in the Revier. Dr. Korn was supposed to give injections of phenol to those the Germans wanted to put to death. He refused. Dr. Korn was one of the first and last Jewish doctors to refuse to do this.[5]

As a result he was imprisoned in Block 11 from where no one ever came out alive. He was there for several days and was released, probably because the Lagerfuehrer was replaced. It was one of the miracles that took place in the Lager. Dr. Korn returned to work in the Revier. There, he also cleaned the floors and washed the clothes and linen for the sick.

At that time, Dr. Weber was looking for qualified people and took Dr. Korn to help organize the Hygiene Institute. He needed a Kapo and thought that he would be the right person. Dr. Korn was desperate, but he was afraid not to cooperate. He agreed to become the Kapo under the condition that he would not have to wear the armband. Others would do anything to become a Kapo because of all the privileges that came with that function, but Dr. Korn did not want it. However, the camp's underground organization was interested; they thought decent people should take functions like this one. He was told to undertake this difficult task for the good of the prisoners. From that day on, he was being punished every day not only because he was not helping the SS-men in beating the prisoners, which was supposed to be his most important task, but also because he was trying to protect them in any way he could.

One day I saw Dr. Korn hanging from a telegraph pole, punished for defending a prisoner accused of stealing a tomato from a vegetable garden. Despite the fact that he was a Kapo, he was starving just like anybody else. We women had many possibilities to "organize" food. Those who had been in the camp for some time already had contacts in the kitchen and with Poles who received food packages from their families. I had so much that from time to time I could help others. Once I sent something through one of the prisoners to Dr. Korn. Then, next time I sent him two sandwiches; he refused to take them. I was able to exchange a few words with him then. He told me that he could not accept help from a woman who needed help herself. "Woman, or not woman, it does not matter here," I told him, "I have more than I can eat myself; instead of helping some other prisoner, I would like to help you." Anyway, he declined.

My conversation with Dr. Korn had somehow reached the Institute. Sometimes the prisoners and the SS-men would exchange a few words. We always tried to find a way to talk to them. One day, I was thrown out of the Institute by Dr. Weber. I was supposed to stay in Block 10 to which we always would return from Rajsko for the night. When the SS-men came to take us to work in the morning, they announced, "Hygiene Institute…antreten! Nur die Pola nicht, die bleibt!"

Everyone knew the reason for this was my contact with Dr. Korn; there could not be another reason. Several weeks passed. I knew that I would be put either on a list of future guinea-pigs or would be sent to Birkenau. I was terrified. In the meantime, I worked as a Pflegerin. I was looking for some kind of solution. I met a French woman in Block 10, Dr. Adelaide Hautval. Her story is a chapter in itself. She was very noble. We became friends; she liked when I sang Hanka Ordanowna songs for her even though she did not understand the words. She was very dedicated and the best person in the whole of Block 10. She had been sent to Auschwitz because she had walked in the streets of Paris with a sign stating that she was opposed to the persecution of Jews. She was very disappointed that not everyone in Block 10 was like her. Days and nights she would take care of the sick. In Block 10, many hundreds of women were experimented on. Dr. Adelaide was supposed to remove the uteruses of these women, but she refused after the first operation. She did not care what was going to happen to her. Consequently, she was sent to Birkenau.

Dr. Samuel was brought in her place; he had to perform the operations on all these women. He did what he could not to hurt them too much. After a period of time, he was shot and killed by the SS-men.

Liquidation of Block 10. Stay in Rajsko

In the summer of 1944, Block 10 was liquidated and we were moved to another block. There, we lived with girls who came from the Stabsgebaeude in block number one. From there, the SS-men would take us to Rajsko. After the first bombardment of Auschwitz, Dr. Weber moved us to Rajsko, to the Pflanzenzucht. Here, unqualified women worked in the Gaertnerei and those more qualified, such as biologists and botanists, in the Pflanzenzucht.

The name of our Obersturmbannfuehrer was Caesar. The conditions here were not that bad. One could steal vegetables from the garden. I again worked in the Hygiene Institute. Dr. Weber was constantly fighting with the lower rank SS-men. There was always something going on. Those that Dr. Weber tried to "reward" they would persecute, and the other way around.

The SS-men created a very difficult atmosphere in Rajsko, persecuting anyone they could. Dr. Weber attempted to improve the situation, but they would not let him. Several times a day they would storm into the laboratory and we would shake with fear.

The Front is Coming

It was the beginning of 1945. Dr. Weber threw my future husband out of the Institute because of the constant incidents with the SS-men, who would not leave us alone. They could not tolerate that Jewish prisoners felt like human beings. Also, Dr. Korn was a thorn in their side. They did not like a Kapo who treated prisoners like human beings. They sent Dr. Korn to Birkenau with instructions not to let him work as a doctor but as an outside worker. Being an experienced Haeftling, he was able to survive there. After a period of time, Dr. Weber brought him back to Rajsko. The front was coming closer. The SS-men did not resist too much anymore. There was one doctor from Belgium, Dr. Delmotte, among the SS-men. He talked very openly, "I wonder how you will be treating me when I become your prisoner. You know that I was decent." It was obvious they were scared.

Dr. Weber had supposedly two doctoral degrees. He was a talented man. Some of the prisoners said that he knew every branch of medicine. He knew what was going on in every laboratory. However, after the war no one ever heard of him. There was one Dr. Muench among the Hitlerites who was such a good man that he was acquitted during the Cracow trials of 1947.

Evacuation of Auschwitz

The evacuation of Auschwitz began in 1945. We were still in Rajsko. On the 18th of January, 1945, we came to the laboratory although the male prisoners had remained in the Lager. We talked openly about the defeat of the Germans. We asked Dr. Muench to let us hide, but he said that was too dangerous, that it would be better to leave the camp because the Russians were very close and were going to be here any day now to free us.

We left the camp and this was a terrible mistake because a few days later the Red Army freed Auschwitz. We, however, had to spend several more months in fear during the infamous death march that was so much written and talked about.

Dr. Seeman was recovering from Heine-Medina disease (polio) and survived thanks only to the help of other prisoners. She had to be in a wheel-chair. She was a woman of strong will. After the war, she left Czechoslovakia for Canada. I met her in Prague. Dr. Umschweif died during the death march; his wife Nusia died of spotted fever one day before the final liberation. Dr. Ena took their son. She now lives in Australia. The Meisels stayed in Poland.

Sometimes during the walk, the Hitlerites would let us rest in someone's stables or in the open. During one of such rests, I took my shoes off in the stables and hid them, knowing that if I would lose them I would lose my life. Then, being extremely tired, I fell asleep and when I woke up I could not find one of the shoes and could not put the other one on my swollen foot. The Germans were already calling, "Raus, raus! marsch, marsch!" and I did not have my shoes. I decided that I had no other option but to hide under the hay. And when I was trying to cover myself with the hay, I found a pair of shoes that were about five sizes larger. I put them on and was ready to continue with the walk. I do not know; maybe if I would have hidden in the hay, they would not have found me. But at the time, I was convinced the other pair of shoes saved my life.

We continued with the walk; people were dropping dead, day after day. When we finally reached Ravensbrueck, I had an eye inflammation because of all the dirt and cold. I went to the Revier and suddenly noticed Dr. Adelaide Hautval. I was convinced that she would help me, that she would do anything for me, but she treated me like any other patient. She did not care about us anymore. After a few days, the condition of my eye improved.

Then they led us to Malchow. We were starving there. One was ready to trade one's hand for a few potato peelings.

During the liquidation of that Lager, a number of prisoners remained and so could we with our Hygiene Institute group. But I decided to leave because Mila, with whom I had been together since Ravensbrueck, could not stay and we were inseparable. We walked a little and then we rode in a train, which was bombed later.

Next, we reached Leipzig where we stayed for a short time. They gave us something to eat and told us to go on. The SS-men were afraid of going to the front and that is why they held on to us as long as they could. They were fleeing in fear of the Americans, then the Russians and then the British: This was the end of the death march.

Liberation

It was April 1945. The days were warm but the nights were rather cold. We did not have any warm clothes to wear. Sometimes we had to walk during the night. Some of the SS-men deserted. One night we were resting in a meadow. When we woke up in the morning, not even one SS-man was left. People started to part. Some went west. A few kilometers ahead they were liberated by the Americans. Mila and I went east and were liberated by the Russians. I wanted to go back to Poland.

A New life

Dr. Korn and I had decided that after the war we would meet in Slovakia. The last time I saw him was in the afternoon of January 17, 1945. The next day, January 18, the men were not brought to work and we left Auschwitz that day. I wanted to be back in Poland as soon as possible and to start looking for my family. I knew that my brother who ran away to Russia would probably write to our village and this would be the only way to get in touch with him.

I joined a large group of Polish prisoners who were returning to Poland. Women were among them. I wanted to get closer, but they were avoiding me. Some of the prisoners attacked me. It was very difficult for me to be alone. They walked about four kilometers an hour; I could not walk so fast. I was also afraid. I went to the leader of the group and asked him for help. He told me, "You do not need to worry anymore. From now on, two men will take care of you, like two knights would."

Every night we would rest in a village or a German country-estate; we would wash and eat and go on. And so we reached Breslau. From there I went to Cracow the first chance I had. And from Cracow to Tyczyn. In the local administration office, I found a letter from my brother and his address in Russia. I contacted him immediately.

Then, I left everything in Poland and decided to go illegally to Czechoslovakia where I met Dr. Korn. However, I had to return to Poland to get my documents to be able to get married. We married in 1946, and our son, Milan was born in 1947. In 1956, when the situation in Poland improved and the government became more liberal, a group of former political Auschwitz prisoners invited us to Poland. They knew about the activities of my husband in the camp; they knew he did not lose his dignity for a moment. The group organized a series of receptions for us in Cracow. Dr. Rejman of the group became one of my husband's best friends.

The Czech Press about Dr. Korn

A number of articles about my husband appeared in the fifties. In a daily Prague newspaper, *Rude Prawo*, Otto Krause, a former Auschwitz prisoner, wrote about my husband in an article entitled: "A look at the history of the underground organization in Auschwitz."

Another article entitled: "Unknown Heroes" appeared in 1967, right after the death of Dr. Mikolasz Korn.

During the Hitlerite trials in Frankfurt, one of the witnesses, his name was Fabian, talked about the behavior of Dr. Korn in Auschwitz. At that time, an article entitled: “Human Massacres” appeared in which my husband was again glorified.

Dr. Korn died in 1967 at the age of 58. He did not live to see the “Prague Spring” nor the possibility to leave Czechoslovakia, where we were very unhappy because of the political situation there.

In 1968, I emigrated to Israel; the borders were “open” then. My son, Milan, now a Doctor of Chemistry, joined me.

❖

Appendices

APPENDIX A
Correspondence with Former SS-Physician Dr. Hans Muench

Dr. Hans Muench was born on May 14, 1911 in Freiburg.

From 1943 until the evacuation of Auschwitz, he worked in the Hygienic Institute in Rajsko as bacteriologist with the rank of SS-Untersturmfuehrer.

He was acquitted in the Cracow Auschwitz trial on December 22, 1947.

After his acquittal, Dr. Muench returned to his home in Southern Germany and practiced medicine in a small town.

In his study of Nazi doctors, Lifton calls him "A Human Being in an SS Uniform."

▼

I believed that Dr. Muench would be able to furnish valuable information from his side of the fence and asked him to answer a few questions about the Hygienic Institute. A part of this interview in letters is given below.

September 5, 1988

Dear Dr. Muench:

I received your address from Dagmar Ostermann, a comrade of mine from Auschwitz, who recently worked together with you in Vienna and am writing to you on the following matter.

I am Jewish and worked from 1943 until the evacuation of Auschwitz in the Political Section of the camp. In 1986, a book was published which contained thirty eyewitness account of former prisoners of the work detail Politische Abteilung/Standesamt which I have compiled, translated and edited.

There was quite a bit of interest in the book and I was asked to also report about other groups. That's why I am preparing at present a manuscript about the Institute of Hygiene and about the experimental Block 10.

Since you worked in both, I would appreciate it if you could send me a report about your activities in both of these institutions.

🖂

November 5, 1988

Dear Mrs. Shelley,

At first an explanation why you are only receiving an answer today to your letter of two months ago. Every spring and fall we live in a remote part of Greece. Lots of letters are being lost there; that's why we do not have anything forwarded to us. We only returned three days ago.

I am certainly qualified to report about the Institute of Hygiene as well as about Block 10...at least from about June 1943 until the end. Since my acquittal in Cracow I consider it my absolute duty to do my best to shed light about Auschwitz. I, therefore, agree with your proposal. In addition, I would like to mention that my acquittal was not only based on my refusal to do ramp service (i.e. perform selections) but above all because of the circumstances and motivation for the experiments I did in Block 10.

There is little to report about the Institute of Hygiene which could contribute to the clarification of doubtful inhuman activities. That the director (Dr. Weber) was persuaded to participate in criminal experiments because his boss in Berlin (Dr. Mugrowsky) did the same has nothing to do with the idea of installing a bacteriological laboratory and an institute of hygiene in Auschwitz. The Institute of Hygiene was installed in Auschwitz because the camp physicians were incapable of stemming the rapid growth of epidemics. In 1942, typhus had broken out among members of the SS as well. For example, Mrs. Caesar had died from it.[1]

Primarily, the Institute of Hygiene had nothing to do with Block 10. During the winter of 1943/44, large quantities of sputum were needed in the laboratory for experimental purposes in order to examine the concentration and suitability of blood type antigens. It was discovered that saliva of normal prisoners could not be used since they did not produce enough due to the weakened immune system. That's why Weber took the relatively well-nourished Clauberg inmates in Block 10 as subjects. It worked. A saliva collection point was established in a room and the prisoner physician, Dr. Alina Brewda, was charged with supervising this task. This activity was continued after Clauberg's experiments had been completed. The women destined for the gas chamber could thus survive for the moment.

In the fall or winter 1943, I came to Block 10 for the first time and had no complaints. The accompanying SDG (SS orderly) told me about the fate of these women, i.e. as bearers of secrets they had to be gassed. It was generally assumed that the experiments would not have to be continued for a protracted period of time. I realized that I (who had, meanwhile, been advanced to the position of deputy of the director who was frequently absent) would be morally responsible for the planned liquidation of these prisoners in case we should give up the laboratory in Block 10. The Kommandantur urged us, they did not like to have women in the men's camp. It was clear that the continuation of experiments in Block 10 had to be thoroughly justified and established with irrefutable arguments. That was not easy. We only succeeded in a roundabout way.

If you think that this story could be a topic for your report, I'll participate. There are enough details. It's a little bit more difficult to talk about the blood taken from prisoners for the Institute of Hygiene to produce test sera for blood groups against special food rations. It might be better if you would get these stories from the inmates. I don't remember much more. From your point of view, this might be different.

Please write to me. I hope your other informants will not keep you waiting for an answer as long as I did. I am sorry.

With all good wishes for your work.

✉

November 20, 1988

Dear Dr. Muench,

I thank you for your letter and your readiness to participate in our project and would appreciate if you could describe the events in Block 10 and in the Institute of Hygiene from your point of view in as much detail as possible

✉

A) Block 10

Question 1: Describe the experiments that were performed by SS doctors:

a) Clauberg...sterilization through injection into the oviducts.
b) Schumann...sterilization through irradiation and verification by oopherectomies
c) Wirths...cervical cancer experiments on women who did not suffer from cancer.
d) Weber...blood-type experimentation
e) others ... ?

Answer: About Clauberg, Schumann, Wirths and Weber, I could tell you a little which I learned from hearsay, but that would be of scant use to you because I do not know more, and probably less, than many prisoners whom you already interviewed. I had no direct contact with either Clauberg or Schumann. I cannot even remember ever having seen Schumann. Clauberg I saw perhaps twice or three times when he appeared in his Revier, i.e. the lower floor of Block 10, probably in the spring of 1944.

I had no special contact with Wirths, but I knew that he had tissue specimen removed from the uterus. He either did it himself or had it done by inmate physicians. I also know that Samuel played a big role here...but I'll discuss this aspect later.

I discussed the removal of this tissue with Wirths. There was nothing criminal in this procedure and nothing unpleasant for the patient if the operation was performed correctly. The pieces taken were so extremely small that they were insignificant. Of course, the cervical wound was bleeding a little but it always healed normally. And this procedure is nowadays (microscopic and colposcopic examinations of cervical and uterine cancer are far more advanced) more or less routine for every woman suspected to suffer from cancer of the uterus. In Germany, it is being done in at least 50% of these cases. Thus, one cannot consider it as an uncommon manipulation.

Wirths needed these tissue specimens in order to train himself in the microscopic diagnostic of uterine cancer. He availed himself of the expertise of Dr. Samuel, and I believe that most of the cervical specimens were removed by Samuel and not by Wirths. The colposcope was an excellent optical instrument which contained a very strong lens. It had only been introduced in the forties and Wirths was interested in it.

In regards to Weber: I have never seen blood transfusions of intentionally not matching blood donors, not in the Institute of Hygiene, nor in Block 10 and not by Weber. It never even occurred to me to ask Weber about it because nobody ever mentioned it.

I did not know any other physicians who made experiments in Block 10.

Question 2: How was the attitude and the behavior of the four SS doctors toward the prisoners?

Answer: As already mentioned, about Schumann and Clauberg I cannot speak. I never heard that Wirths acted cruelly. His behavior toward prisoners was always correct...he adhered to his guidelines. I can't say any more...except, perhaps, his relationship with Samuel...and to this we'll come later.

Question 3: What do you know about the selection of about thirty women in July 1943 in Block 10 who were later gassed in KL-Struthof-Natzweiler for the skeleton collection of Professor Hirt of Strassburg University?

Answer: I cannot tell you anything about it because I hear now from you about it for the first time.

Question 4: You write: "In the fall or winter 1943 I came for the first time to Block 10 and had nothing to complain about." Please explain this sentence. You came to this block of horrors described by survivors as a "nightmare between inferno and lunatic asylum" and found nothing to object to?

Question 5: What did your experiments in Block 10 consist of?

Question 6: You wrote that during the absence of Weber you felt morally responsible for the planned liquidation of the prisoners if the lab in Block 10 would be given up.

a) Did the women remain solely because you did not give up the laboratory?
b) Which "doctors" did you take to continue the laboratory?

Answer: Your questions 4, 5 and 6 are connected and I'll answer them together:

Let's start with the motivation. I already told you that I made these experiments because the women in Block 10 were threatened to be gassed. I had heard about it through Paul Reichel, a prisoner in our "kommando" who came from Karlsbad in Czechoslovakia. He was the first secretary in our office and I had very good, personal contact with him. He told me that it would be inevitable that the Institute of Hygiene work squad in Block 10 would be liquidated. There would not be any more justification for experiments since the blood type research had been terminated. He implored me whether I could do anything to keep this kommando because otherwise it would be sent to the gas chamber. He knew a woman he liked among them and that was the reason that he begged me. Simultaneously, I had heard the same story from Weber. Weber had trouble with Wirths, and Wirths, in turn, had had trouble with the Kommandantur, because it was known that Clauberg was supposed to have completed his experiments. But he had never stated this clearly...he always claimed that it could be, that further experiments would have to be performed and that Block 10 would have to be kept.

Block 10 was a thorn in the side of the camp Kommandantur. There was talk about a big disorder, and great difficulties in keeping the male prisoners out of Block 10 and of maintaining proper camp discipline. There might have been some substance to these rumors. I did not know anything for sure. It was certain, however, that the Kommandantur urged to liquidate the block. They could not do anything against Clauberg because Clauberg had received his research instructions personally from Himmler.

The person responsible for Block 10 was Wirths...he was the go-between between Clauberg and the Kommandantur. Wirths was not interested in keeping Block 10...he was more interested in having good relations with the camp commandant. I personally overheard a conversation between him and Weber in which he down-played his own experiments and claimed that he could obtain the same material from the women's camp in Birkenau.

Objectively speaking, Weber was also not interested in maintaining Block 10. The saliva experiments were finished and there was no sensible reason to keep the kommando in Block 10. However, in reality things were different. Weber was very ambitious and seldom let go of something he had his hands on. He wanted to keep the laboratory in Block 10. One never could know what might happen; and that what you have you don't give up. That was his motto.

Well, I was charged with finding out what was going on in Block 10. That was the reason why I went there. As already mentioned, I did not discover any difficulties and had nothing to object to. I reported back to Weber that the only possibility of keeping Block 10 was to continue doing experiments. He said: "O.K. See what you can come up with, hopefully something which takes a long time so that we won't have trouble immediately again."

This was the motivation why I had closer contact with Block 10 in the first place. I searched for ideas and came up with some suggestions. Weber did not bother at all with it. He stated: "I have no time to take care of this. I'll promise that Berlin...i.e., The Supreme Institute of Hygiene under Mugrowsky...will approve it. You don't have to worry. Everything will be O.K. for sure. I am on good terms with him and I can present it to him the right way. Let me have a proposal. I'll go to Berlin anyway and will settle it there."

In the first place, I selected a subject which was quite interesting and could have produced proper results. Secondly, the experiments could be prolonged ad infinitum, and thirdly, I found a prisoner in our kommando who was a specialist in the field I had chosen and with whom I had a good relationship. We understood each other well and I could entrust him with the real motivation for the experiments. He was Dr. Ernest Pollak of the pathological laboratory, who was specialized in internal medicine and had considerable experience in the area of allergies and rheumatism. When I confided in him, he made it unmistakably clear that this project would turn into an unpleasant situation for me. Like all prisoners in our kommando, he knew that my reputation in the eyes of the Kommandantur was not the best because of favoritism toward prisoners and similar accusations I enjoyed a good reputation among the inmates and we would have to handle this experiment in such a way that it could not be interpreted as favoring prisoners.

Thus, it would only work if I would not behave in a similar fashion toward the "delinquents," i.e. the experimental subjects, as I normally related to prisoners in the Institute or with other inmates in camp with whom I had contact. His (Pollak's) head would be in danger as well as mine. One never could be safe from informers. There was a lot of talk about intrigues in Block 10. He did not know any details, but he wanted to draw my attention to them. He did not want to dissuade me, but he asked me to be cautious and to use a tone that would preclude all kinds of favoritism.

I followed his advice and did not establish any personal contact with the subjects; even with Dr. Alina Brewda, I conversed only in an official manner. I, therefore, believe that neither Pollak nor I were ever suspected of favoritism toward inmates by the camp authorities.

It was not easy to convince the Kommandantur or Wirths of the necessity of our project and only through the strict and decisive intervention of Mugrowsky, the director of the head Institute of Hygiene, did we receive the required permission from the camp to proceed. Well, I had to give this long introduction in order to explain how the experiment was conceived.

I'll attempt to describe the research project in layman's terms because the medical intricacies are rather complex and in hindsight they are obsolete...although at that time they were a correct topic. In the thirties and forties, and even later, there was discussion among medical researchers that rheumatism might be traced to several other diseases or seats of infections in the body, for example to chronic appendicitis, to chronic tonsillitis, or to encysted seats of infections at the root of teeth. It was assumed that these infections would trigger the mechanism via allergic reactions in the body that would finally lead to rheumatism, a disease whose real causes are not well known even today, and which was much discussed at that time. This was the field I wanted to investigate.

Pollak already had some experience from his studies at the university and we investigated the subject and started with preliminary tests. We had to be faster than the Kommandantur because we feared that they might come to an agreement with Clauberg in the meantime. We began with skin tests with saline solutions and completely harmless substances to observe the skin reaction to extracts from infection seats. We pre-tested all our extracts on rabbits, guinea pigs and even ourselves to be sure that there would not occur any shock reactions. This lasted until approximately spring 1944, since all the extracts had to be produced at the Institute and this took many weeks.

Pollak had...as far as possible...a good relationship with the human subjects in Block 10. I left him alone there many times; but I had to personally take him to the block and pick him up again. Intentionally, I avoided closer contact with the women prisoners. However, we demonstrated these allergic reactions on our own skin, mostly on our backs, to show that the experiments were not dangerous, and I believe the patients were convinced of this. All these experiments were extensively deliberated on during the Cracow Auschwitz trial of 1947, and I owe my acquittal in great measure precisely to these tests. It might be useful if I send you a photocopy of the sentence which I received in a German translation from the Central Office of War Crimes in Ludwigsburg.

However, I sensed and was supported in my belief by Ludwig Woerl, the camp elder of the men's camp, that our activities in Block 10 did not contribute to improve the difficulties the camp direction had with the experimental block. Also, Dr. Fejkiel, the elder of the Revier in the Stammlager, had voiced the opinion that our experiments could be performed somewhere else in camp, for example in his sickbay. An additional factor had to be taken into consideration: I could not help but notice...and Pollak had mentioned it to me...that these poor women, who did not know what we were doing to them and, who in spite of our assurances that the experiments were harmless, were in a horrible mental situation.

Nevertheless, everything ran smoothly. In the meantime, I had made good contact with Ludwig Woerl, the camp elder. I soon noticed that this was a man I could trust and I tried to tell him…not everything…but at least the reason behind our experiments.

Question 7: Lifton writes that you saved specific prisoners (for example wives of inmates of the Institute of Hygiene)

a) How did this happen?
b) Whom did you save in this fashion?
c) A part of the wives worked in the Institute of Hygiene anyway, for example Dr. Anna Seemann, Ernestine Fleck, Natalie Umschweif, Helena Meisel and Pola Beck, the friend and later spouse of the kapo, Dr. Mikolaj Korn.

Question 8: Lifton mentions further that you had women declared dead and had them smuggled out of Block 10 with the assistance of or through bribing the kapo of the bordello.

a) How did the women leave the men's camp (because the bordello-kommando stayed in the Stammlager)?
b) Did you free these women?
c) Did you provide these women with a new camp identity, if so which one?
d) Were other persons (SS men or prisoners) involved in this mission?

Answer: In the summer of 1944, Ludwig Woerl offered to smuggle some women out of Block 10, either through death certificates, hospital transfers or other manipulations. He told me: "It will be easiest to do this through the bordello kommando. Here, women are being constantly transferred. It won't be noticeable if one will be mixed in because of unsuitability. We'll be able to manipulate it to take her out of Block 10." In this way, he managed to get a few women out, and, because I was endangered, I did not help at all in this undertaking. I knew everything was in good hands.

After my release in 1947, I met Woerl here in Munich and we got along very well with each other. He also confirmed then that the smuggling had been done through the bordello.

The women who worked in the Institute of Hygiene had nothing to do with Block 10. These were women who marched into camp...so it might have been that they slept in Block 10. I can't say this with certainty since I never looked into this. They were colleagues in the Institute and had a good kommando.

Question 9: What was the task of the laboratory in Block 10 apart from the collection of saliva and the research on blood groups?

Question 10 Which prisoners worked in this laboratory in addition to Dr. Slavka Kleinova (Dorota Lorska)?

Question 11: Re: Sputum collection point; For what type of research did you need the saliva?

Answer: I remember Dr. Slavka Klein quite well. She was the physician who had been allocated for our experiments by her boss, Dr. Brewda. I talked to her a few times and gave her some information about our research...of course, not the true reason for our experiments. Whether or not Pollak did so, I have no idea, but I doubt that he confided in her.

In regard to the drawing of 42 Quaddeln (skin pricks), these injections into the back the size of flea bites, made by a former subject of Block 10 which you sent to me, I would like to point out the following. It does not make any sense since we had no reason to give a maximum of injections to a minimum of inmates. Our problem was to involve, with the relatively small amount of extract we had, as many subjects as possible. For a normal allergy experiment, 10-20 Quaddeln were required. I don't know why there were 42...I cannot prove it, but I believe it was improbable. I certainly did not do it, and if it was done by Pollak for any unfathomable reason, then solely in order to demonstrate that we did not experiment on humanitarian grounds. And if he did it, he surely did not use any substances that would cause inflammation. However, I doubt that it really occurred.

The sputum collection stemmed from the question whether it would be possible to determine a person's blood type through a simple and easy analysis of the saliva, or, in other words, would it be feasible (since it was a generally acknowledged fact that blood-groups could be found out by examining sputum) to improve the procedure so that it would be comparable to the blood-type test based on a blood sample. This would have constituted an essential simplification for practical purposes and Weber had decided to pursue this question. One would avoid potential infections which might occur if blood was drawn from a finger or the ear lobe. It was not very important...but we had enough experts who could occupy themselves with this problem. Furthermore, Weber was specialized in the production of sera for testing blood groups and never gave up when he sensed the possibility of new discoveries in this field. I'll talk later about the importance of the production of test sera for blood types.

That was the reason we required these large quantities of saliva. Nevertheless, the research was unproductive and was discontinued.

Question 12: Lifton states that Dr. Alina Brewda had opportunity to select some women in Block 10 for your harmless tests and to protect them in this way from Clauberg's sterilization experiments. Two of the eyewitnesses who participated in our project received injections from you and were also used as guinea pigs for Clauberg. Did you know that your tests were absolutely no protection from being sterilized?

Answer: All women who had survived Clauberg's experiments were irrevocably destined to be gassed according to our knowledge. An assignment as my research subjects was intended to prevent this. I already reported that for security reasons I was not personally engaged in this undertaking. I, therefore, left the choice of subjects to Mrs. Alina. In my and Mr. Pollak's view she knew best who was most endangered. I cannot now reconstruct how such "double experiments" occurred. I regret them very much.

Question 13: According to accounts by prisoners, the experiments were continued after the women were transferred in the summer of 1944 to Block 1 of the camp extension. Supposedly the block was equipped with new apparatuses for additional experiments which did not seem to hint at the planned liquidation of the entire block.

a) Do you have other information in this respect?

b) Did your laboratory continue to exist after the transfer?

Answer: I don't understand the question very well. The women who were transferred to Block 1 were obviously still needed by Clauberg. I don't know anything about the new apparatuses.

Our experiments were continued in the room on the first floor of Block 10.

Question 14:

At the Cracow trial there were witnesses who testified that you saved the lives of some women in Block 10. Could you please let me know the names of these women?

Answer: I can't tell you much in regard to this question. I know that several testified in Cracow that they were able to leave Block 10 because of the experiments I performed on them. I do not know who they were.

Question 15:

Prof. Maximilian Samuel was a rather controversial figure...condemned by many not only as a collaborator but also as an informer. Nevertheless, some survivors of Block 10 venerate him and make every effort to have him inscribed as a "Righteous" person in Yad Vashem.[2] Slavka Kleinova once devised a scale in regard to the attitudes of prisoner physicians in connection with the pseudo-scientific experiments in Block 10: 1) Those who refused to collaborate; 2) Those who did not execute harmful instructions for co-prisoners without categorically declaring so; 3) Those who executed them; and 4) Those who executed them eagerly. Under Number 1, she placed Dr. Adelaide Hautval, who refused to participate in experiments and under Number 4 she put Dr. Wladyslaw Dering, who boasted about his skills in performing oopherectomies in record time (a few minutes). Please tell me about Samuel and how you would assess him.

Answer: Samuel was a protege of Wirths. Wirths was interested in gynecology. He had written his doctoral dissertation in this field. He was engaged in a colposcopic examination of the cervix and uterus and took Samuel, who was experienced in this area, to help or teach him.

Listening a few times to conversations between Weber and Wirths, I heard that he was not too happy with Samuel. He could not check him because his own knowledge was insufficient, but he had the impression that the examinations and results Samuel made for him were manipulated in some way. He was quite skeptical and asked us whether or not we had anybody who could control Samuel.

Later in August 1944, I remember it well, I talked to Wirths about this subject because I knew somebody who could help him. And then Wirths told me, "Well, it is too late. Samuel already went through the chimney. I could prove to him that he cheated me and I sent him into the gas."

B) The Institute of Hygiene

Question 16: You write that the Institute of Hygiene came to Auschwitz because the spotted fever epidemic of 1942 could not be stopped with the means Hoess applied...extermination of lice together with the sick.

a) What was the contribution of the Institute of Hygiene in fighting this epidemic?
b) Had not the epidemic pretty much petered out by the time the Institute was opened in Rajsko?

Question 17: What was the main task of the Institute?

Answer: It was not spotted fever but a typhus epidemic which had already broken out in 1941 and was spreading all over camp which mainly brought the Institute of Hygiene to Auschwitz. Mrs. Caesar, the wife of the director of the agricultural enterprises, had died of typhus. This institute was charged with the gathering and utilization of dandelion plants which secrete a substance used for the manufacture of rubber. Caesar had grown these dandelions on vast plantations in the Ukraine.

When it became too dangerous in the Ukraine they gave him fields and a building in Auschwitz for his cultivation. Well, his wife had died of typhus and since Caesar was one of the highest ranking SS men in Auschwitz, he was able to complain in high places. They were forced to do something and the Institute of Hygiene was opened in Auschwitz...not over the direct protest of the camp administration, but they certainly were not enchanted with it.

It started as a field laboratory. The Institute of Hygiene had five or seven so-called field laboratories. Every military establishment has these installations...a bacteriological and also a modest serological laboratory which...under conditions of field hospitals...can perform bacteriological examinations. These field laboratories consisted of one or two trained bacteriologists, serologists and lab technicians respectively, and personnel for the motor vehicles and office work (the latter were dispatched to pick up specimens from field hospitals, etc.). A normal field laboratory consisted of a crew of approximately ten persons.

Mugrowsky was happy to avail himself of the opportunity to send a laboratory to Auschwitz because he realized that he needed far less personnel there since the lab technicians could be replaced by prisoners. Moreover, he had the possibility of doing scientific research on a much larger scale, since plenty of equipment was available, but above all, the concentration camp had a multitude of highly qualified first-class scientists whom Mugrowsky could employ...since he had a shortage of people.

Mugrowsky had the Institute for Spotted Fever in Sachsenhausen under the direction of Ding-Schuler[3] (with whom we were in contact) and he had the responsibility of doing experiments on human beings in Ravensbrueck, experiments in his field of bacteriology and serology. He performed a lot of experiments and was sentenced to death as a result of them after the war. It was a good opportunity for him that Auschwitz was added to his list. He was on good terms with Weber, who had received a first-class training and was an excellent organizer. He enjoyed the chance of building an institute for scientific research. He was actually not interested in basic scientific investigation but rather in the production of the most favorable test sera for blood groups. Even nowadays, test sera for blood groups can only be obtained from human blood and are very perishable if they are not concentrated in solid form. Test sera for blood types were far more in demand for the

SS than in other military hospitals because all members of the SS were tattooed with their blood group and for this purpose they required vast amounts of test sera for blood types in a form which could be kept for a long time without refrigeration or other conservation. This was very difficult and was the major task of the Institute in Rajsko.

That was the background...but the actual cause for the opening of the Institute was the typhus epidemic. They had to examine who had typhus, who was a typhus carrier, etc. Many bacteriological tests had to be performed by this bacteriological field laboratory, the forerunner of the Institute of Hygiene South-East.

Spotted fever did, of course, play a large role in Auschwitz, but to combat it one did not necessarily need a laboratory. One had to take general hygienic measures. This, regrettably, was not possible in camps. One could not continue to use the same method the camp administration had employed, i.e., gassing the lice together with the people, because the spotted fever spread even faster this way. We were supposed to devise measures against it, but the camp administration did not allow us to do so. They always cited Wirths, who had jurisdiction over all camps and there was a constant controversy between the Kommandantur, Wirths and us as to who was really in charge. Later on, there was agreement that the Institute of Hygiene was responsible for all the bacteriological and serological tests. The authority for spotted fever remained with Wirths. Over time, the incidence of spotted fever went down, so it was not so important for us.

Some of the major tasks of the Institute of Hygiene were the bacteriological diagnoses in camp, first of all for the SS troops, but also for the prisoners, to prevent epidemics. The diagnostic specimens and preparations were sent to us and examined. We made bacteriological tests of sputum for tuberculosis, stool, urine, etc., everything which might be connected with infectious diseases. Our equipment and our personnel were really tops.

Question 18: What were the tasks and research areas of the SS physicians...you, Dr. Weber[4] and Dr. Delmotte?

Answer: Except for Weber, who was charged with producing test sera for blood groups, there were no research areas assigned from headquarters. It was regarded with approval if one of us managed, in the little time he had, to pursue additional studies, but it was largely left up to us. That's why I was able to perform the aforementioned experiments. On my own initiative I did other research as well. They are not worth mentioning because they did not involve human beings but were purely experimental tasks in bacteriology done with guinea pigs and rabbits.

Delmotte did his doctoral dissertation at the Institute. I don't know too much about his work but I would like to talk more at length about him. He is an important figure to illustrate the special position the Institute of Hygiene occupied in Auschwitz.

The Institute of Hygiene received its orders directly from the head Institute of Hygiene of the Waffen SS in Berlin. It also had to follow the commands of the Kommandantur of Auschwitz and had to work closely with Wirths, the camp Physician-in-Chief. This close collaboration was not as ideal in practice as in theory, simply because physicians don't like to have their designs discovered and also because the Institute of Hygiene had been compelled to come to Auschwitz in order to teach hygiene to the not quite competent camp physicians (as rumor had it then). Well, this tense relationship was heightened when I refused to participate in selections and when Mugrowsky prevailed upon the Kommandantur, and especially upon Wirths, for me in this respect...although I was subordinate to Wirths. In spite of the fact that Mugrowsky had too much personnel at the front he refused to transfer anybody to Auschwitz to assist...among other tasks...in selections which I had refused to do. That's when he was assigned a well-trained young man, namely Hans Delmotte. He was a graduate of the highest SS leadership college and belonged to those young people who had received the best national socialist training destined only for the elite. He surfaced in Auschwitz, arrogant as could be, with family and relatives in the highest SS echelons, and looked down upon me. He was very surprised when suddenly he received an order from Wirths to report for selection duty.

And now comes the strange part...as a highly qualified SS officer Delmotte did not know what a selection was. He had never heard of extermination camps, not of Auschwitz and not of those already liquidated in the Generalgouvernement. He was stunned and did not know the meaning of the term "selection." When he returned early in the morning from his first selection, he was completely destroyed. Never again since have I seen as severe a nervous breakdown as he suffered. For many days he could not eat anything, was completely beside himself, did not sleep, ran around all night long and was entirely incapable of doing anything systematically. He fiercely endeavored to get away from Auschwitz. He not only beseeched Mugrowsky but mobilized all the connections he had since childhood and especially his influential relatives for this purpose. Nobody supported him and it was impressed upon him that as a highly qualified young man he would have to stand up and participate in that which Hitler, and above all Himmler, had preached right from the beginning, namely the extermination of the Jews and everything else coming his way out of racial necessity.

In view of the very difficult situation, the following was decided. For a start, he would work for half a day with Dr. Thilo as camp physician. After a few days or weeks (it was not precisely defined) he should be introduced, at first, to the customary selections in the hospital and later, of course, to the Great Selection. An additional concession was granted...his young wife, whom he had married some time ago and with whom he had hardly lived because of his training, was allowed to move to Auschwitz. All of these measures bore some fruit. After two weeks he was a normal person again, he kept apart from Weber and me, but the arrogance with which he had arrived was totally gone. He now associated with camp physicians. After about four weeks he did selections routinely. His wife stayed for quite some time and Delmotte was soon so integrated into Auschwitz life that nothing was visible any more on the outside. After his wife was gone, he lived a while next to my apartment and I noticed that he often ran around outside at night because he could not sleep. That was all that was noticeable...otherwise he had everything under control again.

Delmotte did not spend too much time on his dissertation. He worked on some bacteriological-pharmacological topic and constantly got advice from the prisoner physician, Prof. Mansfeld. He had a good personal relationship with him. And I knew from Mansfeld, with whom I, too, was on good terms, that he was well-informed about Delmotte's mental state. Prof. Mansfeld really liked the young man.

It is well-known that Delmotte committed suicide in April or May 1945. I believe that he and his dilemma were indicative of the strange exceptional position the Institute of Hygiene occupied in Auschwitz.

Question 19: What were the tasks and attitudes of Unterscharfuehrers Fugger, Zabel, Pargner and others?[5]

Answer: This is a vast area and can sometimes be answered in a speculative way only.

Unterscharfuehrer Zabel was a primitive person with an exaggerated sense of self-confidence. He was inordinately proud of the fact that he was a licensed disinfector and SDG, the only one in our crew. This was the reason that he claimed the privilege of checking and harassing the prisoners of the laboratory. Also, in his capacity as boss of the cultural media kitchen, he endeavored to instill authority. He was the only one of the SS crew who looked for contact with the other SDGs and Unterfuehrers (non-commissioned officers of the camp).

Unterscharfuehrer Fugger was a clever Austrian with black market contacts with the civilian population in town. His attempts to instill authority in the crew failed, mostly because his subordinates knew or suspected too much about his business deals. He was not ostentatiously brutal toward the inmates.

Unterscharfuehrer Pargner was secretary and manager of the depot. He emulated Zabel in attempting to instill "order" and authority vis-à-vis the prisoners of the outside work details, such as animal caretakers, cleaners, tailors and gardeners. This compensated for his underimmersion in his assigned task as secretary (his work was performed by the inmates of the office). He was sentenced in Cracow, the only one of the crew. I do not know when he was released. He came from East Germany as far as I can remember.

Schumacher had no specific function at the Institute. Probably Berlin had too many men at their disposal and had sent him to Auschwitz. Weber always attempted to convince Mugrowsky that his Institute was understaffed (Parkinson effect).

About ten or twelve years ago, Schumacher came to see me. He was scared because they had found out in his home town that he had been stationed in Auschwitz. He wanted to know from me what he could expect if he were to be extradited to Poland. I could assure him that he did not have to fear extradition because the Polish authorities only requested people who had been guilty of personal brutality. This was the case up to the highest ranks and functions. A case in point was Caesar. He had been together with me in the transportation camp to be extradited but was not sent to Poland. There had been too many witnesses who had testified in his favor.

Festweber was in charge of the motor vehicles of the Institute (Fahrbereitschaft).

Rottenfuehrer Kapmeier was a Volksdeutscher, conscripted by force, perhaps from Hungary. He was very young and thoughtless and had been requisitioned by Weber as a courier to the SS hospital in Cracow. That was the right job for him...black market deals in Cracow, the opportunity to drink and "amore." On his courier trips by railroad he also transported Kassibers for the inmates of the Rajsko Kommando. It did not last long. He was too affable and fond of drinking, as Dr. Nieta told me after my release in Germany.

Kapmeier was with me in an American POW camp. He was soon released and took along a letter to my wife. Regretfully, I have had no opportunity to thank him for that.

Question 20: What type of research was done by the different laboratories...serological, histological, bacteriological, entomological, chemical, biological, parasitological, pharmacological, pathological, etc.?

Question 21: What were the research problems of the prisoner personnel, e.g., Dr. Mikolaj Korn, the kapo, from Slovakia; Dr. Janusz Makowski, histopathologist, from Poland; Dr. Jakub Lewin, serologist, from Paris; Prof. Antoni Jakubski, hydrobiologist, from Poland; Prof. Vaclav Tomasek, bacteriologist, from Bruenn; Prof. Artioli, from Saloniki; Prof. Geza Mansfeld, pharmacologist, from Hungary; Prof. Ludvik Fleck, from the Weigl Institute in Lwow; Prof. Marc Klein, histologist, from Strassburg; Dr. George Lewy-Coblence, histopathologist, from Paris, and many others?

Answer: We needed bacteriologists, serologists, histologists and chemists in order to diagnose the specimens and preparations we received from camp, and also from SS-troops stationed in Cracow and other SS-hospitals. We were very busy. A courier came three times a week with material from Cracow to be examined in our laboratory. Of course, we had highly qualified people who normally would never have occupied themselves with these technical tasks.

We employed as many specialists as possible to solve the task given to Weber of producing a dry serum for blood group test sera. Everybody who could contribute to this goal through his field of expertise was accepted. It was one of the best jobs one could find as prisoner in Auschwitz. I can't add much to the names you have mentioned.

Dr. Levin was certainly one of the best serologists. In addition, Arthur Korn deserves to be mentioned. He was the kapo and was responsible for everything that had to do with the organization of prisoners. He was very eager and took care of everything to the satisfaction of his co-prisoners as well as of Weber. It was an ideal collaboration between Korn, the kommando and the direction of the Institute of Hygiene. A hydrobiologist, i.e., Prof. Jakubski, was really not required in the laboratory, but it was good that we had him because we had to check the hygienic conditions of the water in the different camps. He had quite a bit of work and was also important in the lab.

Prof. Mansfeld was a pharmacologist. He came relatively late with the Hungarian transports and always worried whether he could remain in the kommando because he actually was not needed. At certain intervals, the camp administration protested that our kommando of about 100 persons (it was increasing steadily) was much too large. There were constant difficulties. Every prisoner knew about them and everybody was desperately attempting to keep his job.

Prof. Mansfeld was continually searching to make himself useful. I talked to him about the experiments in Block 10. He had no proposals in that respect but he suggested we should investigate the efficacy of sulfonamides on bacteria. He had worked on that subject in Budapest and wanted to continue in that field at the Institute if I would give him the possibility of doing so. And so he began in that area. I was under the impression of having helped him to survive camp since he was already quite old. I did not know his exact age, but he was in the upper sixties. Later he had the possibility of working together with Delmotte.

Question 22: Which discoveries were made in the various fields investigated by the Institute of Hygiene: blood-type research, malaria, typhus and spotted fever, efficacy of sulfonamides, syphilis, noma, etc.?

Question 23: Is it true that Weber wrote his "scientific" papers based on the results of prisoner scientists?

Question 24: Is it true that Dr. Lewin and his colleagues from the serological lab succeeded in finding a dry globulin for fast determination of blood types and Weber attributed the discovery to himself?

Answer: As mentioned previously, the main focus was the production of blood group test sera. Weber collected the results of everybody and went with them to Berlin. There they were written up and published by Mugrowsky and Weber.

Noma was not really investigated. In Auschwitz there existed the rare opportunity to research noma bacteriologically. It was a disease which nobody had ever seen before, which had disappeared long ago and which had re-surfaced only under the catastrophic conditions which had temporarily existed among the children in the Gypsy camp.

I have not seen anything about syphilis research, but Prof. Mansfeld was occupied with sulfonamides.

Prof. Fleck investigated spotted fever, which was his specialty. It was a continuation of work done at Buchenwald. Buchenwald under Ding-Schuler was a branch of the Institute of Hygiene in the KL-Buchenwald. Here, Fleck had already worked for more than a year as a special prisoner who was entitled to live together with his wife before he came to Auschwitz. Mugrowsky later transferred him to Auschwitz because the laboratory possibilities were better there. However, by the summer of 1944 he was returned to Buchenwald.

We also analyzed some malaria preparations...not too many...there was not too much of a possibility. Once, in the summer of 1944, it was believed that a malaria epidemic had broken out in the vicinity of Cracow. Some cases had been reported and mass examinations of the population were ordered.

I was sent together with two non-commissioned officers and two women...one of them was an actress...to Zartoy, a rural area between Auschwitz and Cracow. It was a swampy terrain and we did malaria mass screenings. I believe Zabel and Schumacher were the two Unterscharfuehrers. The women had to be initiated into taking blood from a finger. The screening lasted for about 2-3 weeks. Not much came of it.

Question 25: Marc Klein often asked himself what actually was the purpose of the South-Eastern Institute of Hygiene. He later asserted that all investigations were lacking a plan and originality. What is your opinion?

Answer: Marc Klein is absolutely right. This state of affairs stemmed from the fact that the capacity of the field laboratory was highly strained. The situation was the following: Mugrowsky, Weber and I were properly trained bacteriologists. Weber was also a serologist. We were surrounded by men who were the top authorities in their field, having specialized in their particular areas for many years. So there was an immense supply of brilliant scientists but there was no possibility to supervise and coordinate everything and to spawn truly original work. Mugrowsky's major concern was the production of a dry serum for blood groups. So that was center stage and was forced upon us. If somebody had a particular research project he was given a free hand to investigate it. But there was no coordination and no original planning, exactly as Prof. Klein stated. There were too many possibilities that could not be explored.

Question 26: Klein further asserted that there was a lot of sabotage which was not discovered by the SS. Do you agree?

Question 27: Histological and bacteriological diagnoses were often forged in order not to jeopardize prisoners by positive results (in the cases of Koch bacilli for tuberculosis, malaria, typhus, etc.). Did you know about it and did you quietly look the other way? By the way, Langbein reports how Mrs. Rohde, the wife of an SS-physician, forced inmate physician Dr. André Lettich to declare her diphtheria slide as negative because she wanted to get rid of the bothersome quarantine.

Answer: Yes, of course there were forged results. It was completely impossible to control everything. We had a multitude of preparations to examine and we could not supervise every single analysis. There were many possibilities of mixing up, concealing or manipulating items...even a top-notch expert would not have been able to have his eyes on everything. Naturally, we were aware of this and did not attribute much importance to it. If one tuberculosis case was diagnosed as negative although it was positive...that did not play a big role for conditions in the hospitals of Birkenau or Auschwitz. It was clear to us that the prisoners of our kommando did not report too many misleading results for an epidemic to break out. We were sure, and I am still convinced today, that none of those who worked in the community of the Institute of Hygiene would have permitted anybody to be harmed healthwise by the Institute of Hygiene.

He who knows conditions in Auschwitz would realize that certain quid pro quo diagnoses and certificates were unavoidable...that was inherent in the omnipresent corruption. A case in point was the false diphtheria result for Mrs. Rohde to shorten her quarantine. This was the order of the day and could not be controlled. The possibilities for manipulation were always available and not difficult to realize. But sabotage on a large scale did not exist and, according to me, would not have made any sense. It would have been absurd to supply the prisoner hospitals with incorrect diagnoses and to confuse everybody. Neither the inmates nor the community of inmates would have been helped by this.

Editor replies: You are right...most of the analyses made at the Institute were, of course, correct. The sabotage reported by Marc Klein referred only to Weber's research, i.e., the prisoners were absolutely not interested in developing a dry serum for blood groups for the SS.

Answer. Yes.

Question 28: Did you never have any scruples about using human flesh as a cultural medium for bacteria in your laboratory?

Answer: I must confirm that this happened twice and I want to give an explanation. Once, during the time of the Hungarian transports, we needed a large quantity of cultural media because a typhus epidemic had broken out in the military hospital in Cracow. The soil for cultural media had always been in short supply because the deliveries from the slaughterhouse were very meager and much of the meat from these sparse deliveries disappeared in the cultural media kitchen for "business."

Unterscharfuehrer Zabel knew the SDGs (SS-hospital orderlies) of the camp Revier well. He needed their assistance when he had to take blood from prisoners for the serological laboratory doing the research on blood group test sera. Bread and sausages were distributed and volunteers could donate blood to "make themselves useful," as the saying went. Thus, Zabel complained about the shortage to the SDGs and they persuaded him to simply take the meat which was lying around in large quantities in front of the crematoria. Zabel listened and cut out human flesh from the corpses. He told me about it and said that the same had been done earlier, before he joined the Institute. He had heard this from the prisoners. It simply had been an emergency...and that had been dealt with properly. However, I know that he did the same thing a second time, shortly after the first occurrence. The prisoners of the cultural medium kitchen informed me.

You will probably ask what I did with Zabel, who did not follow my orders. Well, I have to admit that for reasons of prudence and design I did not do anything because I knew it would only backfire. The prisoners would have been in trouble. He would have denied it if I had confronted him and I did not have any proof except to refer to the prisoners. Zabel would surely have found ways and means to make them suffer. And I decided to check better in the future and as far as I know it did not happen again.

Question 29: Langbein mentions your studies about the complete indifference toward their environment and the shockingly blind confidence of Muselmaenner. Were these based on observations and interviews with real Muselmaenner or did you write them down later in your cell in Cracow when you were provided with research material from your institute?

Answer: You are right. My studies concerning Muselmaenner were done while in custody in Cracow. These are the antecedents:

One day I was called to the examining magistrate. He told me that he had a special task for me. He liked me and had assured me previously that most certainly there would not be a big indictment against me. The story was the following:

For half a year, an old man, called Kurt von Burgsdorf, who had been handed over by the Americans to Poland, was sitting in a solitary cell. He had occupied an enormously important position, since he had been the last governor of Cracow. And after the aegis of Hans Frank, von Burgsdorf turned out to be a completely different person. During the six months that he had been in custody, not a single accusation against him had been received…not from Poland and not from anywhere else. On the contrary, the examining magistrate had a thick file of documents from the Polish population testifying to his integrity. Von Burgsdorf had had a Bible while he had been in solitary confinement, and, unfortunately, had become so confused through the constant Bible study that mentally he was completely run down. The magistrate was a humane person and decided to transfer me to his cell so that I could help and counsel him a little to improve his state of mind.

Well, I established a good rapport with him and advised the magistrate to help von Burgsdorf further by occupying his time with something he would be interested in. He was a typical civil servant type and I suggested that we could make order among the many thousands of diagnostic notes that had remained in the Institute of Hygiene. They delivered several cases of medical records and we began to sort them out and to catalogue them. Von Burgsdorf was very eager. I myself had for a long time felt the need to find out at what point an Auschwitz prisoner would reach the limit, i.e., when the state was attained when he would turn into a Muselmann.

In our laboratory we had examined the soup and the entire nutrition provided to prisoners by contents and by calories, and it had been established that the normal prisoner would vegetate at around 1500 calories. It followed that one could stand this as normal nutrition for a limited time only. I had already started to occupy myself with this problem. But now I had the time and opportunity to check the figures statistically.

I searched for those notes which showed diagnoses of people who did not have long to live any more, i.e., who were already in the Muselmann stage. There were those suffering from diarrhea without any bacteriological cause or disease, simply a shortage of albumin. The prison number was also listed on those notes and from the prisoner number I knew how long the prisoner had been in camp. In this way, I arrived at my statistics. One could calculate these dates exactly, taking as a point of departure the physiological knowledge that every physician possesses, ignoring all other possibilities of deficient nutrition, such as a shortage of vitamins, calcium and minerals, and concentrating only on calories. With 1500 calories one obtained a life expectancy curve of four months, i.e., somewhere between three and five months. The span is so large because there are different types, good and bad food utilizers. Anyway, the curve that can be drawn coincides completely with the statistics.

I put all of this together with an introduction giving a physiological explanation to the examining magistrate, who had not been a prisoner himself and who was not well-informed about camp life and conditions for prisoners in camp. I had the impression that he did not really believe some of the material, the way it is with many people who have not seen it with their own eyes.

In my description of Muselmaenner I did not restrict myself to the purely physical symptoms but also discussed the mental state which characterizes this stage, for example, this indifference to the environment. This state of resignation did not actually alleviate the lot of these poor people or improve their chances for survival, just the contrary. But it made them bear the end more easily than it might have looked from the outside.

This paper was published in 1967 in a prominent place of the Polish Medical Journal, "Przeglad Lekarski" in a special Auschwitz edition. Prof. Olbricht from Cracow and also other prisoners whom I knew from Auschwitz participated and I was very pleased and proud that this had been done.

Question 30: Did you have an official residence in the Institute of Hygiene or did you live in the town of Auschwitz?

Answer: Yes. I had an official residence in the Institute of Hygiene and lived there. I never lived in the town of Auschwitz. Later in the fall of 1944, I had a little house built by prisoners of our kommando on the road exactly opposite the Institute. I felt better there as far as this was possible than in that close contact with Delmotte, who was not on good terms with me and who avoided me.

Question 31: The biologists and chemists of the women's Pflanzenzucht detail in Rajsko came sometimes to the Hygienic Institute...officially, in order to use the centrifuge for their latex samples...in reality, however, in order to keep up contact with the male prisoners and to organize. They brought tomatoes, onions, carrots, etc., and received blood from which they made blood sausage. Was there also non-human blood at the Institute?

Answer: Normal slaughterhouse blood was required at the Institute as a cultural medium for streptococci, according to my estimation, about two liters every two weeks, twice as much as was requested and probably also delivered precisely because of the blood sausage.

Question 32: Do you remember the name of the Jewish woman laboratory assistant at the Institute who made drawings from photographs of the families of the SS officers and men?

Answer: I remember well a congenial, dark-haired woman from the laboratory of the agriculture kommando who came to us for a short period of time as draftswoman for graphic designs. She produced very nice sepia drawings from photos. I do not remember her name. She was nameless...but in her case...-unshorn.[6]

C) Personal Questions

Question 33: You told Lifton that in Auschwitz everybody had "Dreck am Stecken" (dirt on his walking stick). Are you willing to report about your dirt?

Answer: The corruption among the SS increased tremendously, especially during the last half year. There was hardly anybody who did not try to "organize" something illegally for himself. It was a foregone conclusion that everybody who could had a tailor sitting in some corner to sew uniforms or other things. The organizing from "Kanada" took astronomic proportions...an investigative commission was supposed to arrive in Auschwitz to stem the flow of goods.

I had a little house built right across the street from the Hygienic Institute. And why shouldn't I? The prisoners of our kommando, which had too many men anyway, worked on it and it was certainly not to their disadvantage. Anyway everybody who acted humanely behaved illegally. I was quite tainted in this respect...one only has to remember the experiments in Block 10. And there were other things in this respect. I could bear it without too much anxiety because I knew that nobody could easily touch me. I avoided everybody who wanted to take me to task in this respect...except for high superiors. In hindsight, I regret this avoidance. I might have known Caesar better, about whom I learned later that he was an especially interesting and remarkable human being as far as humane behavior toward prisoners was concerned.

Question 34: You mentioned to Lifton that one of the reasons you admired Dr. Mengele was his readiness to openly oppose whatever he felt was wrong, a characteristic you had equally admired in your father and which gave you the strength to behave decently in Auschwitz. How then was it possible for you not to protest...unless you agreed with the atrocious conditions there?

Answer: A lot could be said in this respect, but it is very difficult because it could easily lead to misunderstandings. It is being rumored...I don't know why, perhaps Langbein is the source...that Mengele was my friend. If I remember correctly, Lifton reported the same. One cannot look at it this way. I have always stressed and am still stressing the point that Mengele was the only one among the camp physicians with whom one could have a candid discussion, taking into account arguments and counterarguments. It is true that I admired him, because whenever he felt that something was done incorrectly from the point of view of his Weltanschauung or religion...which consisted in demanding that the extermination of Jews had to be executed extremely consistently and precisely...then he voiced his opposition openly. None of the others did that. But I would like to emphasize once more that Mengele never opposed the system of gassing or the annihilation of Jews, i.e., the principle of Auschwitz in general...but what he objected to sometimes were procedural questions. This is often misunderstood.

Now we come to the question of why I did not oppose the horrible occurrences in Auschwitz if I did not agree with the principle. How else could I have protested than by refusing to participate in inhumane actions? It became very relevant when they wanted to force me to do selections. I really put everything in motion in order to be exempted from it. I would not have done it under any circumstances, which, of course, I cannot prove now. In any case, I protested in this way. Whatever else they demanded from me in Auschwitz was not inhumane and I had ample opportunity to help prisoners.

A protest against Auschwitz and against the entire system of the NSDAP within Auschwitz would not have led to anything. It was entirely outside the realm of reality.

Question 35: Is painting...which you once wanted to pursue as a career...still a hobby of yours?

a) Did you paint in Auschwitz?
b) Do you still paint today?

Answer: I gave up painting a long time ago. I always had difficulties with colors. Moreover, my creations became too abstract, which was not beneficial to the mind. I found ample compensation through sculpturing...without it, I cannot function. As long as I was still working and had little leisure time for this hobby I was often quite unhappy about this lack (of time). During the last few years I have worked almost exclusively with clay, doing mostly children's portraits.

Question 36: How would you have acted under the same circumstances with reversed roles, i.e., if you would have been a prisoner physician in a concentration camp where it had been decided to exterminate all Germans as vermin?

Answer: Left unanswered in reply.

D) Tying Up Some Loose Ends

Some of the replies necessitated additional questions and answers during the months of December 1988 to March 1989 which are being dealt with in the following section.

Question 37: *Prof. Geza Mansfeld*

Danuta Czech writes that he was predominantly occupied with three studies which he did in Block 20 of the Stammlager:

a) Extermination of malaria. He was presented with one hundred thousand blood samples of subjects which SS men had collected in the vicinity of Auschwitz.

b) Coordination and study of 120 protocols of patients suffering from spotted fever on orders of Delmotte.

c) Examination of sixteen thousand prisoners for syphilis.

At the Hoess trial Mansfeld and Dr. Leon Landau stated that the examinations and analyses of the Institute were not performed out of worry for the health of the prisoners but served the purposed of, on the one hand, showing success measured by the great number of analyses. On the other hand, the results of these tests could at a future time serve in the Third Reich as justification in front of the world of having systematically murdered malaria patients.

Were you familiar with the examinations mentioned and do you agree with the assessment of Mansfeld and Landau?

Answer:

a) At the request of the civilian government (district Auschwitz) the Hygienic Institute was, in the summer of 1944, requested to do malaria testing in the vicinity of Zator, a larger village in the swampy terrain not far from Auschwitz. The entire population of this area was suspected to suffer from malaria and was to be examined by blood tests and the carriers would be restored to health.

I organized these examinations and had three SS-men from our institute: Fugger, Zabel and a third one at my disposal. In addition, we were assigned two Red Cross women and, for a short time, there was also a young physician from the civilian hospital in Auschwitz. He was a Pole from Cracow and served mainly as interpreter.

According to my recollections, the action lasted 2-3 weeks. It was only reluctantly accepted by the population. The maximum number of blood samples we collected per day was three hundred. The total number we gathered was certainly not higher than three thousand.

It is correct. The blood samples were examined by Prof. Mansfeld in Block 20. At that time, Prof. Mansfeld was so weakened by bleeding ulcers that he would not have been able to stand the march to Rajsko. He requested an occupation in the block in order to avoid a transfer to the Revier. The study of 100,000 preparations is absolutely unrealistic.

b) During his turn as camp physician (he had been assigned to Dr. Thilo) Delmotte occupied himself a lot with spotted fever. Besides, he was always searching for a topic for his doctoral dissertation. He did not like the subject proposed to him by Mugrowsky...also because he intensely endeavored to get away from the Institute of Hygiene.

c) I don't know anything about the 16,000 examinations of inmates for syphilis. The serological tests could only have been performed in Rajsko and I would have learned about them. I can only imagine that this was a statistical evaluation of examinations that had accumulated over the years in Rajsko.

Perhaps it was a study by Delmotte inspired by Mugrowsky. Delmotte complained bitterly that his capabilities were not properly utilized in Rajsko. Maybe Mugrowsky wanted to "occupy" him this way.

Question 38: *Dr. Delmotte*

Some regard Delmotte as one of the most decent and responsible SS doctors in Auschwitz (and not only in regard to the Hippocratic Oath). He was the only one who protested openly against the selections and stated that he did not want to be in a slaughterhouse. He considered it was his duty as a physician to save lives and not to destroy them. Other "healers," Dr. Kremer, for example, made diary entries such as the following: "This night participated in "Sonderaktion" 6 and 7. Had dinner at 20 hours with Obergruppenfuehrer Pohl in the Fuehrerheim, a real feast: baked pike, genuine coffee, excellent beer and sandwiches."

It is well-known that Liebehenschel, Wirths and Weber worked out a therapeutic program for Delmotte which had the desired effect and consisted of three points:

a) Mengele became his mentor and convinced him ideologically of the necessity of the extermination of Jews.

b) His wife could live with him in Auschwitz.

c) A prison doctor assisted him with his doctoral dissertation.

Do you agree with the assessment of Delmotte? It might not be easy for you to judge objectively in view of the fact that you told Lifton you had a guilty conscience in regard to Delmotte since he had to perform the selections which you had successfully managed to shift to others.

Answer: I can confirm that Delmotte was a man of integrity who openly protested against the order of participating in selections to Wirths and Mugrowsky, to whom he had been assigned after completing his training as an active medical SS officer.

He came from a family of high-ranking NS functionaries and SS-Fuehrern and he believed that by mentioning these "good connections" (namedropping his family contacts) he would easily win his protest. However, the opposite occurred. From several conversations about his problems I learned that the authorities were not willing to grant his request precisely because of his training in Ordensburgen and his family connections. His petition to be allowed to go to the front was also denied.

In the beginning, I did not want to believe him that during his training he had never heard anything of the reality of the "Final Solution." In time, I had to change my view in this respect.

a) Mengele did not become his mentor but Dr. Thilo instead. Mengele's special subject on which he elaborated at every opportunity (in contrast to all other camp physicians) was the justification to participate in selections. That's why it is understandable that the impression was created Delmotte had been assigned to Mengele.

b) It is true, Mrs. Delmotte was induced to come and remain in Auschwitz by Weber. It had been arranged by the Kommandantur.

c) I only know about Prof. Mansfeld. But it is also possible that Delmotte approached Dr. Thilo...the camp physician he had been assigned to for assistance with his doctoral dissertation.

In view of the tragic conflict Delmotte had to struggle with, I, of course, had a guilty conscience toward him...and still have today. There are quite a number of former prisoners (as I learned from many conversations) who suffer because they survived thanks to their special position and had sufficient nutrition at the expense of the masses. Certainly, I was lucky that Mugrowsky accepted my refusal to select, but rest assured it was not easy to settle this affair with Wirths and the Kommandantur. It just so happened that Delmotte was unlucky in the same situation in which I had luck. But it is not true that I shirked the selection at Delmotte's expense.

Question 39: *Human Bouillon*

You write that human flesh was used only twice for cultural media. There are a number of persons who dispute this.

a) **Mieczyslaw Kieta** (former prisoner in the Hygienic Institute) reports that SS men wrote officially with colored chalk "Human Bouillon" on the glass containers in the cultural media kitchen (Kieta, 1987, p. 216).

b) **Filip Mueller** (former prisoner in the Sonderkommando) recounts: "From time to time SS doctors came to the crematorium, mostly Hauptsturmfuehrer Dr. Kitt and Obersturmfuehrer Dr. Weber. On those days it was like a slaughterhouse. Before the executions the two physicians fingered like cattle dealers the thighs and calves of the still living men and women in order to select the best pieces. After the shooting, the victims were laid out on a table. The doctors cut out large chunks of still warm flesh and threw them into buckets. Only later did we find out that this flesh was taken to the Hygienic Institute in Rajsko where it was used for bacteria cultures" (Mueller, 1979, pp. 46-47).

c) **Dr. Stanislaw Klodzinski** (former prison doctor), co-founder and editor of "Przeglad Lekarski Oswiecim," tells about a visit of Mugrowsky in the Hygienic Institute in Rajsko. Weber told him about the human bouillon and both started to snicker and laugh.

He also mentions that, initially, there were fat problems with human flesh which, however, later were overcome. Furthermore, Klodzinski noted that you yourself were interrogated on this subject in 1967 in Salzburg (Klodzinski, 1969, p. 69).

d) **Imre Goenczi** worked personally in the cultural media kitchen and asserts that he sometimes found human skin in the meat which the SS-man had forgotten to remove (personal communication).

All these accounts seem to imply that "Menschen-bouillon" (human bouillon) was routinely used at the Institute. Please let me have your point of view.

Answer: During my time, and above all during the time that I was deputy of the Institute, there was only the episode with human bouillon which I have described. When Zabel suggested to get meat from the crematoria he mentioned that this had been done previously. The accounts of former prisoners whom you list under a, b, c and d do not contradict my story. As far as I can remember, I declared the same in Frankfurt (not Salzburg).

Editor replies: The depositions by former prisoners seem to point to a long established custom of using human bouillon as a cultural medium. This would mean that the Hygienic Institute participated not insignificantly in the general Auschwitz practice of desecration of corpses and necrosyly of the murdered victims, such as the utilitization of gold teeth, hair, ashes, fat, etc. This would contradict your initial statement that the Institute was not engaged in inhuman activities.

Answer. Unfortunately, I cannot quantify the use of human flesh for the cultural media kitchen since I cannot exclude the possibility that Zabel continued with this practice even after my prohibition. In addition, I do not know how this matter was taken care of under Weber before my time.

Question 40: *Male Subjects*

Lifton writes that you also experimented on male prisoners where the altruistic motives that might have existed in Block 10 did not apply. What were your reasons in these cases?

Answer: It concerned: 1) pre-tests for the series of experiments in Block 10; and 2) the trials for new tattoo stamps to tattoo the blood type into the armpits as prescribed for the SS. For volunteers there were large sausage and bread rations from the SS kitchen. There was a great rush but I could only use 5-10 persons. The blood groups had been determined in advance. I can imagine that after the liberation some difficulties might have arisen for these volunteers.

Question 41: *Doctoral Dissertations in Auschwitz*

The women prisoners in the Pflanzenzucht wrote the doctoral dissertation (in chemistry) for Ruth Weiman, the second Mrs. Caesar. The subject of Dr. Kitt's dissertation was silicosis and Delmotte received assistance from former professors and other coryphaei (leaders) in their field at the Institute. Was it common practice in Auschwitz to have these papers produced by prisoners?

Answer: I can only talk about Delmotte in this matter. His doctoral advisor was Prof. Mugrowsky. I don't remember the topic, which he did not like anyway.

The temptation to have protracted experiments, in chemistry, for example, or the compilation of medical diagnoses done by expert prisoners was, of course, very great. A control over the independent execution of a study...the way it is required for a doctoral dissertation...was not possible in Auschwitz.

Question 42: *Obsession with large dogs*

What was the reason that SS-men in Auschwitz and their family members who did not belong to the dog squad (Weber and Mrs. Delmotte, for example) frequently surrounded themselves with large dogs? Do you have an explanation for this?

Answer: Weber was very fearful...or perhaps subconsciously frightened. He was sick and died shortly after the war. He was suffering from renal insufficiency and knew that he had only a short life expectancy.

It was a different story with Mrs. Delmotte. She was a strikingly attractive woman, very slender, almost frail and pale. She cultivated these looks very adroitly by consistently wearing black and white. This outfit was especially emphasized through a huge black and white Great Dane. The dog was completely degenerated and could not be used as a guard dog. According to my recollections, she was not fearful.

Question 43: *Prof. Zeiss*

What role was played by Prof. Zeiss of the University of Berlin in the foundation of the Hygienic Institute in Auschwitz?

Answer: Prof. Zeiss was the director of the Hygienic Institute of the University of Berlin. Mugrowsky was the number two man there, i.e., Extraordinarius, and he kept that function when he moved in his capacity as head hygienist of the Waffen SS to his own institute in the Knesebeck Strasse. I do not know whether Prof. Zeiss also had an SS title or function. The SS liked to adorn themselves with prominent persons by conferring honorary ranks on them. In Mugrowsky's case this was, of course, different.

Question 44: *Thies Christophersen*

You wrote that since your acquittal in Cracow you considered it your unconditional duty to bear witness about Auschwitz.

In 1973 the former SS-man Thies Christophersen of the Pflanzenzucht in Rajsko, your immediate neighbor, who worked under Caesar and Dr. Schattenberg, published a book called *Die Auschwitz Luege (The Auschwitz Lie)* in which he denies that there were gas chambers and crematoria in Auschwitz.

Did you ever do anything to dispute these lies or those of other neo-Nazi authors?

Answer: I did not read his book. But from experience I am familiar with his influence on the approximately 590 neo-Nazis in this country. People frequently ask me about it, not only during discussions but also spontaneously. A few months ago he wrote to me from his exile in Denmark. He cannot live in Germany because he was indicted. On advice of the Prosecutor-in-Chief at the War Criminals' Court in Frankfurt I did not answer his letter. Previously, I also had an opportunity to discuss private problems with him while inquiring about Auschwitz. Experience has shown that every discussion with him is only being used to conjure up evidence for the assertions he pulls out of his magic hat.

However, if he runs out of fabricated arguments...something which occurs only rarely...then the circumstance which he cannot dispute is the best proof that one (meaning I) has bought one's acquittal through the dissemination of falsehoods, i.e., the Auschwitz lie. With this argument, they rendered ineffectual the most important document for enlightenment, namely the transcripts of the interrogation of Hoess.

I have 40 years' experience with the most intense efforts for clarification and cannot object to the stance of the Prosecutor-in-Chief in Frankfurt. Until now, only a few dared to accuse me openly of having purchased my acquittal. In Germany, dissemination of *The Auschwitz Lie* is punishable by imprisonment. Skepticism about the facts while citing the purchased acquittal when this is being spread in the circle of comrades has become especially effective through the threat of a jail sentence. That is also one of the reasons why I do not attend neo-Nazi gatherings out of my own initiative. My activity is concentrated on schools. About ten years ago, it was the trade union youth that was interested. Unfortunately, the interest of the young people has markedly decreased. At present, it is mostly the journalists who are interested, regrettably, less in the facts about Auschwitz than in the sensation to show off an acquitted SS doctor from Auschwitz.

In this connection it might interest you that against my decision to be cautious in regard to NS circles, I was tricked a few weeks ago by a very aggressive group. The "Institute for Austro-German Contemporary History" (DOIZ)[7] wrote to me (AU 6911, Lochau, P.O.B. 5) on officially printed stationery. They stated having received my address from the Documentation Center for War Criminals in Ludwigsburg and asked me for a precise description of the process of gassing in Auschwitz. They claimed not to have an authentic deposition in their files, only from prisoners and sometimes there were doubts about them. It was a rather strange request...but I was used to unusual propositions from Austrian institutions. So I wrote a long letter. From the reply I learned that this "Institute" was a rehabilitation organization for war criminals. They virulently insulted me and demanded that I not spread my lies publicly any more.

As proof they sent me, by registered mail, the so-called "Leuchter Document," a thick brochure until then unknown to me. In it, engineer Fred Leuchter, from Madden, Massachusetts, an expert for gas chambers, proves through chemical and personal tests in Birkenau that if all the power during the entire existence of Birkenau had been used, only a maximum of 105,688 persons could have been gassed. This scientific-looking pamphlet is far more dangerous and cannot be invalidated with the claim that things were quite different. For this reason, I have not yet answered in spite of the offensive insults...I first want to discuss it with Frankfurt and also with the Documentation Center in Ludwigsburg.[8]

Question 45:

a) Do you have regular or sporadic contact with your former SS comrades?
b) Do you participate in their gatherings?
c) Do you feel solidarity with this group?

Answer: The question has been answered in part by the previous question. Of course I do not feel solidarity with neo-Nazis.

Editor replies: I don't doubt that you do not feel solidarity with neo-Nazis but what about the old Nazis, your former colleagues? Are there many among your ex-comrades who honestly abandoned their former views through genuine human growth?

Answer: I cannot tell you much about comrades who honestly converted. Even beforehand, I did not have contact with convinced Nazis. Except for the youth, the majority were not genuinely convinced admirers of Hitler, especially in Catholic Bavaria. Most of them were opportunistic camp-followers who did not mind being governed "dictatorially" because they had been used to it under the monarchy.

It seems to me unimportant how many "old Nazis" there are. Soon they will have died out. The education of the young has been a failure from the beginning and the results can be seen in the undeniable increase of conservative and N. S. (national-Socialist) tendencies among the youth. Democracy exhausts itself in bureaucratic administration. This was especially discernible when the Leftists were in power. The centrist parties...ripe to be voted out of office...have no conception of the difficulties looming ahead in overpopulated Europe.

The young people...as far as they were still willing to participate in solving the problems of the future...are drifting to the "Gruenen" or to the slogans and myths of the glorious German past propagated by the Neo-Nazis (especially camouflaged as "Republicans").

I don't have much hope that the situation is going to change and revert to something similar to the pre-Hitler era in Germany or Austria.

Question 46: You claim *a posteriori* that under no circumstances would you have participated in selections. Did you have any contingency plans in case Mrugowsky would not have decided in your favor?

Answer: There were only two alternatives: the revolver or desertion. The easiest way out: to volunteer for front service or to ask for a transfer had been denied by Mrugowsky. Even for Delmotte that had not been possible, in spite of vastly more favorable pre-conditions.

I never considered the revolver. Also, now in hindsight, I would not have opted for it.

Regarding the second possibility, I was convinced that I had to count on the arrest of my entire family. We had been indoctrinated in that fashion through the so-called Waffeneid (loyalty oath) after military basic training. During the "political training" which we had to undergo every three months, we were constantly reminded of it. There was no reason to doubt this state of affairs.

In my case, it would have been relatively easy to take my wife and the two children (four and two at that time) via Austria or Italy to Switzerland. I could hope that the six-months-old infant would not be touched. My wife lived with the children only 15 km. from the Austrian border. The Swiss border was not farther than approximately 100 km. I, myself, would not have had any difficulties because, as deputy director of the Institute, I could initiate an official trip (not only to Berlin) at any time. The risk for desertion would not have been inordinately great.

But, I believe hypothesizing about my past situation is senseless. In all critical situations of my long life, I have always acted purely for emotional reasons. This might be associated with the inevitable degeneration of persons who have been comfortably off for many generations without financial difficulties and who grew up in a non-religious environment...But this, again, is speculation...

▼

Editor's note:

Dr. Muench's testimony is represented without any comment or interpretation. However, in conclusion, two excerpts about the Hygienic Institute are given below which indicate that Dr. Muench, the deputy director of the Institute, claimed unawareness of some of the events that appeared to have been common knowledge among the SS men and prisoners.

The first description is by Pery Broad, a former Unterscharfuehrer of the Auschwitz Political Section, whose accounts of camp conditions were corroborated by others:

> Even after the execution in the crematoria or in Block 11, the dead were not left alone. An SS doctor, mostly SS-Hauptsturmfuehrer Dr. Kitt or SS Obersturmfuehrer Dr. Weber, pounced upon the still warm corpses and cut pieces of flesh out of the thighs and buttocks. They were used for bacteriologic cultures in the Institute of Hygiene. The Institute was located at some distance from the camp on the road leading to Rajsko, and SS Obersturmfuehrer Dr. Weber was its manager (Smolen et al., 1965, p. 38).

The second quote is by Danuta Czech, the former director of research of the Auschwitz Museum:

> SS-Hauptsturmfuehrer Dr. Weber was director of the SS Hygienic Institute in Rajsko near Auschwitz and chief of the branch section in Block 10 of the men's camp, where numerous bacteriological and hematological research and experiments were conducted. Weber determined blood groups on certain inmates and injected some with blood from different groups in order to study the degree of the resultant harmful agglutination of blood cells—with catastrophic consequences. Besides, blood was collected from prisoners in Block 10 for use in transfusions for German personnel. Robert Lifton writes "Not only was the blood at times collected from very weak inmates, but it was sometimes done cruelly or even murderously, by entering the carotid artery in a few prisoners and causing them to bleed to death." The deadly injection with phenol belonged under Weber

equally to Block 10 as did the experiments with hallucinogenous drugs in order to extort confessions about resistance in camp from Polish prisoners at the request of the Gestapo (Czech, 1989, p. 1020).

APPENDIX B
Biographical Notes on the SS

Ackermann, Fred

Unterscharfuehrer in the Kommandantur. On April 20, 1943, he received a medal in Auschwitz, the Kriegsverdienstmedaille.

Armbruester, Michael (Ludwig?)

Born on August 4, 1914, in Radautz. SS-Unterscharfuehrer in the adminstration of prisoners' possessions. He died on September 7, 1974, in Stuttgart.

Aumeier, Hans

Born August 20, 1906, in Amberg. Since 1938 Hauptsturmfuehrer, Lagerfuehrer in Auschwitz. He came from Sachsenhausen and was transferred in August 1943 as commandant to Riga concentration camp. He received a death sentence in Cracow on December 22, 1947.

Baer, Richard

Sturmbannfuehrer, born on September 9, 1911, in Floss/Oberpfalz. Worked in 1933 in Dachau and was later adjutant of Pohl in Oranienburg. Since May 11, 1944, he was commandant in Auschwitz. His wife reported him deceased after the war. He lived as Karl Neumann in Dassendorf. In December 1960 he was arrested and died in prison in Frankfurt on June 17, 1963.

Baretsky, Stefan

Unterscharfuehrer, born March 24, 1919, in Czernowitz. Blockfuehrer 1942-1945 in Birkenau. Lived in Plaidt (Eifel) after the war. Was arrested in 1960 and sentenced in the Frankfurt Auschwitz trial.

Becker, Dorothea (married name Pritzkoleit)

Born October 10, 1912, in Saarbruecken. She was first Aufseherin in Ravensbrueck and from fall 1942 onwards in Auschwitz. At the Cracow trial she was sentenced to five years in prison. She lived (or lives) in Hamburg-Bergedorf.

Berger

Unterscharfuehrer in the office of the Landwirtschaft.

Bischoff, Karl

Sturmbannfuehrer. Born August 9, 1897, in Neuhausbach/Saarpfalz. From October 1941 until autumn 1944 he was the second in command at the Bauleitung in Auschwitz. Afterwards, he became director of construction of the Waffen SS and police in Silesia with headquarters in Kochlowice. He died on October 2, 1950, in Bremen.

Bodmann, Dr. Franz von

Born March 23, 1908, in Munich. SS-Standortarzt in Auschwitz, fell ill in August 1942 and was transferred. Died on May 25, 1945, in a military hospital in Pongau (Salzburg) as per death certificate, presumably suicide.

Boehm, Martin

From the Erzgebirge. Rottenfuehrer and ambulance driver.

Boehme

Dr. Boehme was director of the botanical laboratory in Rajsko. He died in Poland after the war.

Boger, Wilhelm

Oberscharfuehrer, born on December 19, 1906, in Stuttgart. In 1922 he was already a member of the Nazi youth movement. "Ich war ein alter Hase in der nationalsozialistischen Bewegung." After business training, a few apprenticeships, unemployment, service as an auxiliary policeman and attendance at the police academy, he worked for the criminal police and later for the Gestapo.

In Auschwitz he was in charge of the escape detail and excelled in barbarism and sadism beyond anybody's imagination. The prisoners were terrified of him. It was Boger who introduced the torture instrument, called the Boger-Schaukel after him, which he used during his interrogations. His specialty was to torture recaptured prisoners who had attempted to escape.

Boger participated eagerly in the shooting of prisoners with small caliber weapons in the death block. He took part in the mass gassing of Jews. He also organized informers among the prisoners.

In June 1945, he was arrested by American military police and in November 1946 was supposed to be handed over to Poland. However, Boger escaped and for three years lived underground near Crailsheim, not far from Stuttgart. "Da zeigte sich noch, dass die Deutschen zusammenhielten, denn sie kannten mich alle." (This shows that the Germans did stick together, because all of them knew me.)

In 1958 he was arrested once more and was sentenced to a prison term in the Frankfurt Auschwitz trial of 1964-65. He died in the prison hospital of Ziegenhain on March 4, 1977.

Boger had been married twice and was the father of five children, three daughters from his second marriage and two sons from his first.

Bormann, Juana (Hanna)

Born September 10, 1893, in Birkenfelde, Eastern Prussia. From May 5, 1943, onward, she was in Auschwitz, also in Babitz and Budy. On November 17, 1945, she was sentenced to death in the Bergen-Belsen trial and was executed on December 13, 1945.

Broad, Pery

Rottenfuehrer, born on April 25, 1921, in Rio de Janeiro, son of a Brazilian businessman father and a German mother. Shortly after his birth his mother took him to Germany while the father remained in Brazil. Broad attended school in Berlin and, because of his early membership in that organization, received the gold medal of the Hitler Jugend. After graduation from high school he studied at the Technische Hochschule in Berlin. In 1941 he volunteered for service in the Waffen-SS.

In June 1942, Broad came to the Politische Abteilung in Auschwitz. He did general interrogations and was in charge of selecting women for the camp bordello. "Bei uns arbeitet jeder in seinem Beruf, d.h. ein Musterlager." (Here everybody works according to his calling; that's what I call a model camp), he was fond of saying.

Later he was responsible for the Gypsy camp in Birkenau until its liquidation in the summer of 1944. He was one of the most cultured SS-men of the Politische, spoke German, French and English, and studied Polish and Russian in camp. He loved to read classical authors and was a fine musician. In Birkenau he had organized what he used to call "the finest Gypsy orchestra in the world" and afterwards participated in the mass gassing of the entire Gypsy camp.

In May 1945, he was taken prisoner by the British. While in prison he wrote his reminiscences of Auschwitz, highly critical of the camp and the atrocities committed there. However, as a defendant in the Frankfurt Auschwitz trial, solidarity with his old cronies prevailed. He was sentenced to a prison term and now lives in Kaarst.

He was married twice. Both marriages were childless.

Brose, Anton

Born September 26, 1909, in Braunsberg, Eastern Prussia. Before and after his activity at the Political Section in Auschwitz, he worked for the Gestapo of Kattowitz. After the war he worked for Kieserling and Albrecht in Solingen. His address was (or is) Drosselstrasse 2, Solingen. Hermann Langbein's request of August 2, 1965, for criminal investigation was not acted upon.

Brunner, Luise (née Kalb)

Born August 25, 1908, in Aidhausen/Unterfranken. Aufseherin since October 1, 1942, in the Stabsgebaeude in Auschwitz. She was formerly in Ravensbrueck and returned there in October 1944.

On July 28, 1948, she was sentenced by a British court to three years in prison. On September 15, 1960, she was arrested by German authorities. On October 10, 1960, she tried to commit suicide. On December 27, 1960, she was released.

Buehning

SS-Unterscharfuehrer and SDG. A former barber, who performed sterilizations on Clauberg's orders in Block 10 in Auschwitz.

Burger, Wilhelm

Born April 19, 1904, in Dachau. From June 1942 until May 1943 he was in charge of administration in Auschwitz. On April 9, 1952, he was sentenced in Poland and released on May 21, 1955. He lives in Munich, Hilblerstrasse 31.

Caesar, Dr. Joachim

Born May 30, 1901, in Boppard. SS-Obersturmbannfuehrer. An agronomist who worked for the SS-Rassen-Siedlungshauptamt. From March 1942 until the evacuation in January 1945, he was the director of the agricultural enterprises in Auschwitz. He was a witness at the Nuernberg trial and was imprisoned until January 30, 1949. He was equally a witness ad the Frankfurt Auschwitz trial. He died in Kiel on January 25, 1974.

Christophersen, Thies

He came from Schleswig-Holstein. SS-Sonderfuehrer at the Pflanzenzucht in Rajsko from January to December 1944.

For many years he has been active in the neo-Nazi movement. After having been sentenced by the German Federal Republic, he escaped to Denmark, from where he was not extradited.

Author of *Auschwitz...Truth or Lie*, An Eyewitness Report (in German, *Die Auschwitz Luege*).

Cichon, Flora

SS-Aufseherin in Rajsko.

Clauberg, Carl, M.D., Professor of Gynecology.

Born September 28, 1898, in Wupperhof, near Solingen. Honorary SS-Brigadefuehrer. Conducted criminal experiments on women prisoners in Auschwitz on orders of Himmler to find a method for mass sterilization. After the war he was a prisoner of war in the Soviet Union. In 1956 he returned to Kiel. Soon afterwards he was arrested and died in custody on August 9, 1957.

Dejaco, Walter

Untersturmfuehrer. Born September 16, 1909. From 1940 until the evacuation he worked in the Central Construction Company in Auschwitz. The still-existing plan of the large crematorium carries his signature.

In 1950 he was released as a prisoner of war and worked as a master builder in Reutte/Tyrol. At the initiation of Hermann Langbein there was a trial in Vienna from January 18 to March 10, 1972. He was acquitted.

Delmotte, Dr. Hans

Born in 1917 in the Alsace. Camp physician in Auschwitz. Worked in the Institute of Hygiene under Dr. Bruno Weber. In 1945 he committed suicide.

Draser, Hans Andreas

Unterscharfuehrer and an attorney, he was in charge of the Fuersorgeabteilung (welfare section) of the Politische Abteilung. He was a Volksdeutscher from Rumania, spoke German, French and English, and studied Russian in camp. He handled inquiries from the International Red Cross. If an inquiry concerned a non-

Jewish inmate, it was answered, after verification of the card file with a statement that X was in camp, was feeling fine and worked in his/her profession. If it concerned a non-Jewish prisoner who had died, or had been hanged or shot, the reply was that X was not in camp. Inquiries for Jews just went into the waste paper basket. All letters and incoming packages also went through Draser's office. He interrogated prisoners and participated in gassings.

In 1947 Draser was in a sanatorium in Schleswig. On February 8, 1965, Hermann Langbein requested a judicial investigation of his activities. However, the German authorities said they could not locate him.

Drechsler, Margot

Born May 17, 1908, in Nengersdorf (Saxony). Oberaufseherin. She was sentenced to death in the Cracow trial and executed in Poland after the war.

Egersdoerfer, Karl

Born July 20, 1902 in Rosenbach/Bavaria. SS-Unterscharfuehrer, member of the NSDAP since 1934. Membership number in the SS, #289457.

Worked since March 1941 in Auschwitz. From July 1941 he was in charge of the prison kitchen in Auschwitz I. He was acquitted in the trial of the British Military Tribunal in Lueneburg on November 17, 1945, against the crew of the Bergen-Belsen concentration camp. He lives (or lived) in Erlangen, Schillerstrasse 8.

Emmerich, Wilhelm

Born July 2, 1916, in Tiefenbach. SS-Unterscharfuehrer. He supposedly died of typhus in the military hospital of Schwarmstedt.

Erber, Josef (formerly Hustek)

Born October 16, 1897, in Ottendorf, Czechoslovakia. From autumn 1940 until the evacuation he worked in reception of the Political Section of Auschwitz. On February 1, 1944, he became Oberscharfuehrer. Later he worked in Mauthausen. In Frankfurt he was sentenced to life in prison.

Frank, Dr. Willy

Born February 9, 1903, in Regensburg. He worked from March 1943 until August 1944 as dentist in Auschwitz and later, in Dachau. After the war he was in private practice in Stuttgart, Bad Cannstadt. He was sentenced in the Frankfurt Auschwitz trial.

Franz, Anneliese (née Hasse)

Born December 28, 1913, in Goerlitz. She was SS-Aufseherin in the kitchen of the women's camp in Birkenau. After Auschwitz she went to Muehldorf. She died on August 29, 1956.

Fugger, Franz (or Andreas)

Born November 18, 1920, in Mettnitz, Austria. Unterscharfueher. He worked in the Institute of Hygiene. After the war he changed his name to Creigher and lived (or lives) in Friesnach (Kaernten).

Gierisch, Martin

Architect of the Central Construction Company in Auschwitz. He was acquitted in Poland. He died on November 11, 1965.

Glaue (or Claue), Bernhard

SS-Oberscharfuehrer. Came from Pomerania. He was Kommandofuehrer in Harmense. He is said to have fallen during the war.

Goebel, Dr. Johannes

Born October 29, 1891, in Berlin. A chemist (or pharmacologist) who worked for the Schering Company. He was the assistant of Prof. Clauberg in Block 10 in Auschwitz. He died on November 8, 1952, in Bremen.

Grabner, Maximilian

Untersturmfuehrer. A Viennese, he was the director of the Politische Abteilung. He was of medium height and spoke unclearly, as if he had something in his mouth. He loved sports and gymnastics and jogged every morning in a dark blue outfit. Scruples did not exist for him. He participated in the Sondergerichte (special court proceedings which took place in Block 13, and later in Block 11. These sessions occurred every so often at the initiative of the Gestapo in the death block (the name given to the aforementioned blocks) and were parodies of justice administered by the Politische Abteilung. For example, in early spring 1943, when the secret resistance movement was discovered in camp, Grabner randomly selected prisoners from many kommandos, and most of them lost their lives. He especially pursued members of the intelligentsia.

Grabner's abhorrence of the intelligentsia and his lack of education are corroborated by former SS-man Pery Broad: "Grabner's hatred for the intelligentsia, to which he could not be said to belong, not even by the greatest optimist, was limitless" (*Reminiscences of Pery Broad*, p. 84)..."The disconnected sentences of his oration and his vulgar German betrayed his complete lack of education. Nevertheless, he had silver stripes on his uniform. The initiated knew that in his civilian past he used to be a cowherd in the mountains. Now he proudly wore the uniform of the S.D. and was criminal investigator in the Gestapo" (Ibid., p. 16).

Furthermore Grabner was active in the mass gassings of Jews. He himself ordered the shooting of prisoners with small caliber weapons and afterwards faked the causes of death. In the fall of 1943 he was arrested on orders of the SS in Berlin and supposedly sentenced to a twelve-year prison term in Weimar.

After the war, Grabner wrote his memoirs while in a Polish prison. However, these are of questionable value. Not only did he gloss over his own activities, he exaggerated those of his colleagues who had denounced him in Auschwitz during the SS-trial.

He was sentenced to death in the big Auschwitz trial in Cracow and was executed by hanging on December 12, 1947.

Grell, Hermann

Born January 20, 1910, in Siebenbaeumen, County Lauenburg. SS-Rottenfuehrer. Kommandofuehrer in the gardening work squad in Rajsko. He was in Auschwitz from March 1941 until the evacuation in January 1945. He lived (or lives) in Luebeck.

Grese, Irma

Born July 10, 1923, in Wrechen (Mecklenburg). From March 1943 until the evacuation she was Rapportfuehrerin in Auschwitz. Later she came to Bergen-Belsen.

At the British trial in Lueneburg she was sentenced to death on December 12, 1945, and executed.

Hasse, Lisl

Born September 17, 1925, in Goerlitz. Aufseherin in the Arbeitseinsatz in the women's camp in Birkenau. At the end of 1944 she became pregnant through a liaison with SS-man Schippel. Supposedly she has been in custody by the British.

Herpel, Christoph

Born in 1905 in Seeheim an der Bergstrasse. SS-Unterscharfuehrer in the office of the Kommandantur from the beginning of 1943 until the evacuation.

Herpel, Friedrich

Born January 4, 1912, in the Rhineland. SS-Unterscharfuehrer in the kitchen.

Hoess, Rudolf

Born in 1900 in Baden-Baden, SS-Obersturmbannfuehrer. He was the first commandant of Auschwitz from 1940 to 1943. In December 1943, Hoess was appointed chief of Section ID of the SS WVHA. In late June of 1944, he was sent back to Auschwitz, on a temporary assignment, to preside over the murder of the Jews of Hungary. In the operation...Aktion Hoess, as it was named...430,000 Jews were brought to Auschwitz in 56 days to be annihilated there. The Supreme Court in Warsaw, Poland, sentenced Hoess to death and he was hanged in Auschwitz on April 16, 1947.

Hoessler, Franz

Born April 2, 1906, in Kempen. SS-Obersturmfuehrer. He was at first Arbeitsdienstfuehrer and later Lagerfuehrer in Auschwitz. On November 17, 1945, he was sentenced to death by a British tribunal and executed on December 13, 1945.

Hoffman, Hans

Born December 2, 1919, in Yugoslavia. SS-Unterscharfuehrer at the Political Section in Birkenau until the evacuation. At the Cracow trial he was sentenced to 15 years. He was released on July 28, 1956, and lives in Stuttgart-Muffenhausen, working as a locksmith. He was a witness at the Frankfurt Auschwitz trial.

Josten, Heinrich

Born December 11, 1893, in Malmedy.

SS-Obersturmfuehrer. He was second Lagerfuehrer and Arbeitseinsatzfuehrer in Auschwitz I. On December 22, 1947, he was sentenced to death in the Cracow Auschwitz trial and executed.

Jothan, Werner

SS-Obersturmfuehrer. Deputy of Bischoff at the Central Construction Company. He was a witness at the Frankfurt Auschwitz trial.

Kapper, Hans

Born May 4, 1920, in Trachenberg. SS-Unterscharfuehrer in the work allocation center (Arbeitseinsatz). On June 11, 1954, he was declared dead at the request of the Frankfurt District Attorney's office.

Kampmaier, Philipp

Born in 1924 in Uivydek, Hungary. SS-Rottenfuehrer.

Kiefer, Gwendolyn

Came from the Suedsteiermark or Slovenia. He worked in the Kommandantur. His post-war whereabouts are unknown.

Kirschner, Herbert

Oberscharfuehrer, he came from Dresden, was Grabner's right hand man and chief administrator of the Politische Abteilung from 1940 to 1945. On Grabner's orders he shot prisoners in the death block with 5-6 mm. small caliber weapons. He fabricated false documents and fictitious death certificates. The S.B. lists of those prisoners who were gassed immediately upon arrival at the ramp were handled by him. Kirschner participated in the special gassings which took place in the small "farmhouses" and in the mass gassings in the Stammlager in Auschwitz as well as in Birkenau. He sent goods which had belonged to the murdered Jews to his wife, Jesse Kirschner in Dresden, although he had signed an agreement (required of all SS-men) not to touch the property of Jews. Feliks Mylyk packed and dispatched the packages.

Kirschner also participated in the liquidation of the ghetto of Bedzin. After the war, Kirschner could not be located.

Kitt, Dr. Bruno

Born September 8, 1906, in Hamm. From June 1942 until the evacuation he was camp physician in Auschwitz. Then he came to Neuengamme. In May 1946 he was sentenced to death by a British tribunal for crimes committed in Neuengamme. He was executed on August 10, 1946.

Klein, Dr. Fritz

Born November 24, 1888, in Zeiden, near Kronstadt (Rumania). SS-Untersturmfuehrer. From December 1943 until December 1944 he was camp physician in Auschwitz and later in Bergen-Belsen. On November 17, 1945, he was sentenced to death by a British tribunal in Lueneburg and was executed on December 13, 1945.

Klein, Marianne (married name Rendel)

Director of the poultry farm in Harmense.

Kleindienst, Karl

Born February 26, 1903, in Austria. SS-Unterscharfuehrer. He worked in the bookkeeping section of the agricultural offices. After the war he was interned in Glassenbach (Salzburg). He died in Graz on September 2, 1958.

Koch, Hans

Born August 13, 1912, in Tangelhuette. SS-Unterscharfuehrer. SDG (medical orderly) and disinfector (Cyclone-B operator). On December 12, 1947, he received a life sentence in Cracow. He died in prison on July 14, 1955.

Koenig, Dr. Hans Wilhelm

Born May 13, 1912, in Stuttgart. SS-Untersturmfuehrer. He was camp physician in Auschwitz. His last known residence was in Holt-Colnrade. On May 4, 1945, his wife, Mrs. Dagmar Kalling-Koenig, reported him dead. Dagmar is Swedish and lives in Uppsala.

All inquiries as to whether Dr. Koenig is living in Sweden have been unsuccessful, although the likelihood of his living there is very great.

Kopotinski, Josef

SS-Rottenfuehrer, had received an honorary military medal during World War I.

Kramer, Josef

Born November 10, 1906, in Munich. SS-Hauptsturmfuehrer. Worked in Dachau, Struthof-Natzweiler, and in May 1944 as commandant of Auschwitz II...later in Bergen-Belsen.

On November 17, 1945, he was sentenced to death by a British tribunal and on December 13, 1945, he was executed.

Kremer, Dr. Joachim Paul

SS-Obersturmfuehrer, born in 1884. Professor of Anatomy at the University of Muenster. He was camp physician in 1942 in Auschwitz for three months. At the Cracow trial he was condemned to death, but because of his age his sentence was commuted to a prison term. After ten years, he was released in 1958 and returned to West Germany, where he died in the 1960s.

Langefeld, Johanna, née May

Born February 5, 1900, in Essen-Kupferdreh. She was Aufseherin in the first women's camp in Nohringen (county Nordheim). From 1941 unti April 1942 she was Oberaufseherin in KL Ravensbrueck and from April 1942 to October 1942 she was SS woman-in-chief in Auschwitz. In Auschwitz she was sentenced by the SS because of "organizing."

After the war she was extradited to Poland from where she escaped. She is said to have become mentally ill and became very religious. She died in Augsburg on January 26, 1974.

Lettmann

SS-Rottenfuehrer. Born approximately 1923. He worked as a guard in Rajsko.

Liebehenschel, Arthur

Born November 25, 1901. SS-Obersturmbannfuehrer. He worked in the Gestapo headquarters in Oranienburg and was commandant of Majdanek. From November 1943 until May 1944 he was commandant of Auschwitz I. On December 22, 1947, he was sentenced to death in Cracow and executed.

Lolling, Dr. Enno

Born July 19, 1888, in Cologne. SS-Standartenfuehrer. Chief of the Section D III in the WVHA (Wirtschaftsverwaltungshauptamt) in Oranienburg since March 3, 1942. He committed suicide on May 27, 1945, in the military hospital in Flensburg.

Mandel, Maria

Born January 10, 1912, in Muenzkirchen, Upper Austria. She worked at first in Ravensbrueck and later became SS-woman-in-chief of the women's camp in Birkenau. On December 12, 1947, she was sentenced to death in Cracow.

Manger, Herbert

SS-Unterscharfuehrer, born December 12, 1904. He worked in purchasing in the agricultural offices of Auschwitz.

Martin, Rudolf

Born in Burg, near Magdeburg, June 23, 1904. SS-Unterscharfuehrer. He was in charge of the ponds in Harmense. After the war he had been indicted in Poland. The sentence is not known. He lives in East Germany.

Mayer, Dr. Georg Franz

Born September 5, 1917, in Vienna. SS-Obersturmfuehrer. Camp physician in Auschwitz since the middle of July 1942.

In spite of information against him he was not investigated by the Austrian judiciary. He is mentioned in Dr. Kremer's diary. He practices medicine in Vienna 5, Reinprechtsdorfer Strasse 57.

Mengele, Dr. Josef

Born March 16, 1911, in Guenzburg. SS-Hauptsturmfuehrer. Since May 30, 1943, camp physician in Auschwitz.

He escaped to Argentina after the war and later went to Paraguay. Through intervention of Herman Langbein he was deprived of his M.D. and Ph.D. degrees from the Universities of Munich and Frankfurt. On March 23, 1954, he divorced his wife in Duesseldorf. All attempts by the Federal Republic of Germany to have him extradited have been unsuccessful. The mysterious report about his death is rather doubtful in the light of new information.

Moeckel, Ernst Karl

Born January 9, 1901. Obersturmbannfuehrer, director of the SS-Standortverwaltung. On April 20, 1943, he was transferred to Burger. He was sentenced to death in Cracow on December 22, 1947, and executed.

Mokrus, J.

Came from Upper Silesia. SS-Oberscharfuehrer. He was the head of the penal squad in the women's camp and later Kommandofuehrer in Plawy.

Moll, Otto Wilhelm

Born March 4, 1915, in Hohenschoenberg, county Greuesmuehlen. SS-Oberscharfuehrer. He worked in Sachsenhausen and became the chief of the crematoria in Auschwitz. After the war he was sentenced to death by an American military tribunal for killings that occurred during the evacuation of a satellite camp of Dachau. On May 28, 1946, he was executed in Landsberg.

Mrugowsky, Prof. Joachim

SS-Oberfuehrer and chief of the Hygienic Institute of the Waffen-SS. He was sentenced to death during the Nuremberg trial of physicians by an American military tribunal on August 20, 1947, and was executed.

Muelsow

SS-Untersturmfuehrer. Meteorologist in Rajsko.

Muench, Dr. Hans

Born May 14, 1911, in Freiburg/Breisgau. SS-Untersturmfuehrer. From summer 1943 until the evacuation of Auschwitz he worked in the Institute of Hygiene. He was acquitted in the Cracow Auschwitz trial on December 22, 1947. He lives in Rosshaupten, county Fuessen, Allgaeu.

Nebbe, Detlev

Born June 20, 1912. SS-Stabscharfuehrer. From 1941-1944 he worked in the Kommandantur in Auschwitz. Later he worked for the Wehrmachts-Leitstelle in Cracow. On December 12, 1947, he received a life sentence in Cracow. On October 23, 1956, he was pardoned. He lived in Husum and died on April 17, 1972.

Nestroy, Edith

SS-Aufseherin. She was sentenced to three years in prison after the war in Poland. Later she lived in Kaiserslautern.

Opitz, Erna

SS-Aufseherin, born on October 6, 1910. She died on May 16, 1945.

Orlowska, Alice (or Alicia)

Born September 30, 1903. SS-Aufseherin in Auschwitz. She was sentenced to fifteen years in prison in the Cracow Auschwitz trial.

Pach, Josef (or Ludwig)

Rottenfuehrer, he came from Silesia and spoke Polish well. From 1943 he was a guard in the Politische Abteilung. He was cruel and especially hated Poles. He was present as interpreter when prisoners were interrogated and tortured. He also participated in the mass gassings of Jews and appropriated Jewish belongings.

Palitzsch, Gerhard Arno Max

Born June 16, 1913, in Grosspitz nr. Tharandt. SS-Hauptscharfuehrer, member of the SS since March 1933. He worked at first in Sachsenhausen as Arbeitsdienstfuehrer. From May 20, 1940, onward, he was Rapportfuehrer in Auschwitz. On October 1, 1943, he was transferred as Kommandofuehrer to the satellite camp of Brno.

Because of a liaison with the Slovakian Jewish Rapportschreiberin of the women's camp, Katja Singer, he was first put into the bunker, then was court-martialed by the SS and sent to the penal camp in Matzkau and later to the front for probation. He fell in Hungary on December 7, 1944.

Pargner, Karl

Born August 6, 1921, in Kutterschitz, Czechoslovakia. Administrative Unterscharfuehrer in the Institute of Hygiene from June 1943 until the evacuation in January 1945.

On August 31, 1948, he was sentenced to fifteen years in prison in Poland. On June 16, 1956, he was pardoned. He lives in Conweiler, county Calw.

Rohde, Dr. Werner

Born June 11, 1904, in Marburg/Lahn. SS-Untersturmfuehrer and camp physician in Auschwitz. At the end of June 1944 he became SS-Standortarzt (physician-in-chief) in Natzweiler.

On June 1, 1946, he was sentenced to death in the Natzweiler trial by a British tribunal. He was executed on October 11, 1946.

Rosenthal, Guenther

SS-Unterscharfuehrer. He worked in the Landwirtschaft. He fell in February 1945.

Runge

SS-Aufseherin. Kommandofuehrer in the shoe detail and in the penal camp at Budy.

Sauer

SS-Obersturmfuehrer from Ingolstadt. Director of the DAW in Auschwitz.

Schlachter, August

Born January 25, 1901, in Barabein, county Biberach. SS-Hauptsturmfuehrer, director of the Construction Company before Bischoff, i.e., until 1941. He was later in Oranienburg, Natzweiler and Dora. As architect, in 1941 he installed the gas chamber in Crematory I in Auschwitz. After the war he lived as an architect in Biberach, Remminger Str. 17.

Schmidt, Otto

Born March 9, 1906, in Saarbruecken. SS-Oberscharfuehrer. Worked in the Political Section, also in the satellite camps of Blechhammer and Janinagrube.

Schulz, Wilhelm

SS-Scharfuehrer. Worked in the office of the Landwirtschaft.

Schumann, Dr. Horst

Born May 1, 1906, in Halle/Saale. Air Force physician and SS-Sturmbannfuehrer. Director of "Euthanasia" Institutions. In Auschwitz he selected prisoners in 1941 for "Euthanasia" Institutions. He later did sterilization experiments in Birkenau and Block 10 in Auschwitz.

Until 1951 he lived undisturbed under his name in Gladbeck. Then he went to Africa. After long endeavors he was finally arrested in Ghana and extradited to Germany on November 16, 1966. His trial in Frankfurt for having murdered 13,720 mental patients in the "Euthanasia" Institutions of Grafeneck and Sonnestein was discontinued in April 1971 for health reasons. In a separate indictment he was accused of having conducted sterilization experiments on male and female prisoners at Auschwitz. Before the start of the trial, 54 out of 115 witnesses had died.

Schumann died in Frankfurt in September 1983.

Schurz, Hans

Untersturmfuehrer, he came from Vienna and belonged to the S.D., the Sicherheitsdienst. He was Grabner's successor and headed the Politische Abteilung from the fall of 1943 until its liquidation in January 1945. It was during the directorship of Schurz that the mass transports from Hungary arrived. He frequently was present and assisted at the gassings. It was Schurz who gave a premium of two liters of liquor and 150 cigarettes to each SS-man of the Politische Abteilung in reward for the smooth operation in the crematoria.

He has been missing since December 1944 and been legally declared dead.

Schwarz, Heinrich

Born June 14, 1906, in Munich. SS-Haupsturmfuehrer. At first Arbeitseinsatzfuehrer and since November 1943 commandant of Auschwitz III. He later came to Natzweiler. In 1947 he was sentenced to death by a French tribunal and was executed on March 20, 1947.

Sell, Max

Born January 8, 1893, in Kiel. SS-Obersturmfuehrer. Director of the Arbeitseinsatz in Auschwitz. Beforehand he had been in Ravensbrueck and after Auschwitz he was in Dora-Mittelbau. On October 2, 1950, he was officially declared deceased.

Stiwitz, Friedrich

Born May 15, 1910, in Sobernheim, county Kreuznach. SS-Unterscharfuehrer. Rapportfuehrer and Arbeitsdienstfuehrer. In February 1944 he was transferred to Riga. He is said to have fallen during the last months of the war.

Swoboda

From Vienna. SS-Untersturmfuehrer in the Construction Company.

Tauber, Anton

Born February 13, 1922, in Grein (Sudeten). SS-Unterscharfuehrer, Blockfuehrer and Rapportfuehrer in the women's camp of Birkenau. Later he was Lagerfuehrer in Laurahuette. His post-war whereabouts are unknown.

Thilo, Dr. Heinz

Born October 8, 1911. In October 1942 he became camp physician in Auschwitz II. Toward the end of 1944 he was transferred to Gross-Rosen. He died either in May 1945 or in November 1947.

Thomsen, Reinhard

Born February 7, 1901, in Eckernfoerde. SS-Obersturmfuehrer since November 1943. From May 28, 1940, until the evacuation he was in Auschwitz. He worked as Caesar's deputy in the agricultural office. He lived as a farmer in Schleswig-Holstein after the war.

Tietz (or Teitze), Richard

SS-Rottenfuehrer, born February 12, 1902). Secretary of Caesar in the agricultural office. He had a glass eye.

Vetter, Dr. Helmut

SS-Obersturmfuehrer, born March 21, 1910, in Rastenburg. Camp physician in Auschwitz. He had been in Dachau before and was later transferred to Mauthausen. He was sentenced to death by an American military tribunal and was executed on February 2, 1949.

Volkenrath, Elisabeth (née Muehlan)

Born September 5, 1919, in Schoenau nr. Bad Landeck. Originally a beautician. She came to Auschwitz in March 1942 and worked in the distribution of bread and parcels. On November 17, 1945, she was sentenced to death by a British tribunal and on December 13, 1945, she was executed.

Wagner, Rudolf

SS-Haupsturmfuehrer at the Administration. He fell at the front in July 1944.

Weber, Dr. Bruno Nikolaus

Born on May 21, 1915, in Koblenz. SS-Hauptsturmfuehrer. Director of the Institute of Hygiene. He died in Homburg an der Saar on September 23, 1956.

Weimann-Caesar, Ruth

Civilian worker, director of the laboratories in Rajsko.

Wilk

SS-Hauptscharfuehrer from Upper Silesia. He worked as bookkeeper at the Construction Company.

Wirths, Dr. Eduard

Born September 4, 1909, in Wuerzburg. SS-Sturmbannfuehrer. He was SS-physician in Dachau, Neuengamme, and from September 1942 until the evacuation, SS-Standortarzt in Auschwitz. He was arrested by the British and on September 20, 1945, he committed suicide in the camp of Neuengamme.

Wunsch, Franz

Born March 21, 1922, in Drasenhofen (Lower Austria). SS-Unterscharfuehrer. He worked in the Effektenkammer (Kanada). At the end of August 1971, he was denounced and arrested in Austria. On June 27, 1972, he was acquitted in Vienna.

Zabel

SS-Scharfuehrer. He worked in the Institute of Hygiene. He probably fell at the end of the war.

Ziemssen, Wilhelm

SS-Hauptsturmfuehrer, born February 21, 1910. Caesar's deputy in the agricultural offices.

Zimmer, Emma

SS-Aufseherin in Auschwitz. The Frankfurt Court of Justice halted the proceedings against her on August 25, 1961.

Zoller, Viktor

Born June 22, 1912. SS-Obersturmfuehrer and adjutant of camp commandant Hoess. He was sentenced to death by an American tribunal and was executed in Landsberg on July 28, 1947.

APPENDIX C
Synopsis of Major Dates and Events Referred to by Participants

March 26, 1942	The women's concentration camp of Auschwitz came into being with the arrival of a transport of 999 German non-Jewish prisoners from Ravensbrueck and 999 Jewish women from Eastern Slovakia receiving prison numbers 1-1998
August 1942	The women's camp of Auschwitz was moved to camp B I a in Birkenau.
September 1942	A section of the basement of the Stabsgebaeude was used as living quarters for some women prisoners working in Auschwitz-based squads.
November 1942	Dr. Horst Schumann started sterilization experiments of male and female Jewish prisoners in Block 30 of the women's camp in Birkenau.

December 1942	The "Big Selection" took place in the women's camp in Birkenau.
January 1943	Prof. Carl Clauberg commenced sterilization experiments of Jewish women in Block 30 of the women's camp in Birkenau.
January 27, 1943	The only transport of French political women prisoners arrived in Birkenau.
March 1943	Block 10 in the men's camp of Auschwitz, having been remodeled to Prof. Clauberg's specifications, was opened as the experimental block for sterilization experiments.
April 20, 1943	The Neuendorf transport arrived in Auschwitz.
June 1943	Living quarters for the kok-saghyz women prisoners were completed and the Pflanzenzucht (plant cultivation) work detail left the Stabsgebaeude and moved to Rajsko.
August 1943	Thirty women prisoners from Block 10 and 85 men prisoners from Auschwitz were gassed in the Struthof-Natzweiler concentration camp. Their bodies were delivered to the anatomy laboratory at Strassburg University for Prof. Hirt's skeleton collection.
November 10, 1943	Ten oophorectomies were performed in record time by prisoner physician Dr. Wladyslaw Dering on Dr. Schumann's teenage Greek guinea pigs of Block 10.

Summer 1944	The women prisoners of the Stabsgebaeude and of the experimental Block 10 were transferred to the newly constructed camp extension in Auschwitz.
September 1944	One SS block adjacent to the camp extension was destroyed by an air raid and Block 1, housing the former Stabsgebaeude prisoners, was damaged.
October 7, 1944	Uprising of the Jewish prisoners of the Sonderkommando in Birkenau.
January 6, 1945	Four Jewish women prisoners: Alla Gartner, Roza Robota, Regina Saphirstein, and Esther Wajcblum, who had smuggled gunpowder out of the Union factory for the resistance movement, were hanged in the camp extension in front of the prisoners.
January 18, 1945	Auschwitz was evacuated. Approximately 60,000 prisoners started the death march towards the West.
January 27, 1945	The Soviet Army reached Auschwitz and liberated about 7000 prisoners who had been left in camp.

APPENDIX D
Glossary

Abbruchkommando	*(German)* Work squad that destroyed houses
Abitur	*(German)* High school certificate
Ahnenpass	*(German)* Genealogical record to prove "Aryan" descent
AK	*(Polish)* Armja Krajowa, a Polish partisan organization
Aliya	*(Hebrew)* Immigration to Israel
Altweibermuehle	*(German)* Literally old women's mill, legendary rejuvenation process
Amie des Juifs	*(French)* Friend of the Jews
Am Yisrael Chay	*(Hebrew)* The people of Israel will live
Antreten	*(German)* To line up (for roll call or for marching out to work)
Appell	*(German)* Roll call

Arbeit Macht Frei	*(German)* Work liberates—notorious inscription at the entrance gate of Auschwitz
Arbeitsbaracke	*(German)* Work barrack
Arbeitsdienst	*(German)* Labor allocation office
Arbeitsdienstfuehrer	*(German)* SS-man in charge of the division of labor in camp
Arbeitseinsatz-kommando	*(German)* Prisoner kommando which worked in the labor allocation office
Arbeitslager	*(German)* Labor camp
Arisierung	*(German)* Confiscation of Jewish property and business by "Aryans"
Askarah	*(Hebrew)* Memorial service or ceremony
Asozial	*(German)* Anti-social. The term used in camp for the black-triangled prisoners, mostly prostitutes and Gypsies
Auf der Flucht erschossen	*(German)* Shot while escaping
Aufnahmegebaeude	*(German)* Building of the reception
Aufseherin	*(German)* SS-woman
Aufstehen	*(German)* To get up
Auschwitz-Luege	*(German)* Auschwitz-lie, signifying the denial of the extermination process, punishable by law in Germany
Aussenkommando	*(German)* Work squad which labored in the outdoors
Austreten	*(German)* To relieve oneself

Ausweis	*(German)* Identity card
Autobahn	*(German)* Freeway
Baccalaureat	*(French)* High school diploma
Bauleitung	*(German)* Building section
Berufskartei	*(German)* Index file according to occupations
Beth Noar	*(Hebrew)* Youth movement
Bezaubernd	*(German)* Charming
Bibelforscher/in	*(German)* Jehovah's Witnesses
Bituach Leumi	*(Hebrew)* National Insurance
Blockaelteste/r	*(German)* Block senior (an inmate)
Blockfuehrer/in	*(German)* SS-man (or woman) in charge of a block
Blockfuehrerstube	*(German)* The office of a Blockfuehrer, usually near the entrance of camp
Blockova	*(Polish)* Female block senior (inmate)
Blocksperre	*(German)* Curfew during which no prisoner was allowed to leave the block
Buegelstube	*(German)* Ironing room
Buero	*(German)* Office
Bunker	*(German)* The prison block in a concentration camp. In Auschwitz I it was Block 11
Burgenland	Most easterly portion of the Austrian Republic bordering on Hungary

BV-er	*(German)* Befristete Vorbeugungshaft (limited preventive custody); in camp jargon, Berufsverbrecher (professional criminal), i.e., a criminal prisoner with a green triangle
C'est fini	*(French)* It's finished. It's all over
Chaluz/im	*(Hebrew)* Pioneer/s
Chacham	*(Hebrew)* Wise man
Chanoine	*(French)* Canon
Chanukah	*(Hebrew)* Festival commemorating defeat of Syrian Greeks by Maccabees, 165 B.C.E.
Chaver/a/im/ot	*(Hebrew)* Friend, comrade
Chevrah	*(Hebrew)* Group, community, commune
CNRS	*(French)* Centre national de la recherche scientifique, i.e., National Center for Scientific Research
Colposcopy	*(Greek)* Examination of vagina and uterus by means of an apparatus with strong optical lenses
Damenorchester	*(German)* Ladies' orchestra
DAW	*(German)* Deutsche Ausruestungswerke, i.e., German Armament Works
DEST	*(German)* Deutsche Erd und Steinwerke, i.e., German Mineral and Stone Works
Deutsche Gruendlichkeit	*(German)* German thoroughness
Deutsche Staatsbuerger	*(German)* German citizens

Dienstverpflichtet *(German)* Obliged to serve

DP Displaced person

Durchfall *(German)* Diarrhea

Effektenkammer *(German)* Storehouse, section of camp where incoming goods were sorted out and stored

Einbrenne *(Yiddish)* Basic stock for sauces, roux

Entlausung *(German)* Delousing

Entzueckend *(German)* Exquisite

Erez Israel *(Hebrew)* The land of Israel

Erweiterung *(German)* Enlargement, extension

Extraordinarius *(Latin, used in German)* Extraordinary professor

Fahrbereitschaft *(German)* SS motorized vehicle corps in camp

FFI *(French)* Forces francais de l'interieur, i.e., French Forces of the Interior

FFL Forces français libres, i.e., French Free Forces

FIPO *(German)* Acronym for Finanzpolizei, i.e., financial police

FKL *(German)* Frauen-KL signified the Birkenau women's camp

Fleckfieber *(German)* Spotted fever

Flickstube *(German)* Mending room

Forsteinsatzlager *(German)* Forestry labor camp

Frauenlager	*(German)* Women's camp
FTPF	*(French)* Francs-Tireurs et Partisans Francais, i.e., French Freearchers and Partisans
Fuehrer	*(German)* Hitler's title. In camp everything was based on the Fuehrer principle, i.e., each Kommandofuehrer or Blockfuehrer and even Kapo and Blockova was a Fuehrer en miniature.
Fuehrerheim	*(German)* Officers' club in Auschwitz
Funktionshaeftling	*(German)* Prisoner occupying a prominent position
Gaertnerei	*(German)* Gardening, nursery
Gartenbau	*(German)* Horticulture
Gauleiter	*(German)* Nazi district commandant or governor
Gefahr	*(German)* Danger
Geheimnistraeger/in	*(German)* Bearer of secrets
Geist	*(German)* Spirit
Geltungsjude	*(German)* Considered a Jew according to the Nuremberg laws
Generalgouvernement	*(German)* Part of central Poland placed under German control in 1939
Geraetehaus	*(German)* Tool shed
Gestapo	*(German)* Geheime Staatspolizei, i.e., Secret State Police
Gryps	(Polish slang) Illegal, smuggled notes

Gut	*(German)* Manor, large farm
Gymnasium	(Greek) High school in Germany
Hachsharah	*(Hebrew)* Preparatory agricultural education for chalutzim (Israeli pioneers)
Haeftling	*(German)* Prisoner
Haeftlings-beguenstigung	*(German)* Favoritism toward prisoners
Haeftlings-bekleidungskammer	*(German)* Clothing storehouse for prisoners
Haeftlingsschreibstube	*(German)* Inmate secretariat
Halt Deine Schnauze!	*(German)* Shut up!
Haute Couture	*(French)* High fashion
Hazkarah	*(Hebrew)* Memorial ceremony or service
Heimatgefuehl or Heimatverbundenheit	*(German)* Feeling of connectivity and alliance with home
Heim ins Reich	*(German)* Back to the Reich
Herrenmensch	*(German)* Master race specimen
HIAS	Hebrew Immigrant Aid Society, formed in the USA to assist immigrants
Hitlerjugend	*(German)* Nazi youth movement
Horah	*(Hebrew)* Modern Jewish Folk Dance
Hundestaffel	*(German)* SS canine corps in Auschwitz

HWL	*(German)* Hauptwirtschaftslager, previous term for TWL (q.v.)
Hygieneinstitut	*(German)* Hygienic Institute
Interessengebiet	*(German)* The blocked and sequestered area around the camp complex of Auschwitz, a region of approximately forty square kilometers.
Jahrzeitlicht	*(German)* Candle to be lit on the anniversary of the death of close relatives
Jude	*(German)* Jew
Judengasse	*(German)* Ghetto
Judenrein	*(German)* Free of Jews
Juedische Gemeinde	*(German)* Jewish community
Jugendlager	*(German)* One of the areas in Ravensbrueck concentration camp where women prisoners who arrived from Auschwitz in January 1945 were housed
Kaernten	*(German)* Carinthia, Austrian province
Kalfaktor	*(Latin)* Cleaner, heater
Kanada	*(Camp jargon)* Auschwitz kommando in charge of sorting out the belongings of the Jewish arrivals
Kapelusz	*(Polish)* Hat
Karpele	*(Yiddish)* Term for the camp soup in Birkenau
Kapo	(Camp jargon) Prisoner in charge of a work detail
Kartei	*(German)* Card file

Kashern	*(Yiddish)* Verb signifying process of rendering foods and utentils Kosher according to ritual law
Kassiber	*(Hebrew)* Clandestine communication between prisoners, or letters smuggled into or out of camp
KB	*(German)* Krankenbau, i.e., sick bay
Kennkarte	*(German)* Identification card
KL or KZ	*(German)* Konzentrationslager, i.e., concentration camp
Kochanyi	*(Polish)* Boyfriend
Kogel Mogel	(Slang) Food mixture
Koje	*(German)* Berth, three tier mass stone beds in Birkenau
Kol Nidre	*(Hebrew)* Beginning prayer on the Day of Atonement
Kommandantur	*(German)* Command building
Kommando	*(German)* Work squad
Kommandofuehrer	*(German)* SS-man in charge of a kommando
Kommandoruf	*(German)* Order, command
KPD	*(German)* Kommunistische Partei Deutschland, i.e., German Communist Party
Kraeuterkommando	*(German)* Work detail to collect herbs
Kriegswichtiges Unternehmen	*(German)* Enterprise important for the war effort
Kristallnacht	*(German)* The Night of Broken Glass, the pogrom of November 1938

Kronzeuge/in	*(German)* Star witness
Kurhaus	*(German)* Spa hotel, casino, health resort, restaurant
Kvutzah	*(Hebrew)* Group, especially in kibbutzim
Lager	*(German)* Camp, concentration camp
Lageraelteste	*(German)* Camp senior, the highest position a prisoner could occupy in camp
Lagererweiterung	*(German)* Camp extension
Lagerfuehrer/in	*(German)* SS-officer, deputy of the commandant
Lagerkleidung	*(German)* Prisoner clothing, the striped uniform
Lagerkommandant	*(German)* Camp commandant
Lagerstrasse	*(German)* Camp street
Landwirtschaft	*(German)* Agriculture
Lazarett	*(German)* Military hospital
Lehrgut	*(German)* Training farm
Leichenkommando	*(German)* Work squad charged with removing corpses
Liberez!	*(French)* Imperative: Free! Liberate!
Los, los	*(German)* Fast, quickly
Madrich/a	*(Hebrew)* Youth leader
Maquis	*(French)* Resistance movement in France during World War II

Marketenderei — *(German)* Sutlery, dealing with peddlers (sutlers) who sell goods and food to an army

Maslow, Abraham (1908–1968) — Professor of psychology at Brandeis University. He posited a need hierarchy from most to least powerful (see figure below). Only when the basic needs have been sufficiently satisfied can the needs for growth and cognitive understanding become salient.

Self-actualization needs
Esteem needs
Belongingness and love needs
Safety needs
Physiological needs

Meldung — *(German)* Short for Strafmeldung, penal report

Messtruppe — *(German)* Term for land surveyor work squad in Auschwitz

Mischehe — *(German)* Mixed marriage (here usually between a Jew and a Gentile

Mischling — *(German)* Offspring of one Jewish and one Gentile parent

Mishpoche — *(Yiddish from Hebrew Mishpaha)* Relatives

Mittlere Maedchen — *(German)* Intermediate girls, age group category in Gross Breesen

Mittlere Reife — *(German)* Diploma below the level of a high school certificate. Roughly equivalent to 0 level certificate in the United Kingdom

Mitleid	*(German)* Compassion
Mitmenschen	*(German)* Fellow creatures or human beings
Moorsoldaten	*(German)* Moor soldiers; title of first concentration camp song that circulated in Central Europe in the thirties
Muede bin ich geh' zur Ruh'	*(German)* Sleepily, I go to bed; first line of a German children's evening prayer
Muselmann(er)	*(German, inmate slang)* Literally, Moslems, extremely emaciated prisoners, walking corpses
Musterlager	*(German)* Model camp
Mutti	*(German)* Mommie
Nach vorn	*(German)* To the front—refers to prisoners being summond to the camp commandant, Blockfuehrer, SS-woman-in-chief, etc.
Nacht und Nebel or N.N.	*(German)* Night and fog, code word for particular treatment of prisoners; often it signified that the inmates were not supposed to leave the camp alive.
Naehstube	*(German)* Sewing room
Noar Agudati	*(Hebrew)* Religious Jewish youth group
NSDAP	*(German)* Nationalsozialistische Deutsche Arbeiterpartei, movement founded by Hitler
Nuremberg Laws	*(German)* In September 1935, Hitler promulgated discriminatory measures against all German Jews at the annual party congress in Nuremberg

Nummernbuch	*(German)* Book of numbers, prisoner records according to inmates' numbers kept by the work allocation office in Auschwitz
Obere Maedchen	*(German)* Older girls, age group category in Gross Breesen
Obere Naehstube	*(German)* Upstairs fashion studio or tailoring workshop in the Stabsgebaeude
Oberaufseherin or O	*(German)* SS-woman-in-chief
Oberlyzeum	(Germ. from the Greek) High school
Oberschlesische Zeitung	*(German)* Upper Silesian newspaper
Oberschwester	*(German)* Head nurse, matron
Oberwachtmeister	*(German)* Squadron sergeant, German police rank; also in the Schupo
Oneg Shabbat	*(Hebrew)* Social gathering in honor of the Sabbath
Ordensburg	*(German)* SS cadet training school
Ordnungsdienst	*(German)* Privileged prisoners in the Slovakian transports
Organisieren	*(German, inmate slang)* Obtaining a thing or things by some kind of sharp practice
Ostjuden	*(German)* Jews from Eastern European countries
Panzerfaust	*(German)* Rocket used in World War II to fight enemy tanks
Papirosy	*(Polish)* Cigarettes

Pechvogel und Glueckskind	*(German)* The lucky and the unlucky person, a fairy tale by Volkmann Leander
Perennierender Roggen	*(German)* Perennial rye
Personalkartei	*(German)* Card file of inmates by name
Pflanzenzucht	*(German)* Plant cultivation
Pfleger/in	*(German)* Practical nurse
Pflegestube	*(German)* Sick bay
Pfoertner/in	*(German)* Gate keeper
Pilpel	*(Inmate slang)* Young inmate boy who performed various services— including in many cases sexual favors—for a kapo, block elder or other camp functionary
Politische Abteilung	*(German)* Camp Gestapo of Auschwitz
Posten	*(German)* SS-guard
Postenkette	*(German)* Sentry chain. Auschwitz had a kleine (small) and grosse (large) Postenkette.
Primus	Small portable petroleum cooking stove
Protektorat	In 1939, Germany established a protectorate over parts of Czechoslovakia, i.e., over Bohemia and Moravia.
Protektorat-sangehoerige	*(German)* German designation of the inhabitants of Bohemia and Moravia between 1939 and 1945
Quaddel	*(German)* Swelling of the skin
Raeder muessen rollen fuer den Sieg	*(German)* War slogan: wheels have to run for victory

Rampe *(German)* Ramp, platform in Auschwitz where the Jewish transports arrived and the selection for the gas chambers took place

Rapportfuehrer *(German)* The SS-man underneath the Schutzhaftlagerfuehrer and in charge of all the Blockfuehrers.

Rapportschreiber/in *(German)* Inmate functionary helping with the administrative work of the Rapportfuehrer

Rashomon *(Japanese)* A Japanese film produced in 1950, based on two short stories by Akutagawa Ryunosuke. It recounts a crime—rape and murder—from four different points of view: the rapist-murderer bandit's, the raped wife's, her murdered husband's, and that of a witness to the crime. Each story is creditable and the truth, always elusive, is never established.

Rassenforschung *(German)* Race research

Rassenlehre *(German)* Racial theory

Rassenschande *(German)* Disgracing one's race

Rasse-Siedlungsamt *(German)* Government office for settlement and racial affairs

Raus! Raus! *(German)* Get out!

Realschule *(German)* School stressing the teaching of mathematics and natural science

Rechtsabteilung *(German)* Legal section

Registratur *(German)* Registration office

Reichsprotektor	*(German)* Official title of Heydrich
Revier	*(German, inmate slang)* Hospital
Revieraelteste/r	*(German)* Revier senior
Rittergut	*(German)* Manor belonging to titled gentry
Rosh-ha-Shanah	*(Hebrew)* The Jewish New Year
Rotkaeppchen	*(German, inmate slang)* Women prisoners who worked in Kanada and wore red headkerchiefs
RSHA	*(German)* Reichssicherheitshauptamt, Nazi Department of Security, organized in 1939 and headed first by Heydrich and later by Kaltenbrunner
Rusznikarnia	*(Polish)* Weapons arsenal
S.A.	*(German)* Sturmabteilung, i.e., storm troop, Nazi brownshirt organization
Sachsen	*(German)* Saxony, province in Germany
Sammellager	*(German)* Collection point from which Jews were deported to extermination camps
Sammelplatz	*(German)* Square which served as gathering point for deportations
Saujuden	*(German)* Jewish pigs
S.B.	*(German)* Sonderbehandlung, i.e., extermination of Jews
Schloss	*(German)* Castle
Schnell, schnell	*(German)* Fast, hurry

Schreibstube — *(German)* Office

Schroepfkoepfchen — *(German)* Cupping glasses

Schuettelmaschine — *(German)* Shaking machine

Schutzhaftlagerfuehrer — *(German)* SS-man in charge of the camp, directly under the commandant

Schutzpolizei — *(German)* Protective police

S.D. — *(German)* Sicherheitsdienst, i.e., Security Service

SDG — *(German)* Sanitaetsdienstgrad, an SS-man who had received training as disinfector and practical nurse

Seder — *(Hebrew)* Ritual around the table in the home on the first two nights of Passover

Shabat-ha-Gadol — *(Hebrew)* The Great Sabbath preceding Passover

Sheitl — *(Hebrew)* Wig worn by Orthodox women

Siddur — *(Hebrew)* Daily prayer book

Schneidermeister — *(German)* Master tailor

Sonderhaeftling — *(German)* Special prisoner

Sonderaktion — *(German)* Euphemism for murdering Jews

Sonderkommando — *(German)* Special squad working in the gas chambers

Sortierung — *(German)* Selection for gassing

Sperre — *(German)* a) In camp: prohibition of leaving a certain block or area; b) In Holland: being put on a list to delay deportation

Spitzmaeuschen *(German)* Literally, little shrew-mouse. May be used as a term of endearment.

Spritze *(German)* Injection, shot. In Block 10 "die Spritze" usually referred to Clauberg's sterilization.

SS-Ranks

Army Equivalent	SS
Private	SS-Mann
Lance Corporal	Sturmmann
—	Rottenfuehrer
Corporal	Unterscharfuehrer
—	Scharfuehrer
Sergeant	Standartenjunker
Staff Sergeant	Oberscharfuehrer
Warrant Off. Cl. II	—
Warrant Off. Cl. I	Hauptscharfuehrer
—	Standartenoberjunker
Second Lieutenant	Sturmscharfuehrer
—	Untersturmfuehrer
Lieutenant	Obersturmfuehrer
Captain	Hauptsturmfuehrer
Major	Sturmbannfuehrer
Lt. Colonel	Obersturmbannfuehrer
Colonel	Standartenfuehrer
Brigadier General	Oberfuehrer
Major General	Brigadefuehrer
Lieutenant General	Gruppenfuehrer
General	Obergruppenfuehrer
—	Oberstgruppenfuehrer

Staatsoberreal-gymnasium *(German)* State-run high school with emphasis on mathematics and natural sciences

Stabsgebaeude *(German)* Staff building

Stammlager	*(German)* Base camp or the mother camp, e.g., the men's camp in Auschwitz I
Standesamt	*(German)* Recorder's office or civil registry
Standortarzt	*(German)* The SS physician-in-chief of the camp
Standortverwaltung	*(German)* Camp administration
Stichtag	*(German)* Key date
Stinkjuden	*(German)* Stinking Jews
Strafgefangene	*(German)* Prisoner
Strafkolonne or Strafkommando	*(German)* Penal squad
Strohsack	*(German)* Straw mattress
Stubenaelteste or Stubendienst(	Germ.) Inmate who cleaned the block and distributed the food
Sudetendeutscher	*(German)* Ethnic German from the Sudetenland
Sztubowa	*(Polish)* Room senior
Talmud	*(Hebrew)* Comprehensive term for the Mishnah, next to the Bible the main teachings of Judaism
Teichwirtschaft	*(German)* Pool management
Tenach	*(Hebrew)* Acronym for trilogy of Torah, Prophets and Writings (Hagiographa) formed from the initial letters Torah, Neviim, Ketuvim.
Tochus	*(Yiddish, from Hebrew Tahat)* Behind, posterior, arse
Todesmarsch	*(German)* Death march

Torwache *(German)* Gate keeper

Totenkartei *(German)* Card file of the dead

Triangles A prisoner was identified not only by his or her camp number but also by the triangle which preceded it. The colors revealed the reason for imprisonment—red stood for political prisoner, green for criminal, pink for homosexual, purple for Jehovah's Witness, black for prostitute, black with the letter "Z" for gypsy (i.e., Zigeuner, yellow for Jew. However, the Jews wore a double triangle which formed a Star of David. All the RSHA Jews (those sent to Auschwitz for the "Final Solution") had a yellow and red Mogen David. Those admitted for "crimes" wore yellow and green on their number sign. A German non-Jewish inmate accused of Rassenschande (miscegenation) had a yellow and black Star of David.

Trockenboden *(German)* Loft for drying clothes or laundry

Truppenwaesche *(German)* Laundry for the troops

TWL *(German)* Truppenwirtschaftslager, i.e., supply storage for the troops

Uebersicht *(German)* Survey, review

Unter den Linden *(German)* Boulevard in Berlin

Unterkunft *(German)* Storage facility in Auschwitz

Unterkunftskammer *(German)* Specific area in the Unterkunft

Untermencsh *(German)* The counterpart to Nietzche's Superman

Verfuegbar *(German)* Available

Vernichtungslager	*(German)* Extermination camp
Versippt	*(German)* Related
Verwaltung	*(German)* Administration
Volksdeutscher	*(German)* Ethnic German
Volkssturm	*(German)* German military units toward the end of World War II consisting of adolescent boys and old men
Vorzugshaeftling	*(German)* Privileged prisoner
Waescherei or Waschkueche	*(German)* Wash-house, laundry detail
Waffen-SS	*(German)* Armed SS
Wandervogel	*(German)* German youth movement
Wasserpolacken	*(German)* Poles living near the German border
Wegerich	*(German)* Plantain
Wehrmacht	*(German)* All German military forces from 1933-1945
Weisskaeppchen	*(German)* Women who worked in the Weissen Effekten squad in the men's camp in Birkenau, sorting out incoming goods. They wore white headkerchiefs.
Weltanschauung	*(German)* Philosophy of life
Wiedergutmachung	*(German)* Popular term for the German legislation concerning individual reparation payments under the German Indemnification Law
Wirtschaftsbetriebe	*(German)* Economic enterprises
Wirtschaftskueche	*(German)* Designation for the kitchen in Malchow camp

Zaehlappell	*(German)* Roll call
Zehnfingersystem	*(German)* Typing with ten fingers
Zentralbauleitung or ZB	*(German)* Central Construction Co.
Z.L.	*(Hebrew)* Of blessed memory
Zugangsliste	*(German)* List of new arrivals
Zurueck!	*(German)* Go back! (imperative)

Notes

PART 1

Chapter 1

1. Nowadays, non-surgical transcervical tubal occlusion methods are sometimes used on a voluntary basis for irreversible female sterilization (Zatuchni et al., 1983).

2 Clauberg induced Dr. Johannes Goebel—an employee of the Schering Co. who provided chemical supplies for his injections—to take up residency in Auschwitz. He had a house not far from camp put at his disposal and entrusted him with the execution of intrauterine injections on his own. Goebel boasted so loudly about his activities that the Schering Co. distanced itself from him. Eduard de Wind characterizes him as follows: "He sticks his nose into everything and forces all women to undergo experiments without pity. While Clauberg could sometimes behave quite properly toward a woman if she objected to receiving an injection for a certain reason, Goebel was gross and sarcastic. He was a typically pusillanimous person suddenly thrown into a position of power without having learnt how to handle the situation" (Langbein, 1972, p. 386).

3 After the war Dr. Goebel had been in custody. He died on August 11, 1952.

Dr. Margita (Manci) Schwalbova

4 On December 28, 1942, Prof. Dr. Clauberg began his sterilization experiments of female prisoners in Block 28 of the hospital complex of the women's camp in Birkenau. For this purpose, several women inmates were housed at his exclusive disposal in Block 27. From time to time he visited the camp and undertook a number of procedures during which he injected a certain liquid into the women's uterus. Subsequently the results were verified by x-rays (Czech, 1989, p. 366).

5 Jiri Beranovsky was an inmate in Auschwitz from September 15, 1941, until his escape during the death march on January 18, 1945. He appeared as a witness at the Auschwitz trial in Frankfurt/Main (Naumann, 1965, p. 158).

6 Orli Reichert, a German political prisoner, had been arrested as a young girl in 1936 for her membership in an illegal youth organization. After her prison term she had been sent to Ravensbrueck from where she was transferred to Auschwitz with the first women's transport. She was camp elder in the women's hospital in Birkenau and in spite of her high position she never forgot that National Socialism was the common enemy. She died from tuberculosis shortly after the war (Langbein, 1972, pp. 247-248).

There exists a different assessment of Orli: "I cannot judge Orli. I will not even try. I really do not understand her. I always saw her in a variety of situations, and in each situation she was a different person. On one occasion she would be defiant to the authorities; on another she would be cruel to the prisoners. At one moment she was filled with compassion for human suffering; at another, without blinking an eye she made sure that not even one of the victims sentenced to the gas chamber would escape" (Nomberg-Przytyk, 1985, pp. 41-42).

7 For more on Gertrud Frinke see Shelley, 1986, pp. 12-17.

8 On March 8, 1990, Cardinal Dr. Hans Hermann Groer initiated the process of beatification for the former nun Cecilia Autsch in the Archepiscopal Palace in Vienna. (Processus Super Martyrio, Sessio Prima, in causa Beatificationis et Canonizationis Servae Dei Sororis Angelae Mariae a Corde Iesu [Mariae Caeciliae Autsch] e Congregatione Sororum SS Trinitatis.

9 Nomberg-Przytyk, who worked in the Birkenau hospital together with Manci Schwalbova, gives a detailed description of life in the Revier in her book *Auschwitz*, 1985.

Sonja Fritz (née Fischmann)

10 The physician Enna Weiss was in charge of the women's Revier in Birkenau. She had been deported from Slovakia, was young (she had not yet completed medical school), pretty and quite self-assured. Opinions as to her behavior in Auschwitz are divided, some praise her actions and others condemn her. After the war, she refused to testify. She is living in Australia (Langbein, 1972).

11 Ria Hans, now Elias, lives in Sao Paulo, Brazil. (See also contribution by Magda Blau.)

12 On January 5, 1945, six prisoners, so-called "bearers of secrets," were being transferred to Mauthausen: five Polish inmates who had worked in the Sonderkommando and the Czech prisoner Stanislaw Slezak (Nr. 39340), who had been in charge of the x-ray machines used for Dr. Schumann's sterilization experiments. All of them were shot in the crematorium of Mauthausen on April 3, 1945 (Czech, 1989, p. 956). See also Langbein, 1972, p. 106.

13 In a deposition in the case against former SS-physician Dr. Horst Schumann made on July 1, 1968, at the Hall of Justice in Presov, Czechoslovakia, Sylvia Vesela, née Friedmann, Prof. Clauberg's former nurse, described the early sterilization experiments of Dr. Schumann in the following way:

> Schumann did sterilization experiments through radiation. The equipment was manufactured by Siemens. The experiments were performed on women and men. The inmates were placed between two heavy x-ray plates for about 3-6 minutes. Dr. Schumann adjusted the intensity of the radiation without regard to the health of the prisoners. About 50 inmates per day underwent this procedure. Schumann also varied the length of time of the radiation exposure. When a prisoner was exposed for 10-15 minutes to the x-rays, severe third-degree burns occurred, visible on the lower abdomen. Shortly after the radiation a very strong reaction took place—vomiting, blood in urine and stool, and unbearable abdominal pains. The prisoners screamed but the staff was not allowed to assist them in any way.
>
> Ria Hansova, from Slovakia, and Marika, from Austria, were working in Dr. Schumann's office at that time. Both were prisoners that had been assigned to him. The inmates that were used as guinea pigs were sent back to their barracks in the camp. They were ordered to return the following day for further treatments. However, we warned some of the girls from Slovakia—Klari Baumoehlova, Lenka Belanova, Eva Farkasova and Magda Herbstova—to mingle in other work assignments, even in very hard outside work squads, in order to escape from the horrible experiments. (Deposition File #SPR 475/68, made by Sylvia Vesela, née Friedmanova, in Presov on July 1, 1968, in front of Judge Vojtech Majoros, for the Central Justice Court Department in Ludwigsburg, DDR.)

14 On May 10, 1943, the well-known French resistance fighter Danielle Casanova (Nr. 31655), a communist, died of typhus in the women's camp of Auschwitz-Birkenau (Czech, 1989, p. 491).

15 Kielar reports inmates had believed that Sonja had left Auschwitz for good: "Sonja F., the beautiful Austrian woman, was not released after her stay at the quarantine

block—contrary to all our assumptions. After a one month stay at the Viennese prison, she returned to camp" (Kielar, 1979, p. 349).

16 He was sentenced to death in the big Auschwitz trial in Cracow and was executed by hanging on December 12, 1947.

Chapter 2

Dr. Alina Bialostocka (née Brewda)

1 On orders of SS-Standartenfuehrer Dr. Enno Lolling, the head of Section D III of the WVHA (responsible for sanitary questions and camp hygiene in all concentration camps), Dr. Alina Brewda was transferred from KL Lublin (Majdanek) to KL Auschwitz on September 21, 1943. She received the number 62761 (Czech, 1989, p. 611).

2 More information about this can be found in *Auschwitz in England* by Mavis M. Hill and L. Norman Williams, Stern & Day, 1965.

Leon Uris wrote his novel *QB VII* about these events but this time, cautiously, prefaced his book with the following note: "The English legal profession adheres to an extremely formal protocol and a rigid etiquette. I have not attempted to bind myself to all these customs but have used a reasonable literary license so long as the novel remains within a framework of basic truth and credibility. The characters contained herein are purely fictitious" (Uris, 1989).

3 Dr. Bialostocka died in the summer of 1988.

Ima Spanjaard (née van Esso)

4 Joop Westerweel (1899-1944) was a Dutch Christian rescuer of Jews. Together with Joachim Simon of the Zionist pioneers, he created an underground movement for concealing Halutsim. He was captured by the Germans while attempting to transfer two young girls to the Belgian border crossing. Despite severe torture, he refused to betray his group. He was executed on August 11, 1944 (Gutman, 1990, pp. 1648-1649).

5 The camp experiences of Louis Micheels are published in his Holocaust memoirs, *Doctor 117641*, Yale University Press, 1989.

6 There is another version of how Adelaide Hautval escaped the execution squad, given in Charlotte Delbo's *Le Convoi du 24 Janvier*:

On the evening of August 16, 1943, Orli Reichert, the Revieraelteste in Birkenau, informed Heidi that she had heard the execution would take place the following day and that they would pick up Dr. Hautval.

She added, "You have to give in."

"No," Heidi replied.

Then Orli made arrangements. "Take this, lie down and don't move!" She gave Heidi a sleeping pill and assigned her to a bed in the Revier.

Next day, when Heidi woke up, everything had been taken care of. Heidi never knew exactly what had happened. She believed that they had given a corpse which they had presented as hers. The judgment could not be executed any more, since she was dead. But what about the number tattooed on the arm which served to precisely identify all corpses? So many bodies were gnawed at by rats—they could have eaten the tattooed arm just as well as another piece—cheating was possible. And the SS-physician in charge of examining the executed prisoners had liked Heidi Hautval. He probably did not investigate too thoroughly.

Adelaide Hautval had quite a bit of experience with rats in the Revier of Birkenau. After the liberation she related:

> We had a tremendous number of rats. Six or seven came to see us every night. It's an infernal round. There is a very fat one whom we believe to be the grandmother. She regularly drank our Lysol as a rejuvenating elixir. It seemed to work perfectly. We were so familiar with the rats that we even gave them names. However, what bothered us is that they eat human flesh. They attacked the women even before they were dead. In order not to be bothered too much by them at night, I fell into the habit of leaving them a free passage close to my head and to reserve the pillow space as their thoroughfare *(Descente Aux Enfers,* by Vladimir Pozner).

7 In January 1944 a course in nursing for women prisoners was given in Auschwitz I, officially under the direction of inmate prisoner Dr. Franciszek Gralla.

As a result of the typhus epidemic, access to the women's camp in Birkenau had been blocked and it had been completely isolated since November 1943. Thus, the members of the camp resistance organization had lost all contact with the women's camp. In order to establish a connection, they decided to arrange a nursing course. The curriculum, worked out by prisoners Dr. Alina Brewda and Dr. Slavka Kleinova, had been accepted by Auschwitz physician-in-chief Dr. Wirths and approved by the WVHA in Berlin. Through a select group of women prisoners sent for this course to Block 10 in Auschwitz, contacts were made. The classes were taught by prison physicians of the men's camp (Czech, 1989, p. 708).

According to Dr. Alina Brewda the women for the nurses' course in Block 10 were selected by Revier elder Dr. Fejkiel together with other prisoners of the underground movement. They went to Birkenau and brought back thirty-six girls, nearly all of them non-Jewish, mostly wives and sisters of resistance fighters. Among them was Countess Romer, a titled Polish nurse (Minney, 1966, pp. 150, 177).

Former Polish prisoner Tadeusz Borowski also describes the nurses' training course which took place in the Stammlager in *Bei Uns in Auschwitz* (Borowski, 1987, pp. 134-185).

8 For more information about Alma Rosé consult *Playing for Time,* by Fania Fenelon. New York: Atheneum, 1977.

Magda Blau (née Hellinger)

9 Nine hundred ninety-nine Jewish women from Poprad in Slovakia were admitted into the women's camp on March 26, 1942. That was the first registered transport which had been sent by Section IV B 4 of the RSHA. The head of this section in charge of Jewish affairs was Obersturmbannfuehrer Adolf Eichmann. The Jewesses received the uniforms which had belonged to the murdered Russian prisoners-of-war (Czech, 1989, p. 190).

10 On December 5, 1942, in the women's camp B I a in Birkenau, a large selection was held by the SS among the prisoners which lasted all day. After the selection, about 2000 young and healthy women, capable of work, were taken to the gas chambers (Czech, 1989, p. 351).

11 There was a marked difference in the reaction of the SS as a result of the singing of the Marseillaise by the French women prisoners entering Birkenau and the singing of the Dutch national anthem by Jewish women from the Netherlands during their arrival at Birkenau in 1942. Most of them drowned in a ditch where they had to stand all night for punishment (eye witness account of Helen Kuban).

12 About 20 women of different nationalities were taken from the women's camp B I a in Birkenau on April 3, 1943, to the experimental Block 10 in the men's camp of Auschwitz to work as physicians and nurses (Czech, 1989, p. 458).

13 See also contribution by Sonja Fritz.

14 Regarding the "mask experiments" see entry on prisoners gassed for Prof. Hirt at the KL-Natzweiler in Czech, 1989, p. 521.

15 The Drechsler woman, whose mere name spelled terror, was called "zubata" (the one with the mouthful of teeth) by the Russian prisoners (Szmaglewska, 1947, p. 154). Other nicknames for SS woman Drechsler, also called "Drekslerka," were "Smierc" (death) and "Kostucha" (reaper), because of her cruelty (Jagoda, Klodzinski and Maslowski, 1987, p. 255) Band II.

16 Stanislawa Staroska, known in camp as "Stana the Flogger," was, together with former SS members, among the accused prisoners at the Bergen-Belsen trial in Lueneburg, which was held from September 17 to November 17, 1945. She was given the status of agent of the camp administration and was sentenced to ten years' imprisonment. The Foreign Office files offer conflicting evidence on her further fate. Either she committed suicide on May 10, 1946, or her sentence was reduced to five years; the latter is probably correct (Gutman, 1990, pp. 1499, 1796).

17 The C-Lager in Birkenau is described by the former Polish prisoner Tadeusz Borowski, who referred to it as the "Persian Market" ("Und Sie Gingen. . . .," 1987, pp. 186-203).

18 The deceased Hungarian physician, Dr. Gisella Perl, gave an account of Magda's activity as camp elder in an article, "Magda—Lageraelteste des C. Lagers in Auschwitz-Birkenau," published in the Hungarian paper *Uj Kelet,* 1952, Tel Aviv.

19 Magda Blau has been active in defending the reputation of Slovakian survivors who were the first Jewish women sent to the concentration camp of Auschwitz in the spring of 1942. She feels that many of these veterans—who occupied prominent positions in camp like herself—have been unjustly accused of collaboration.

Orli Reichert-Wald, herself a former camp elder of the Revier in Birkenau, pleaded for better understanding in her report, "Jackelis Mutter," the story of Fela Dreksler (an ex-room elder in Auschwitz), who had been denounced by fellow inmates after the war and sentenced by a French military tribunal to ten years' imprisonment (Steger & Thiele, 1989, pp. 115-118).

It was the great humanist, writer and Auschwitz survivor, Primo Levi, who investigated the "gray zone" in camp, i.e., the "intricate and stratified microcosm of the 'protekcja' inmate." He stated that "privileged prisoners were a minority within the Lager population. Nevertheless, they represent a potent majority among survivors." However, he also asserted that "the privileged prisoner par excellence did not bear witness at all for obvious reasons" (Levi, 1988, pp. 18, 20, 40).

Chapter 3

Aliza Barouch

1 Dr. Zvi Koretz, the chief rabbi of Salonika (born in Rzeszow, Galicia), was made president of the newly created Judenrat by the Germans in December 1942. His role as head of the Jewish community is controversial. Some historians criticized his seeming lack of leadership, others have tried to revise the picture. He was deported to Bergen-Belsen and died there in May or June 1945 (Gutman, 1990, pp. 819, 1326).

2 On April 9, 1941, Germany conquered Salonika and its fifty thousand Jews. Between March 20 and August 18, 1943, at least 43,850 Jews from Salonika arrived in Auschwitz-Birkenau, where the majority was gassed. After the war, in 1945, the Salonikan community numbered 1,950. Many of them had survived hiding in the mountains or fighting with the partisans. Only a few had returned from concentration camps (Gutman, 1990, p. 1326).

3 In a paper entitled "Carcinoma of the Large Bowel After a Single Massive Dosage of Radiation in Healthy Teenagers," published in *Cancer* (57:728-731) in 1986 by Siegfried Rotmensch, et al. about some of Aliza Barouch's co-prisoners in Block 10, they reported: "Three healthy teenagers were exposed to a single pelvic x-ray irradiation as part of sterilization experiments performed in the Auschwitz concentration camp in 1943. Single and multiple carcinomas of the colon and rectum developed 40 years later in the radiation field. ... These women had not undergone repeated courses of radiation, had no known co-existing disease that might raise the risk for colonic and rectal malignancies and had an extremely long and remarkably similar latency period ... Since thousands of teenagers were subjected to similar

sterilization experiments, awareness of the association might help in the early diagnosis of additional cases."

Renée Duering

4 Most probably, the blood was required for the SS-Hygiene Institute in Rajsko and not for transfusions for German soldiers.)

5 Karl Lill, Nr. 60356, a German political prisoner, was in charge of the herbal work squad. Precisely for this purpose, he had organized and studied a medicinal herbs book and had received permission from Dr. Wirths (in whose SS-Revier he worked) to take over the kommando for a few weeks. He started in May 1944 and managed to provide some relaxation and respite on some beautiful spring days in the sun-drenched green meadows near the Sola River for about 50 women of Block 10, who hopped and sang like children, i.e., like people who had not seen a ray of sun for a long, long time (the windows of Block 10 were covered with boards to prevent the inmates from watching the executions that occurred at the Black Wall between Blocks 10 and 11). (Lill,, 1978, pp. 142-144.)

6 The women of Clauberg's experimental Block 10 were transferred to Block 1 in the new Auschwitz women's camp (Schutzhaftlagererweiterung) on May 22, 1944, on the same day when the women of the Stabsgebaeude were moved to Block 6 of the same camp (Czech, 1989, p. 781 and Skodova1962, p. 146).

7 On January 6, 1945, in the evening, the following four Jewish female prisoners were hanged in the Auschwitz women's camp: Ella Gartner, Roza Robota, Regina Safir and Estera Wajsblum. They had been sentenced to death for aiding the uprising of the members of the Sonderkommando in the crematoria of Birkenau on October 7, 1944. The help had consisted of supplying the Sonderkommando with dynamite and ammunition from the warehouse of the Weichsel-Union Metal Works, where three of those condemned to death had been working. The execution occurred in two stages. Two women prisoners were hanged during the evening roll-call in the presence of the men and women who worked the night shift in the Weichsel-Union Metal Works. The two other women were hanged after the return of the day shift. The sentence was read by Hoessler, the First Schutzhaftlagerfuehrer in Auschwitz. He screamed that all traitors would be exterminated this way (Czech, 1989, p. 958).

On October 7, 1944, some Jewish prisoners of the Sonderkommando revolted. They armed themselves with hammers, axes, stones and some self-made grenades, threw their kapo and an SS-man into the burning oven, burned down Crematorium IV and attacked the SS. However, since some of the prisoners had been threatened with immediate extermination, there had not been sufficient time to coordinate the uprising with all members of the work squad. Only Kommandos 57B and 59B were involved. Kommandos 58B and 60B did not participate because some of them had not been informed about the plan and also because the SS had the situation pretty much under control in their area. Two hundred and fifty prisoners were killed during the fighting, among them the organizers of the uprising: Zelman Gradowski of Suwalki, Josef Warszawski of Warsaw, Josef Deresinski of Luny, Ajzyk Kalniak of Lomza, Lajb Langfus of Warsaw, and Lajb Panusz of Lomza. Two hundred additional inmates of the Sonderkommando were shot the evening of October 7, 1944. The three SS-men killed during the revolt were Unterscharfuehrers Rudolf Erler, Willi Freese and Josef Purke (Czech, 1989 pp. 898-900).

Eva Golgevit

8 During her stay in Block 10, Eva was also a member of the herbal work squad which collected medicinal herbs for the SS and which was led for a short time by political prisoner Karl Lill, who writes in his memoirs: "Our women overcame death marches, new camps, hunger and epidemics. May I hope that those short weeks of our 'spring hikes,' the ample rests in the glades, those hours of 'feeling like a human being' have contributed to surmount the trials of the last year. Eva Goldgewicht, Dédé, Irene, Mother Gutnic, Perelka (little pearl), didn't all of you continue our good fight? We haven't reached our goal yet by a long stretch" (Lill, 1978, p. 145). (See also Kraeuter kommando under Renée Duering.)

9 Slavka Klein wrote about her underground activities in Block 10: "When a group of political women prisoners from France, to whom I also belonged, arrived at Block 10, a new chapter in the history of this block started. Through contacts with members of the resistance movement we succeeded to change the personnel of the block and to exert a beneficial influence upon the others.

At the request of the underground movement, I provided a detailed and systematic description of the experiments to which the women of Block 10 were subjected, emphasizing especially the names of the SS men and other persons responsible for these procedures.

This report, the first account of the events in the only women's block in the Stammlager Auschwitz, was smuggled out of camp at the end of 1943 through the comrades Tadeusz Holuj and Stanislaw Klodzinski. With satisfaction I discovered after the war that at that time a complete summary of the report had been forwarded to London. It is kept at the Polish Documentation Centre of WW II in London"' (Lorska, 1987, pp. 209-211).

Karl Lill reports in his memoirs that Slavka Kleinova (Dorota Lorska) was a beautiful young woman who had been a clever and courageous comrade-in-arms and surgeon during the Civil War in Spain. Immediately after her arrival in Auschwitz, she had met inmate Rudi Goebel from Freudenthal, who also had fought in the Spanish war and from whose foot she had extracted a bullet after the battle on the Ebro. In camp she tried to provide food items for herself and her party comrades. Slavka succeeded in saving herself and a group of about 17, mostly French women, from Clauberg's experiments (Lill, 1978, p. 142).

10 Slavka Klein reported about the attempts to help change the atmosphere in Block 10: "There were quite a number of gifted women at the block. Under the direction of Hadas Lerner from Lwow, real concerts with songs, recitations and dances were arranged. Thus, besides the moaning and crying and shooting (from the Black Wall between Blocks 10 and 11) you could hear folk songs of many European countries after the block had been locked at night. The introductory words of Hadas/Dédé awakened interest and, gradually, human feelings of mutual understanding and good will returned together with laughter. Hearts that had become petrified in face of the inhuman cataclysm began to thaw and to re-discover that a person does not have to behave like a wolf towards another and that you prosper if your fellow human being is like a sister to you" (Lorska, 1987, p. 211).

11 Lill remembers that he learned in the summer of 1944 that all women without exception, even those that had previously been protected by Slavka, should now be sterilized. The comrades decided to go to the extermination camp of Birkenau rather than become Clauberg's victims. Perhaps, they would be able to survive (Lill, 1978, p. 144).

Friedel de Wind of Block 10, who worked in the Kraeuterkommando (herbal work detail), described re-encountering the women who had formerly stayed at Block 10: "Yesterday, I finally was allowed to join the Kraeuterkommando. At 8 a.m. we left the camp and marched a long way. We also reached the vicinity of Birkenau. There, I saw some of the 70 girls who had left the block last month. For some the experiments had been terminated, for others they had been unsucessful, and then there were the French communists who had refused to undergo the experiments (see contribution of Renée Duering on this subject). It is dreadful to see the women in Birkenau. How they have changed, completely shaved and barefoot, just a piece of jute around their body tied together with a string. These are no more women, they are sexless beings..." (de Wind, 1979, p. 176).

PART II

Chapter 4

Dr. Claudette Kennedy

1 Claudette Kennedy is a grand-niece of Emile Durkheim, the father of modern sociology, and a cousin of Marcel Mauss, the famous French anthropologist who never recovered from the mental breakdown caused by the brutalities of the German occupation.

2 SS Hauptsturmfuehrer Theodor Dannecker (1913-1945) was a young Bavarian lawyer from Munich who became one of Adolf Eichmann's indispensable agents in the implementation of the "Final Solution." He was in charge of the deportation of Jews from France (1942), Bulgaria (1943) and Italy (1944) to Auschwitz. Dannecker headed the French bureau and Judenreferat (Jewish section) of the RSHA, receiving his orders directly from Eichmann. He was a fanatic Nazi who went into a trance every time the word "Jew" was mentioned and claimed credit for being the first to propose continuous Jewish deportations from France to the East. Dannecker committed suicide in an American prison camp in Bad Toelz on December 10, 1945 (Wistrich, 1982, pp. 44-45).

3 On September 15, 1942, the Polish prisoner Janina Kukowska (#7453) died of typhus in Birkenau. Together with the other women prisoners she had worked as botanist at the Pflanzenzucht in Rajsko. Caesar, the director of the agricultural enterprises, feared that the other women prisoners who worked at the laboratory and came in close contact with members of the SS might spread typhus at their work place. He, therefore, obtained permission to lodge them in the Stabsgebaeude in Auschwitz (Czech, 1989, p. 301).

4 Dr. Claudette Bloch-Kennedy was in the bunker from May 21-May 29, 1943 (Czech, 1989, p. 501).

5 On June 12, 1943, the women of the gardening work squad who used to come daily from Birkenau and the women of the plant cultivation detail who commuted from the Stabsgebaeude moved to the newly erected satellite camp of Rajsko (Czech, 1989, p. 519).

Dr. Marie-Elisa Cohen

6 Stenia Staroska of Tarnow, the spruce and pretty camp senior, is a Polish girl appointed to the highest post a prisoner may attain. She runs through camp spilling the precious water with a kick of her high boot, thrusting the bowl and the clothes in it into the mud, and scattering the washing women. In a hoarse voice she calls after the women who have scattered in all directions, "Du Mistbiene!" (You dung fly!) "Du alte Kuh!" (You old cow!) "Du Krematoriumfigur!" (You crematory figure!) (Szmaglewska, 1947, pp. 227-228.)

7 The Polish prisoner Stanislawa Staroska, called Stenia, was initially block-elder at the women's camp in Birkenau and later advanced to camp elder. In the post-war Bergen-Belsen trial she was accused together with members of the SS. To defend herself she asserted, "If I as camp elder wanted to help the prisoners, I had to win the confidence of the German authorities. I had to fight for every compromise, and this was more difficult for me than for German prisoner functionaries." (Langbein, 1972, p. 192).

8 On May 12, 1942, five female prisoners were transferred from Ravensbrueck to Auschwitz. Among them were the engineers Wanda Dutczynska, Maria Raczynska, Emilia Goszkowska, M.A., and Janina Kukowska, M.A. SS Obersturmbannfuehrer Dr. Joachim Caesar, the director of the agricultural enterprises, had requested highly qualified prisoners in biology, chemistry, agriculture and horticulture from Ravensbrueck to research the caotchouc containing Kok-saghiz plant for the Pflanzenzucht (Czech, 1989, pp. 209-210).

9 On September 11, 1943, Lili Toffler (Nr. 4738), who works at the Pflanzenzuchtstation in Rajsko, secretly gives a letter for a friend to Abraham Solarz (Nr. 101028), a Jewish prisoner, who had been sent to Rajsko together with the Pole Waclaw Gniazdowski (Nr. 102331) in order to pick up flowers. Solarz

delivers the flowers at the Political Section and loses the letter. An SS man finds it, an investigation is started and the two prisoners are thrown into the bunker of Block 11. During the interrogations Abraham Solarz does not reveal the name of the prisoner to whom the letter is addressed. Gniazdowski does not even know anything about the letter. The sender of the letter is identified through her signature and also thrown into the bunker, but does not betray the name of the intended recipient of the letter. (The editor, who worked at that time at the Political Section, remembers that all secretaries of the work squad, including herself, had to give a handwriting sample.) After a selection of the bunker, all three were shot on September 21, 1943 (Czech, 1989, pp. 604-605).

10 Obergruppenfuehrer Oswald Pohl, the chief of the Economic Administration Head Office (WVHA), constantly inspected all the concentration camps and, next to Dachau, Auschwitz received his special attention (Hoess, 1949, p. 252).

11 On February 25, 1944, commandant Liebehenschel informed the SS men in Auschwitz that the Reichsfuehrer SS had promoted Dr. Joachim Caesar, the director of the agricultural enterprises, to Obersturmbannfuehrer (Czech, 1989, p. 729).

12 Berthe Falk was sent on July 5, 1944, for three months to the Strafkompagnie. However, Obersturmbannfuehrer Caesar's wife took her out frequently and returned her to the laboratory to help with her doctoral dissertation (Czech, 1989, p. 813).

13 In 1968, Dr. Marie-Elisa Cohen received the Legion of Honor.

Madeleine Odru

14 Madeleine Odru was decorated with the Croix de guerre and earned the honor of sublieutenant of the FFI.

Hélène Parreaux

15 Paul Langevin was a French physicist born in Paris in 1872. He was the author of books about ions, magnestism and the relativity of ultra sound. In 1934 he became a member of the Academie des Sciences. He died in 1946 (Larousse, 1947, p. 1483).

16 Wermacht General Hans Speidel was Rommel's last Chief of Staff in France. He became involved in the plot against Hitler, was interrogated by the Gestapo and acquitted. After the war Speidel became Adenauer's military adviser. He represented the Federal Republic of Germany in NATO and from April 1957 to September 1963 he was commander of all NATO forces in Central Europe. He retired in 1964 (Wistrich, 1982, pp. 292-293).

17 On January 27, 1943, 230 female political prisoners from France received the numbers 31625-31854. They had been transported from Romainville to Auschwitz. Among them were: Danielle Casanova (31655), Maie Politzer, Hélène Solomon-Langevin, Yvonne Blech, Henriette Schmidt and Raymonde Salez (Czech, 1989, p. 394).

Chapter 5

Jozefa Kiwalowa

1 Concerning Wanda Dulczynska, see endnote in contribution by Marie-Elisa Cohen.

2 For some time now the women's camp has been harrassed by Aufseherin Bormann, a petty, stupid woman who has a flair for finding the best-hidden treasures. It was at her suggestion that the famous inspection in Rajsko took place, among the workers of the botanical laboratory. The women were ordered to take off their clothes and underwear, put on gray dresses, congregate before the barracks and not budge. Before their very eyes everything was removed under Bormann's supervision from the residential barracks and from the laboratories, every tiniest bit of their belongings were found, even the letters concealed in the trees or in the garden under the leaves. Even the garbage heap was searched. Most prominent in their eagerness in the inspection were Camp Commandant Kramer and his chauffeur, Lagerfuehrerin Mandel, Aufseherin Milan-Volkenrat. All the things they found were segregated into two piles. The inspection lasted all day. In the evening trucks drove up and carried off all the confiscated property. The day after the inspection, Wanda, the Capo of Rajsko, was transferred to Birkenau as a punitive measure.

It was rumored later that the SS men who carried out the inspection in Rajsko, in their servile zeal burned down, among other things, the priceless files and records on research work concerning a plant called kok-sagiz, which was raised on a large scale in Rajsko and with which experiments were being made for the production of artificial rubber. In addition, all the personal effects of the wife of the chief of Rajsko were burned, which started a feud between him and Aufseherin Bormann (Szmaglewska, 1947, pp. 312-313).

3 Anton Mencner is also spelled Mecner or Metzner.

4 On January 20, 1945, during the footmarch from Wodzislaw in Silesia, a few women prisoners succeeded in escaping. Among them were Jozefa Kaleta-Kiwalowa, Irena Glowacka-Zakrzewska, Wanda Blachowska-Tarasiewicz and Zofia Augustyn-Pajerska (Czech, 1989, 981-982).

Riva Krieglova

5 Film director Wanda Jakubowska, number 43513, made two movies about Auschwitz: In 1948, "Ostatni Etap" ("The Last Stop"), and in 1964 "Koniec Naszego Swiata" ("The End of Our World"). (Czech, 1989, p. 480.)

6 Slang for former Petchek bank in Prague taken over by the Gestapo as their headquarters.

7 The Czech physician Dr. Zdena Nedvedova was among the group of women prisoners who, early in 1943, started an underground movement in the women's camp of Birkenau; among them were also Hélène Solomon-Langevin-Parreaux, Anni Binder-Urbanova and Herta Soswinski (Garlinski, 1975, pp. 124-125).

Chapter 6

Wanda Ladniewska

1 Gideon Hausner (1915-1990) was Israel's Attorney General from 1960-1963 and in that capacity he became the prosecutor in the Eichmann trial in Jerusalem. His opening speech was one of the highlights of the trial: "I do not stand alone here in denouncing this man. Beside me stand the six million who can no longer stand here to accuse him" (Gutman, 1990, pp. 649-650).

Inge Schlesinger

2 Concerning Wanda Jacubowska, see footnote in contribution by Riva Krieglova.

3 Author of *Auschwitz—Ein Tatsachenbericht,* Lettner Verlag, Berlin, 1956.

4 The Polish prisoner Eugenia Halbreich, number 29700, was the only woman who succeeded in staying in Rajsko when all other inmates went on the death march on January 18, 1945. She hid in the attic of SS-man Grell's house, remained there for three or four days, and then went to the village of Rajsko, where the inhabitants gave her asylum (Czech, 1989, p. 971).

5 Concerning Berthe Falk see footnote in contribution of Marie-Elisa Cohen.

Chapter 7

Pola Plotnicka

1 Graetz, Heinrich (1817-1891), a German Jewish historian.

2 In June 1942, twelve thousand Jews from the vicinity were forced into the ghetto of Rzeszow, mostly from the towns of Tyczyn, Lancut, Lezajsk, Kolbuszowa, Sokolow Malopolski, Strzyzow and Blazowa, raising the ghetto population to 23,000 (Gutman, 1990, p. 1316).

3 Concerning Dédé and Perelka, see footnote in contribution by Eva Golgevit.

4 Mieczyslaw Kieta (1920-1984) No. 59590, a Polish political prisoner, was a member of the camp resistance movement, "Fighting Group Auschwitz." He worked as secretary in the Hygiene Institute. After the war, he published works about Auschwitz, among them *Das Hygiene Institut der Waffen SS und Polizei in Auschwitz.*

5 Langbein recounts that Dr. Korn refused to administer lethal phenol injections into the heart: "The SS-orderlies needed willing, skillful and tireless helpers. This could not be achieved through coercion. Dr. Mikulas Korn proved that there was a possibility to refuse to 'spritzen' (give these shots). When Panszczyk had left Auschwitz, Korn was told by SS Hantl to continue his work. Korn declared that he would not do it although as a Jew he had to be more afraid than the 'Aryans' of the consequences of such a refusal. However, nothing happened to him. He did survive Auschwitz" (Langbein, 1972, p. 213).

Appendices

Hans Muench

1 On October 13, 1942, SS Obersturmbannfuehrer Joachim Caesar, the head of the agricultural enterprises in Auschwitz, fell ill with typhus. A few days earlier his wife had died from typhus (Czech, 1989, p. 319).

2 In a personal communication Dr. Hautval had this to say about Dr. Samuel: "To inscribe the name of Dr. Samuel in Yad Vashem would not only be nonsense but veritable mockery. Personally, without bearing a grudge against him for what he did to me, I consider him a wretched person without even the most elementary dignity. With exaggerated zeal, often without necessity, he executed the orders of the SS. He was also ambitious and loved to show off his surgical skills. It might well be that once or twice he did some good. Why not? At times, some of the more notorious SS men did show a human gesture, among others even Mengele."

3 Sturmbannfuehrer Ding-Schuler was at first camp physician and later did spotted fever experiments for the Hygienic Institute in Buchenwald. Kogon wrote that he was one of the few higher SS functionaires who had been won over by the inmates not only through corruption but through genuine political persuasion. Ding-Schuler kept seven Jewish researchers (among them Dr. Fleck) in block 50 in Buchenwald to which he referred jokingly as "ultimum refugium judaeorum" (last refuge of Jews). In September 1945 he was arrested and committed suicide before Kogon and the other prisoners were able to provide testimony in his favor (Kogon, 1974, pp. 176-177, 318-320).

4 Re: Weber, see Micheels, 1989, p. 101.

5 Re. Fugger, Zabel, Pargner and others, see Micheels, 1989, p. 102.

6 The young Jewish woman laboratory assistant was the Slovakian prisoner Eva Gabanyi, Claudette Kennedy's draftswoman in Rajsko, who died a number of years ago. According to Lifton, Robert Jay Lifton, Dr. Muench was fascinated by this very "primitive" young person who was able to alter her drawings from crude ones for crude SS-men to "marvelous" and "tasteful" renditions for more cultivated SS officers like himself (Lifton, 1986, pp. 316-317).

7 Deutsches Oesterreichisches Institut fuer Zeitgeschichte, i.e., German-Austrian Institute for Contemporary History. In 1984 the Institute was reportedly a front for the USA-based NSDAP-AO Nazi group.

8 For a rebuttal of the Leuchter report, see Wellers (1990) and Bailer-Galanda (1991).

Bibliography

Adelsberger, Lucie. *Auschwitz, Ein Tatsachenbericht*. Berlin: Lettner, 1960

Adler, H.G.; Langbein, Hermann; and Lingens-Reiner, Ella (Eds.). *Auschwitz, Zeugnisse und Berichte*. Koeln & Frankfurt/M: Europaeische Verlagsanstalt, 1979.

Allainmat, Henri. *Auschwitz en France*. Paris: Presse de la Cite, 1974.

Augé, Claude & Augé, Paul (Publ.). *Nouveau Petit Larousse*. Paris: Librairie Larousse, 1947.

Bailer-Galanda, Brigitte. "Der Leuchter Bericht," in *Information der Gesellschaft fuer Politische Aufklaerung*, Nr. 29, Juni 1991, pp. 1-2.

Bauer, Yehuda. "Danger Signals." *London Jewish Chronicle*, pp. 34-35. July 8, 1988.

Bauer, Yehuda. "The Danger of Distortion." *The Jerusalem Post*, International Ed., Sept. 30, 1989, p. 7.

Berger, Karin; Holzinger, Elizabeth; Podgornik, Lotte; and Trallori, Lisbeth (Eds.). *Ich geb Dir einen Mantel, dass Du ihn noch in Freiheit tragen Kannst*. Vienna: Promedia, 1987.

Bettelheim, Bruno. *The Informed Heart* (Autonomy in a Mass Age). New York: Avon, 1979.

Bezwinska, Jadwiga; and Czech, Danuta (Eds.). *KL Auschwitz in den Augen der SS*. Katowice, Poland: Krajowa Agencja Wydawnicza, 1981.

Bialowna, Irena. "Aus der Geschichte des Reviers im Frauenlager in Birkenau." In *Die Auschwitz-Hefte,* Band I. Weinheim & Basel: Beltz, 1987, pp. 173-184.

Bielecki, Jerzy. *Kto Ratuje Jedno Zycie...* Ludowa Spoldzielnia Wydawnicza, 1990.

Borowski, Tadeusz. *Bei Uns In Auschwitz*. Muenchen: Piper, 1987.

Brewster, Eva. *Vanished in Darkness*. Edmonton, Alberta: NeWest Publishers, 1984.

Broad, Pery. *Reminiscences of Pery Broad, SS-Man in the Auschwitz Concentration Camp*. Oswiecim: Panstwowe Museum, 1965.

Buber-Neumann, Margarete. *Milena*. New York: Seaver Books, 1988.

Christophersen, Thies. *Auschwitz: Truth or Lie*? P.O. Box 156, Verdun 19, Quebec, Canada.

Czech, Danuta. "Kalendarium der Ereiguisse im KL Auschwitz-Birkenau." In *Hefte von Auschwitz 4,* 1961, p. 4.

Czech, Danuta. "Die Rolle Des Haeftlings Krankenbaulagers im KL Auschwitz II." In *Hefte von Auschwitz 15,* pp. 5-112. Auschwitz, Staatliches Museum, 1975.

Czech, Danuta. *Kalendarium der Ereignisse im Konzentrationslager Auschwitz-Birkenau 1939-1945*. Reinbek bei Hamburg, Rohwolt, 1989.

Delbo, Charlotte. *Aucun De Nous Ne Reviendra*. Paris: Les Editions de Minuit, 1970.

Delbo, Charlotte. *Le Convoi du 24 Janvier.* Paris: Les Editions de Minuit, 1965.

De Wind, Eduard. "Der Experimentierblock." In *Auschwitz, Zeugnisse und Berichte,* M.G. Adler, Hermann Langbein and Ella Lingens-Reiner (Eds.). Cologne: Europaeische Verlagsanstalt, 1979.

Fejkiel, Wladyslaw. "Ethisch-Rechtliche Grenzen Bei Experimenten In Der Medizin—Und Der Fall Prof. Clauberg." In *Hefte von Auschwitz 2,* pp. 33-87. Wydawnictwo Panstwowego Muzeum W Oswiecimiu, 1959.

Friedmann-Vesela, Sylvia. Depositions in the case against Dr. Horst Schumann made before Judge Vojtech Majoros at the Hall of Justice in Presov, Czechoslovakia on July 1, 1968.

Garlinski, Josef. *Fighting Auschwitz: The Resistance Movement in the Concentration Camp.* Glasgow: Fontana/Collins, 1975.

Gutman, Israel (Ed.). *Encyclopedia of the Holocaust.* New York: Macmillan, 1990.

Hamburger Institut fuer Sozialforschung (Eds.). *Die Auschwitz Hefte.* Weinheim: Beltz, 1987.

Hartman, Geoffrey H. "Learning From Survivors." In *Remembering for the Future,* Theme II, pp. 1713-1717. Oxford: Pergamon Press, 1988.

Hautval, Dr. Adelaïde. *Médecine et Crimes contre L'Humanité.* Arles: Actes Sud, 1991.

"Heroes of the Jewish Resistance Honored for the First Time in Germany." *The Voice,* 1985, 31: 9-10, July/August.

Hill, Mavis M.; and Williams, L. Norman. *Auschwitz in England.* New York: Ballantine, 1966.

Hoess, Rudolf. *Commandant of Auschwitz.* Cleveland: The World Publishing Co., 1959.

International Auschwitz Committee. *Nazi Medicine, Doctors, Victims and Medicine in Auschwitz.* New York: Howard Fertig, 1986.

Jagoda, Zenon; Klodzinski, Stanislaw; and Maslowski, Jan. "Bauernfuss, goldzupa, himmelautostrada." Zum "Krematoriumsesperanto, der Sprache polnischer KZ-Haeftlinge." In *Die Auschwitz Hefte,* Band II. Weinheim und Basel: Beltz, 1987.

Jagoda, Zenon; Klodzinski, Stanislaw; and Maslowski, Jan. "Das Ueberleben im Lager aus der Sicht ehemaliger Haeftlinge von Auschwitz Birkenau." In *Die Auschwitz Hefte,* Band I. Weinheim und Basel: Beltz, 1987.

Kagan, Raya. *Nashim B'lishkat Na 'Gehennom.* Sifrat Poalim, Palestine, 1947.

Keesling's *Reference Publications.* "The Radical Right." London: 1987.

Kielar, Wieslaw. *Anus Mundi: Fuenf Jahre Auschwitz.* Frankfurt (Main): S. Fischer, 1979.

Kieta, Mieczyslaw. "Das Hygiene-Institut der Waffen-SS und Polizei in Auschwitz." In *Die Auschwitz Hefte,* Band I, pp. 213-217. Weinheim and Basel: Beltz, 1987.

Klodzinski, Stanislaw. "Laboratorium Instytutu Hiegieny SS w Oswiecimiu, Bulion z miesa ludzkiego." In *Przeglad Lekarski,* Nr. 1, 1969, pp. 67-71.

Koelbl, Herlinde. *Juedische Portraits.* Frankfurt/M: S. Fischer, 1989.

Kogon, Eugen. *Der SS-Staat.* Muenchen: Kindler, 1974.

Langbein, Hermann. *Menschen in Auschwitz.* Vienna: Europaverlag, 1972.

Laska, Vera (Ed.). *Women in the Resistance and in the Holocaust: The Voices of Eyewitnesses.* Westport: Greenwood Press.

Lengyel, Olga. *Five Chimneys.* Chicago: Ziff-Davis, 1947.

Levi, Primo. *The Drowned and the Saved.* New York: Summit, 1988.

Lewinska, Pelagia. *Vingt Mois a Auschwitz.* Paris: Editions Nagel, 1945.

Lifton, Robert Jay. *The Nazi Doctors.* New York: Basic Books, 1986.

Lill, Karl. "Erinnerungen." In *Hefte von Auschwitz 16,* pp. 137-157. Auschwitz: Staatliches Museum, 1978.

Lorska, Dorota. "Block 10 in Auschwitz." In *Die Auschwitz-Hefte,* Band I, pp. 209-212. Weinheim und Basel: Beltz, 1987.

Michalak, Wanda. *Auschwitz, Faschistisches Vernichtungslager.* Warsaw: Verlag Interpress, 1981.

Micheels, Louis J. *Doctor #117641, an Auschwitz Memoir.* New Haven: Yale University Press, 1989.

Minney, R.J. *I Shall Fear No Evil.* London: William Kimber, 1966.

Mitscherlich, Alexander; and Mielke, Fred. *Medizin Ohne Menschlichkeit.* Frankfurt a. M.: Fischer, 1981.

Muller, Filip. *Eyewitness Auschwitz.* New York: Stein and Day, 1979.

Naumann, Bernd. *Auschwitz: Bericht ueber die Strafsache Mulka und andere vor dem Schwurgericht Frankfurt.* Frankfurt/M: Athenaeum, 1965.

Nomberg-Przytyk, Sara. *Auschwitz, True Tales From a Grotesque Land.* Chapel Hill: University of North Carolina Press, 1985.

Nyiszli, Dr. Miklos. *Auschwitz, A Doctor's Eyewitness Account.* Geneva: Ferni Publishing House, 1979.

Ourisson, Dounia. *Les Secrets du Bureau Politique d'Auschwitz.* Paris: Amicale d'Auschwitz, 1947.

Perl, Dr. Gisella. *I Was a Doctor in Auschwitz.* New York: International University Press, 1948.

Piper, Franciszek. *Zatrudnienie Wiezniow KL Auschwitz.* Oswiecim, Poland: Panstwowe Museum, 1981.

Poliakov, Leon; and Wulf, Joseph. *Das Dritte Reich Und Die Juden.* Berlin: Verlags GmbH, 1955.

Pozner, Vladimir. *Descente Aux Enfers*. Paris: Juillard, 1980.

Rotmensch, Siegfried; Avigad, Itamar; Soffer, Eddy; Horowitz, Ada; Bar-Meir, Simon; Confino, Ronit; Czerniak, Abraham; and Wolfstein, Isidor. "Carcinoma of the Large Bowel After a Single Massive Dosis of Radiation in Healthy Teenagers." *Cancer,* 57:728-731, 1986.

"Schwester Angela—Der Engel von Auschwitz." In *Der Dom*. Kirchenzeitung fuer das Erzbistum Paderborn. 42 Jahrgang, Sept. 27, 1987, Nr. 39.

Sehn, Jan. "Carl Claubergs Verbrecherische Unfruchtbarmachungsversuche An Haeftlings-Frauen In Den Nazi-Konzentrationslagern." In *Hefte von Auschwitz 2,* pp. 3-32. Wydawnictwo Panstwowego Muzeum W Oswiecimiu, 1959.

Shelley, Lore. *Auschwitz—The Nazi Civilization*. Lanham: University Press of America, 1991.

Shelley, Lore. *Jewish Holocaust Survivors' Attitudes Toward Contemporary Beliefs About Themselves*. Ann Arbor, MI: University Microfilms, 1983.

Shelley, Lore. *Secretaries of Death*. New York: Shengold, 1986.

Sherwin, Byron. "Primo Levi and Arnost Lustig on Moral Implications of the Holocaust." *Shoah I,* No. 4, 1979, pp. 24-29.

Skodova, Julia. *Tri Roky Bez Mena*. Bratislava, Czechoslovakia: Osveta, 1962.

Smolen, Kazimierz (Ed.). *Problemes Choisis de l'Histoire du KL Auschwitz*. Oswiecim, Poland: Edition du Museé d'Etat, 1979.

Smolen, Kazimierz; Bezwinska, Jadwiga; Brandhuber, Jerzy and Czech, Danuta (Eds.). *Reminiscences of Pery Broad, SS-Man in the Auschwitz Concentration Camp*. Auschwitz: Panstwowe Muzeum Oswiecim, 1965.

Sobanski, Tomasz. *Fluchtwege aus Auschwitz*. Warszawa: Sport i Turystika, 1980.

Steger, Bernd & Thiele, Guenther. *Der Dunkle Schatten,* Leben mit Auschwitz, Erinnerungen an Orli Reichert-Wald. Marburg: SP Verlag Norbert Schueren, 1989.

Svalbova, Margita. *Vyhasnute Oci*. Bratislava, Czechoslovakia: Nakladatelstvo Pravda, 1948.

Szmaglewska, Seweryna. *Smoke Over Birkenau*. New York: Henry Holt, 1947.

The Leuchter Report, Decatur, Alabama: Samisdat Publishers, 1988.

Tichauer, Eva. *J'etais le numero 20832 a Auschwitz*. Paris: L'Harmattan, 1988.

Uris, Leon. *Exodus*. New York: Bantam, 1986.

Uris, Leon. *QBVII*. New York: Bantam, 1989.

Wellers, Georges. "A propos 'Rapport Leuchter' und die Gaskammern von Auschwitz." In *Informationen der Gesellschaft fuer Politische Aufklaerung*. Innsbruck: Nr. 24, Maerz 1990.

Wistrich, Robert. *Who's Who in Nazi Germany*. New York: Bonanza Books, 1982.

Zatuchni, Gerald I.; Shelton, James D.; Goldsmith, Alfredo & Sciarra, John J. *Female Transcervical Sterilization.* Proceedings of an International Workshop on Non-Surgical Methods for Female Tubal Occlusion, held June 1982 at Northwestern University, Chicago. Philadelphia: Harper & Row, 1983.

Zieba, Anna. "Das Nebenlager Rajsko," *Hefte von Auschwitz,* 1966, Verlag Staatliches Museum, Auschwitz, #9, pp. 73-108.

Zieba, Anna. "Die Gefluegelfarm Harmense," *Hefte von Auschwitz,* 1970, Verlag Staatliches Museum, Auschwitz, #11, pp. 39-72.

Index

C

D

E

F

G

H

I

J

K

L

M

N

O

P

R

S

Z